Teen Health Series

Diet Information For Teens,
Third Edition

Diet Information For Teens, Third Edition

Health Tips About Nutrition Fundamentals And Eating Plans

Including Facts About Vitamins, Minerals, Food Additives, And Weight-Related Concerns

Edited by Zachary Klimecki and Karen Bellenir

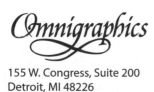

155 W. Congress, Suite 200
Detroit, MI 48226

Bibliographic Note

Because this page cannot legibly accommodate all the copyright notices, the Bibliographic Note portion of the Preface constitutes an extension of the copyright notice.

Edited by Zachary Klimecki and Karen Bellenir

Teen Health Series

Karen Bellenir, *Managing Editor*
David A. Cooke, M.D., *Medical Consultant*
Elizabeth Collins, *Research and Permissions Coordinator*
Cherry Edwards, *Permissions Assistant*
EdIndex, *Services for Publishers, Indexers*

* * *

Omnigraphics, Inc.

Matthew P. Barbour, *Senior Vice President*
Kevin M. Hayes, *Operations Manager*

* * *

Peter E. Ruffner, *Publisher*

Copyright © 2012 Omnigraphics, Inc.
ISBN 978-0-7808-1156-0

Library of Congress Cataloging-in-Publication Data

Diet information for teens : health tips about nutrition fundamentals and eating plans including facts about vitamins, minerals, food additives, and weight-related concerns / edited by Zachary Klimecki and Karen Bellenir. -- 3rd ed.
   p. cm. -- (Teen health series)
  Includes bibliographical references and index.
  ISBN 978-0-7808-1156-0 (hardcover : alk. paper) 1. Teenagers--Nutrition. 2. Teenagers--Health and hygiene. 3. Diet. 4. Health. I. Klimecki, Zachary. II. Bellenir, Karen.
  RJ235.D546 2011
  613.2083--dc23

                          2011031595

Table of Contents

Preface

Part Three: Other Elements Inside Food

Part Four: Smart Eating Plans

Part Five: Eating And Weight-Related Concerns

Preface

About This Book

Today's teens are exposed to an array of technological tools that they can use to connect with information. In fact, the National Heart Lung and Blood Institute reports that children and teens aged 8 to 18 spend 7½ hours a day using media, such as watching television, playing video games, or using computers and cell phones. But, being so connected might be disconnecting them from the healthy diets their developing bodies need.

In the swirl of misleading and confusing nutrition information found in television advertisements and on the internet, it can be difficult for a teen to know what constitutes a proper diet. Rising rates of some health conditions, like diabetes and obesity, make it especially important that teens become educated about their dietary choices because what a teenager chooses to eat can have implications that last a lifetime.

Diet Information for Teens, Third Edition provides updated information about healthy eating patterns and making smart dietary choices, including facts from the recently released *Dietary Guidelines for Americans* and the new MyPlate food guidance system. The book discusses the essential components of a well-constructed diet and explains how major food groups—such as grains, vegetables, fruits, and protein foods—play an important role in providing the vitamins and minerals needed to maintain good health. Dietary elements that may need to be limited, such as caffeine, sugar, fat, and salt, are also discussed along with tips for reducing screen time, staying active, and addressing weight-related concerns. A special section on eating and disease provides information about foodborne illness, eating disorders, and disorders where dietary choices are an essential part of disease management procedures. The book concludes with cooking tips and directories of resources for dietary and fitness information.

How To Use This Book

This book is divided into parts and chapters. Parts focus on broad areas of interest; chapters are devoted to single topics within a part.

Part One: Nutrition Fundamentals looks at the most recently released *Dietary Guidelines for Americans* and explains dietary components. It discusses calorie requirements and energy balance, and it explains how nutrition facts labels can be used to help compare the nutrient contents of food items. Details about the individual food groups that comprise a healthy diet, including grains vegetables, fruits, and proteins, are also included.

Part Two: Vitamins And Minerals offers individual chapters focusing on the major vitamins—A, B, C, D, and E—and calcium, a mineral of special concern to growing teens. Each chapter discusses the role the nutrient plays in maintaining good health and gives examples of foods that are rich sources of the nutrient. Additional chapters provide facts about other important minerals and dietary supplements.

Part Three: Other Elements Inside Food discusses components of foods that are sometimes consumed in excess or that may be monitored carefully for specific purposes. These include salt, carbohydrates, sugars, and fats. Information about food additives and artificial sweeteners is also included.

Part Four: Smart Eating Plans introduces the MyPlate food guidance system and discusses ways to develop eating patterns that support a healthy lifestyle. It also offers suggestions for making healthy food choices in a variety of settings, including eating out, eating in the school cafeteria, and snacking. Facts about caffeine, energy drinks, and sports nutrition are presented, and the part concludes with information for vegetarians and vegans.

Part Five: Eating And Weight-Related Concerns addresses readers who want to identify and maintain a healthy weight. It describes the body mass index (BMI), discusses body image concerns, and provides suggestions for people seeking to achieve weight-related goals. Facts about how physical activity contributes to the success of weight management—and how spending too much time in front of a screen (television, computer, etc.) can disrupt efforts—are also included

Part Six: Eating And Disease explains the link between dietary elements and some specific health conditions, such as dental health, heart health, and obesity, where food choices may either contribute to, or help prevent, disease. It describes situations where careful adherence to a meal plan is an integral part of disease management strategies, such as avoiding gluten in celiac disease, managing blood sugar in diabetes, and avoiding triggers when food allergies or intolerances are present. The part concludes with information about foodborne illness and eating disorders.

Part Seven: If You Need More Information offers a chapter with cooking tips and suggested resources for finding healthy recipes and planning meals. Directories of dietary and fitness resources are also included.

Bibliographic Note

This volume contains documents and excerpts from publications issued by the following government agencies: Centers for Disease Control and Prevention; Federal Trade Commission; Food Safety and Inspection Service; National Cancer Institute; National Diabetes Education Program; National Diabetes Information Clearinghouse; National Digestive Diseases Information Clearinghouse; National Heart Lung and Blood Institute; National Institute of Allergy and Infectious Diseases; National Institute of Child Health and Development; National Institute of Diabetes and Digestive and Kidney Diseases; National Institute of Mental Health; National Institutes of Health, Office of Dietary Supplements; National Women's Health Information Center; President's Council on Physical Fitness and Sports; U.S. Department of Agriculture; and the U.S. Food and Drug Administration.

In addition, this volume contains copyrighted documents and articles produced by the following organizations and publications: A.D.A.M., Inc.; Academy of General Dentistry; American Heart Association; Colorado State University Extension; HealthDay News; International Food Information Council; Nemours Foundation; Ontario Ministry of Agriculture, Food and Rural Affairs; Robert Wood Johnson Center to Prevent Childhood Obesity; and the *Yale Journal of Biology and Medicine.*

The photograph on the front cover is from Corbis Royalty Free Photo/Fotosearch.

Full citation information is provided on the first page of each chapter. Every effort has been made to secure all necessary rights to reprint the copyrighted material. If any omissions have been made, please contact Omnigraphics to make corrections for future editions.

Acknowledgements

In addition to the organizations listed above, special thanks are due to Liz Collins, research and permissions coordinator; Cherry Edwards, permissions assistant; and WhimsyInk, pre-press services provider.

About the Teen Health Series

At the request of librarians serving today's young adults, the *Teen Health Series* was developed as a specially focused set of volumes within Omnigraphics' *Health Reference Series*. Each volume deals comprehensively with a topic selected according to the needs and interests of people in middle school and high school.

Teens seeking preventive guidance, information about disease warning signs, medical statistics, and risk factors for health problems will find answers to their questions in the *Teen Health Series*. The *Series*, however, is not intended to serve as a tool for diagnosing illness, in prescribing treatments, or as a substitute for the physician/patient relationship. All people concerned about medical symptoms or the possibility of disease are encouraged to seek professional care from an appropriate health care provider.

If there is a topic you would like to see addressed in a future volume of the *Teen Health Series*, please write to:

Editor, *Teen Health Series*
Omnigraphics, Inc.
155 W. Congress, Suite 200
Detroit, MI 48226

A Note about Spelling and Style

Teen Health Series editors use *Stedman's Medical Dictionary* as an authority for questions related to the spelling of medical terms and the *Chicago Manual of Style* for questions related to grammatical structures, punctuation, and other editorial concerns. Consistent adherence is not always possible, however, because the individual volumes within the *Series* include many documents from a wide variety of different producers and copyright holders, and the editor's primary goal is to present material from each source as accurately as is possible following the terms specified by each document's producer. This sometimes means that information in different chapters or sections may follow other guidelines and alternate spelling authorities. For example, occasionally a copyright holder may require that eponymous terms be shown in possessive forms (Crohn's disease *vs.* Crohn disease) or that British spelling norms be retained (leukaemia *vs.* leukemia).

Locating Information within the Teen Health Series

The *Teen Health Series* contains a wealth of information about a wide variety of medical topics. As the *Series* continues to grow in size and scope, locating the precise information needed by a specific student may become more challenging. To address this concern, information about books within the *Teen Health Series* is included in *A Contents Guide to the Health Reference Series*. The *Contents Guide* presents an extensive list of more than 15,000 diseases, treatments, and other topics of general interest compiled from the Tables of Contents and major index headings from the books of the *Teen Health Series* and *Health Reference Series*. To access *A Contents Guide to the Health Reference Series*, visit www.healthreferenceseries.com.

Our Advisory Board

We would like to thank the following advisory board members for providing guidance to the development of this *Series*:

Dr. Lynda Baker, Associate Professor of Library and Information Science,
Wayne State University, Detroit, MI

Nancy Bulgarelli, William Beaumont Hospital Library,
Royal Oak, MI

Karen Imarisio, Bloomfield Township Public Library,
Bloomfield Township, MI

Karen Morgan, Mardigian Library, University of Michigan–Dearborn,
Dearborn, MI

Rosemary Orlando, St. Clair Shores Public Library,
St. Clair Shores, MI

Medical Consultant

Medical consultation services are provided to the *Teen Health Series* editors by David A. Cooke, M.D. Dr. Cooke is a graduate of Brandeis University, and he received his M.D. degree from the University of Michigan. He completed residency training at the University of Wisconsin Hospital and Clinics. He is board-certified in internal medicine. Dr. Cooke currently works as part of the University of Michigan Health System and practices in Ann Arbor, MI. In his free time, he enjoys writing, science fiction, and spending time with his family.

Part One
Nutrition Fundamentals

Chapter 1

Dietary Guidelines

Introduction

In 1980, the U.S. Department of Agriculture (USDA) and the U.S. Department of Health and Human Services (HHS) released the first edition of *Nutrition and Your Health: Dietary Guidelines for Americans*. These *Dietary Guidelines* were different from previous dietary guidance in that they reflected emerging scientific evidence about diet and health and expanded the traditional focus on nutrient adequacy to also address the impact of diet on chronic disease.

Subsequent editions of the *Dietary Guidelines for Americans* have been remarkably consistent in their recommendations about the components of a health-promoting diet, but they also have changed in some significant ways to reflect an evolving body of evidence about nutrition, the food and physical activity environment, and health. The ultimate goal of the *Dietary Guidelines for Americans* is to improve the health of our nation's current and future generations by facilitating and promoting healthy eating and physical activity choices so that these behaviors become the norm among all individuals.

Poor diet and physical inactivity are the most important factors contributing to an epidemic of overweight and obesity in this country. The most recent data indicate that 72% of men and 64% of women are overweight or obese, with about one-third of adults being obese. Even in the absence of overweight, poor diet and physical inactivity are associated with major causes of morbidity and mortality. These include cardiovascular disease, hypertension, type 2 diabetes, osteoporosis, and some types of cancer. Some racial and ethnic population groups are disproportionately affected by the high rates of overweight, obesity, and associated chronic

About This Chapter: Excerpted from *Dietary Guidelines for Americans 2010*, U.S. Department of Agriculture, December 2010.

diseases. These diet and health associations make a focus on improved nutrition and physical activity choices ever more urgent. These associations also provide important opportunities to reduce health disparities through dietary and physical activity changes.

Dietary Guidelines for Americans also recognizes that in recent years nearly 15 percent of American households have been unable to acquire adequate food to meet their needs because of insufficient money or other resources for food. This dietary guidance can help them maximize the nutritional content of their meals within their resource constraints. Many other Americans consume less than optimal intake of certain nutrients, even though they have adequate resources for a healthy diet. This dietary guidance and nutrition information can help them choose a healthy, nutritionally adequate diet.

Children are a particularly important focus of the *Dietary Guidelines for Americans* because of the growing body of evidence documenting the vital role that optimal nutrition plays throughout the lifespan. Today, too many children are consuming diets with too many calories and not enough nutrients and are not getting enough physical activity. Approximately 32% of children and adolescents ages 2–19 years are overweight or obese, with 17% percent of children being obese. In addition, risk factors for adult chronic diseases are increasingly found in

What's It Mean?

Calorie Balance: The balance between calories consumed in foods and beverages and calories expended through physical activity and metabolic processes.

Eating Pattern: The combination of foods and beverages that constitute an individual's complete dietary intake over time.

Nutrient Dense: Nutrient-dense foods and beverages provide vitamins, minerals, and other substances that may have positive health effects with relatively few calories. The term "nutrient dense" indicates that the nutrients and other beneficial substances in a food have not been "diluted" by the addition of calories from added solid fats, added sugars, or added refined starches, or by the solid fats naturally present in the food. Nutrient-dense foods and beverages are lean or low in solid fats, and minimize or exclude added solid fats, sugars, starches, and sodium. Ideally, they also are in forms that retain naturally occurring components, such as dietary fiber. All vegetables, fruits, whole grains, seafood, eggs, beans and peas, unsalted nuts and seeds, fat-free and low-fat milk and milk products, and lean meats and poultry—when prepared without adding solid fats or sugars—are nutrient-dense foods. For most Americans, meeting nutrient needs within their calorie needs is an important goal for health. Eating recommended amounts from each food group in nutrient-dense forms is the best approach to achieving this goal and building a healthy eating pattern.

younger ages. Eating patterns established in childhood often track into later life, making early intervention on adopting healthy nutrition and physical activity behaviors a priority.

Balancing Calories To Manage Weight

Achieving and sustaining appropriate body weight across the lifespan is vital to maintaining good health and quality of life. Many behavioral, environmental, and genetic factors have been shown to affect a person's body weight. Calorie balance over time is the key to weight management. Calorie balance refers to the relationship between calories consumed from foods and beverages and calories expended in normal body functions (for example, metabolic processes) and through physical activity. People cannot control the calories expended in metabolic processes, but they can control what they eat and drink, as well as how many calories they use in physical activity.

Calories consumed must equal calories expended for a person to maintain the same body weight. Consuming more calories than expended will result in weight gain. Conversely, consuming fewer calories than expended will result in weight loss. This can be achieved over time by eating fewer calories, being more physically active, or, best of all, a combination of the two.

Maintaining a healthy body weight and preventing excess weight gain throughout the lifespan are highly preferable to losing weight after weight gain. Once a person becomes obese, reducing body weight back to a healthy range requires significant effort over a span of time, even years. People who are most successful at losing weight and keeping it off do so through continued attention to calorie balance.

Understanding Calorie Needs

The total number of calories a person needs each day varies depending on a number of factors, including the person's age, gender, height, weight, and level of physical activity. In addition, a desire to lose, maintain, or gain weight affects how many calories should be consumed. Table 1.1 provides estimated total calorie needs for weight maintenance based on age, gender, and physical activity level. Estimates range from 1,600 to 2,400 calories per day for adult women and 2,000 to 3,000 calories per day for adult men, depending on age and physical activity level. Within each age and gender category, the low end of the range is for sedentary individuals; the high end of the range is for active individuals. Due to reductions in basal metabolic rate that occurs with aging, calorie needs generally decrease for adults as they age. Estimated needs for young children range from 1,000 to 2,000 calories per day, and the range for older children and adolescents varies substantially from 1,400 to 3,200 calories per day, with boys generally having higher calorie needs than girls. These are only estimates, and estimation of individual calorie needs can be aided with online tools such as those available at ChooseMyPlate.gov.

Table 1.1. Estimated Calorie Needs Per Day By Age, Gender, And Physical Activity Level.[a] Estimated amounts of calories needed to maintain calorie balance for various gender and age groups at three different levels of physical activity. The estimates are rounded to the nearest 200 calories. An individual's calorie needs may be higher or lower than these average estimates.

Gender	Age (Years)	Physical Activity Level[b]		
		Sedentary[c]	Moderately Active[c]	Active[c]
Child (Female And Male)	2–3	1,000–1,200	1,000–1,400	1,000–1,400
Female[d]				
	4–8	1,200–1,400	1,400–1,600	1,400–1,800
	9–13	1,400–1,600	1,600–2,000	1,800–2,200
	14–18	1,800	2,000	2,400
	19–30	1,800–2,000	2,000–2,200	2,400
	31–50	1,800	2,000	2,200
	51+	1,600	1,800	2,000–2,200
Male				
	4–8	1,200–1,400	1,400–1,600	1,600–2,000
	9–13	1,600–2,000	1,800–2,200	2,000–2,600
	14–18	2,000–2,400	2,400–2,800	2,800–3,200
	19–30	2,400–2,600	2,600–2,800	3,000
	31–50	2,200–2,400	2,400–2,600	2,800–3,000
	51+	2,000–2,200	2,200–2,400	2,400–2,800

a. Based on Estimated Energy Requirements (EER) equations, using reference heights (average) and reference weights (healthy) for each age/gender group. For children and adolescents, reference height and weight vary. For adults, the reference man is 5 feet 10 inches tall and weighs 154 pounds. The reference woman is 5 feet 4 inches tall and weighs 126 pounds. EER equations are from the Institute of Medicine. Dietary Reference Intakes for Energy, Carbohydrate, Fiber, Fat, Fatty Acids, Cholesterol, Protein, and Amino Acids. Washington (DC): The National Academies Press; 2002.

b. Sedentary means a lifestyle that includes only the light physical activity associated with typical day-to-day life. Moderately active means a lifestyle that includes physical activity equivalent to walking about 1.5 to 3 miles per day at 3 to 4 miles per hour, in addition to the light physical activity associated with typical day-to-day life. Active means a lifestyle that includes physical activity equivalent to walking more than 3 miles per day at 3 to 4 miles per hour, in addition to the light physical activity associated with typical day-to-day life.

c. The calorie ranges shown are to accommodate needs of different ages within the group. For children and adolescents, more calories are needed at older ages. For adults, fewer calories are needed at older ages.

d. Estimates for females do not include women who are pregnant or breastfeeding.

What's It Mean?

Vegetables

Dark-Green Vegetables: All fresh, frozen, and canned dark-green leafy vegetables and broccoli, cooked or raw: for example, broccoli; spinach; romaine; collard, turnip, and mustard greens.

Red And Orange Vegetables: All fresh, frozen, and canned red and orange vegetables, cooked or raw: for example, tomatoes, red peppers, carrots, sweet potatoes, winter squash, and pumpkin.

Beans And Peas: All cooked and canned beans and peas: for example, kidney beans, lentils, chickpeas, and pinto beans. Does not include green beans or green peas. (See additional comment under protein foods group.)

Starchy Vegetables: All fresh, frozen, and canned starchy vegetables: for example, white potatoes, corn, and green peas.

Other Vegetables: All fresh, frozen, and canned other vegetables, cooked or raw: for example, iceberg lettuce, green beans, and onions.

Other Food Groups

Fruits: All fresh, frozen, canned, and dried fruits and fruit juices: for example, oranges and orange juice, apples and apple juice, bananas, grapes, melons, berries, and raisins.

Whole Grains: All whole-grain products and whole grains used as ingredients: for example, whole-wheat bread, whole-grain cereals and crackers, oatmeal, and brown rice.

Enriched Grains: All enriched refined-grain products and enriched refined grains used as ingredients: for example, white breads, enriched grain cereals and crackers, enriched pasta, and white rice.

Dairy Products: All milks, including lactose-free and lactose-reduced products and fortified soy beverages; yogurts; frozen yogurts; dairy desserts; and cheeses. Most choices should be fat-free or low-fat. Cream, sour cream, and cream cheese are not included due to their low calcium content.

Protein Foods: All meat, poultry, seafood, eggs, nuts, seeds, and processed soy products. Meat and poultry should be lean or low-fat. Beans and peas are considered part of this group, as well as the vegetable group, but should be counted in one group only.

Foods And Food Components To Reduce

Currently, very few Americans consume diets that meet *Dietary Guideline* recommendations. Certain foods and food components are consumed in excessive amounts and may increase the risk of certain chronic diseases. These include sodium, solid fats (major sources of saturated and trans fatty acids), added sugars, and refined grains. These food components are consumed in excess by children, adolescents, adults, and older adults. In addition, the diets of most men exceed the recommendation for cholesterol. Some people also consume too much alcohol (and anyone younger than the legal drinking age should not consume any alcohol).

Excessive intake of these foods and food components replaces nutrient-dense forms of foods in the diet, making it difficult for people to achieve recommended nutrient intake and control calorie intake. Many Americans are overweight or obese, and are at higher risk of chronic diseases, such as cardiovascular disease, diabetes, and certain types of cancer. Even in the absence of overweight or obesity, consuming too much sodium, solid fats, saturated and trans fatty acids, cholesterol, added sugars, and alcohol increases the risk of some of the most common chronic diseases in the United States. Discussing solid fats in addition to saturated and trans fatty acids is important because, apart from the effects of saturated and trans fatty acids on cardiovascular disease risk, solid fats are abundant in the diets of Americans and contribute significantly to excess calorie intake.

Key Recommendations

- Reduce daily sodium intake to less than 2,300 milligrams (mg) and further reduce intake to 1,500 mg among persons who are 51 and older and those of any age who are African American or have hypertension, diabetes, or chronic kidney disease. The 1,500 mg recommendation applies to about half of the U.S. population, including children, and the majority of adults.

- Consume less than 10% of calories from saturated fatty acids by replacing them with monounsaturated and polyunsaturated fatty acids.

- Consume less than 300 mg per day of dietary cholesterol.

- Keep trans fatty acid consumption as low as possible, especially by limiting foods that contain synthetic sources of trans fats, such as partially hydrogenated oils, and by limiting other solid fats.

- Reduce the intake of calories from solid fats and added sugars.

- Limit the consumption of foods that contain refined grains, especially refined grain foods that contain solid fats, added sugars, and sodium.

Foods And Nutrients To Increase

A wide variety of nutritious foods are available in the United States. However, many Americans do not eat the array of foods that will provide all needed nutrients while staying within calorie needs. In the United States, intakes of vegetables, fruits, whole grains, milk and milk products, and oils are lower than recommended. As a result, dietary intakes of several nutrients—potassium, dietary fiber, calcium, and vitamin D—are low enough to be of public health concern for both adults and children. Several other nutrients also are of concern for specific population groups, such as folic acid for women who are capable of becoming pregnant.

Recommendations are based on evidence that consuming these foods within the context of an overall healthy eating pattern is associated with a health benefit or meeting nutrient needs. Guidance on food choices for a healthy eating pattern generally groups foods based on commonalities in nutrients provided and how the foods are viewed and used by consumers. The following recommendations provide advice about making choices from all food groups while balancing calorie needs.

Key Recommendations

Individuals should meet the following recommendations as part of a healthy eating pattern and while staying within their calorie needs.

- Increase vegetable and fruit intake.

- Eat a variety of vegetables, especially dark-green and red and orange vegetables and beans and peas.

- Consume at least half of all grains as whole grains. Increase whole-grain intake by replacing refined grains with whole grains.

- Increase intake of fat-free or low-fat milk and milk products, such as milk, yogurt, cheese, or fortified soy beverages.

- Choose a variety of protein foods, which include seafood, lean meat and poultry, eggs, beans and peas, soy products, and unsalted nuts and seeds.

- Increase the amount and variety of seafood consumed by choosing seafood in place of some meat and poultry.

- Replace protein foods that are higher in solid fats with choices that are lower in solid fats and calories and/or are sources of oils.

- Use oils to replace solid fats where possible.

- Choose foods that provide more potassium, dietary fiber, calcium, and vitamin D, which are nutrients of concern in American diets. These foods include vegetables, fruits, whole grains, and milk and milk products.

Nutritional Goals

Nutritional goals for age and gender groups, based on dietary reference intakes and dietary guidelines recommendations are shown in Tables 1.2 (maconutrients), 1.3 (minerals), and 1.4 (vitamins).

Table 1.2. Macronutrients—Nutritional Goals For Age-Gender Groups, Based on Dietary Reference Intakes and Dietary Guidelines Recommendations.

Nutrient (units)	Source of goal[a]	Child 1-3	Female 4-8	Male 4-8	Female 9-13	Male 9-13	Female 14-18	Male 14-18	Female 19-30	Male 19-30	Female 31-50	Male 31-50	Female 51+	Male 51+
Macronutrients														
Protein (g)	RDA[b]	13	19	19	34	34	46	52	46	56	46	56	46	56
(% of calories)	AMDR[c]	5-20	10-30	10-30	10-30	10-30	10-30	10-30	10-35	10-35	10-35	10-35	10-35	10-35
Carbohydrate (g)	RDA	130	130	130	130	130	130	130	130	130	130	130	130	130
(% of calories)	AMDR	45-65	45-65	45-65	45-65	45-65	45-65	45-65	45-65	45-65	45-65	45-65	45-65	45-65
Total fiber (g)	IOM[d]	14	17	20	22	25	25	31	28	34	25	31	22	28
Total fat (% of calories)	AMDR	30-40	25-35	25-35	25-35	25-35	25-35	25-35	20-35	20-35	20-35	20-35	20-35	20-35
Saturated fat (% of calories)	DG[e]	<10%	<10%	<10%	<10%	<10%	<10%	<10%	<10%	<10%	<10%	<10%	<10%	<10%
Linoleic acid (g)	AI[f]	7	10	10	10	12	11	16	12	17	12	17	11	14
(% of calories)	AMDR	5-10	5-10	5-10	5-10	5-10	5-10	5-10	5-10	5-10	5-10	5-10	5-10	5-10
alpha-Linolenic acid (g)	AI	0.7	0.9	0.9	1.0	1.2	1.1	1.6	1.1	1.6	1.1	1.6	1.1	1.6
(% of calories)	AMDR	0.6-1.2	0.6-1.2	0.6-1.2	0.6-1.2	0.6-1.2	0.6-1.2	0.6-1.2	0.6-1.2	0.6-1.2	0.6-1.2	0.6-1.2	0.6-1.2	0.6-1.2
Cholesterol (mg)	DG	<300	<300	<300	<300	<300	<300	<300	<300	<300	<300	<300	<300	<300

Table 1.3. Minerals—Nutritional Goals For Age-Gender Groups, Based on Dietary Reference Intakes and Dietary Guidelines Recommendations.

Nutrient (units)	Source of goal[a]	Child 1-3	Female 4-8	Male 4-8	Female 9-13	Male 9-13	Female 14-18	Male 14-18	Female 19-30	Male 19-30	Female 31-50	Male 31-50	Female 51+	Male 51+
Minerals														
Calcium (mg)	RDA	700	1,000	1,000	1,300	1,300	1,300	1,300	1,000	1,000	1,000	1,000	1,200	1,200
Iron (mg)	RDA	7	10	10	8	8	15	11	18	8	18	8	8	8
Magnesium (mg)	RDA	80	130	130	240	240	360	410	310	400	320	420	320	420
Phosphorus (mg)	RDA	460	500	500	1,250	1,250	1,250	1,250	700	700	700	700	700	700
Potassium (mg)	AI	3,000	3,800	3,800	4,500	4,500	4,700	4,700	4,700	4,700	4,700	4,700	4,700	4,700
Sodium (mg)	UL[g]	<1,500	<1,900	<1,900	<2,200	<2,200	<2,300	<2,300	<2,300	<2,300	<2,300	<2,300	<2,300	<2,300
Zinc (mg)	RDA	3	5	5	8	8	9	11	8	11	8	11	8	11
Copper (mcg)	RDA	340	440	440	700	700	890	890	900	900	900	900	900	900
Selenium (mcg)	RDA	20	30	30	40	40	55	55	55	55	55	55	55	55

Table 1.4. Vitamins—Nutritional Goals For Age-Gender Groups, Based on Dietary Reference Intakes and Dietary Guidelines Recommendations.

Nutrient (units)	Source of goal[a]	Child 1–3	Female 4–8	Male 4–8	Female 9–13	Male 9–13	Female 14–18	Male 14–18	Female 19–30	Male 19–30	Female 31–50	Male 31–50	Female 51+	Male 51+
Vitamins														
Vitamin A (mcg RAE)	RDA	300	400	400	600	600	700	900	700	900	700	900	700	900
Vitamin D[h] (mcg)	RDA	15	15	15	15	15	15	15	15	15	15	15	15	15
Vitamin E (mg AT)	RDA	6	7	7	11	11	15	15	15	15	15	15	15	15
Vitamin C (mg)	RDA	15	25	25	45	45	65	75	75	90	75	90	75	90
Thiamin (mg)	RDA	0.5	0.6	0.6	0.9	0.9	1.0	1.2	1.1	1.2	1.1	1.2	1.1	1.2
Riboflavin (mg)	RDA	0.5	0.6	0.6	0.9	0.9	1.0	1.3	1.1	1.3	1.1	1.3	1.1	1.3
Niacin (mg)	RDA	6	8	8	12	12	14	16	14	16	14	16	14	16
Folate (mcg)	RDA	150	200	200	300	300	400	400	400	400	400	400	400	400
Vitamin B$_6$ (mg)	RDA	0.5	0.6	0.6	1.0	1.0	1.2	1.3	1.3	1.3	1.3	1.3	1.5	1.7
Vitamin B$_{12}$ (mcg)	RDA	0.9	1.2	1.2	1.8	1.8	2.4	2.4	2.4	2.4	2.4	2.4	2.4	2.4
Choline (mg)	AI	200	250	250	375	375	400	550	425	550	425	550	425	550
Vitamin K (mcg)	AI	30	55	55	60	60	75	75	90	120	90	120	90	120

Notes for Tables 1.2–4

a. *Dietary Guidelines* recommendations are used when no quantitative Dietary Reference Intake value is available; apply to ages 2 years and older.

b. Recommended Dietary Allowance, IOM [Institute of Medicine].

c. Acceptable Macronutrient Distribution Range, IOM.

d. 14 grams per 1,000 calories, IOM.

e. *Dietary Guidelines* recommendation.

f. Adequate Intake, IOM.

g. Upper Limit, IOM.

h. 1 mcg of vitamin D is equivalent to 40 IU.

AT = alpha-tocopherol; DFE = dietary folate equivalents; RAE = retinol activity equivalents.

Sources:

Britten P, Marcoe K, Yamini S, Davis C. Development of food intake patterns for the MyPyramid Food Guidance System. *J Nutr Educ Behav* 2006;38(6 Suppl):S78-S92.

IOM. *Dietary Reference Intakes*: The essential guide to nutrient requirements. Washington (DC): The National Academies Press; 2006.

IOM. *Dietary Reference Intakes for Calcium and Vitamin D*. Washington (DC): The National Academies Press; 2010.

Building Healthy Eating Patterns

Around the world and within the United States, people make strikingly different food choices and have different diet-related health outcomes. Although the study of eating patterns is complex, evidence from international scientific research has identified various eating patterns that may provide short- and long-term health benefits, including a reduced risk of chronic disease. Many traditional eating patterns can provide health benefits, and their variety demonstrates that people can eat healthfully in a number of ways.

Several types of research studies have been conducted on these eating patterns. Considerable research exists on health outcomes as well as information on nutrient and food group composition of some eating patterns constructed for clinical trials (for example, dietary approaches to stop hypertension, an eating pattern known as DASH, and its variations) and traditional eating patterns (for example, Mediterranean-style patterns). Some evidence for beneficial health outcomes for adults also exists for vegetarian eating patterns. In addition, investigators have studied traditional Japanese and Okinawan dietary patterns and have found associations with a low risk of coronary heart disease. However, detailed information on the composition of these Asian diets, and evidence on health benefits similar to that available for the other types of diets, is very limited.

Dietary Approaches To Stop Hypertension (DASH)

DASH emphasizes vegetables, fruits, and low-fat milk and milk products; includes whole grains, poultry, seafood, and nuts; and is lower in sodium, red and processed meats, sweets, and sugar-containing beverages than typical intakes in the United States. One of the original DASH study diets also was lower in total fat (27% of calories) than typical American intakes

Flexibility In Eating Patterns

A healthy eating pattern is not a rigid prescription, but rather an array of options that can accommodate cultural, ethnic, traditional, and personal preferences and food cost and availability.

However, modifications containing higher levels of either unsaturated fatty acids or protein have been tested. In research studies, each of these DASH-style patterns lowered blood pressure, improved blood lipids, and reduced cardiovascular disease risk compared to diets that were designed to resemble a typical American diet. The DASH-Sodium study of hypertensives and pre-hypertensives also reduced sodium, and resulted in lower blood pressure in comparison to the same eating pattern, but with a higher sodium intake. Eating patterns that are similar to DASH also have been associated with a reduced risk of cardiovascular disease and lowered mortality.

Mediterranean-Style Eating Patterns

A large number of cultures and agricultural patterns exist in countries that border the Mediterranean Sea, so the "Mediterranean diet" is not one eating pattern. No single set of criteria exists for what constitutes a traditional Mediterranean eating pattern. However, in general terms, it can be described as an eating pattern that emphasizes vegetables, fruits and nuts, olive oil, and grains (often whole grains). Only small amounts of meats and full-fat milk and milk products are usually included. It has a high monounsaturated to saturated fatty acid intake ratio.

Vegetarian Eating Patterns

The types of vegetarian diets consumed in the United States vary widely. Vegans do not consume any animal products, while lacto-ovo vegetarians consume milk and eggs. Some individuals eat diets that are primarily vegetarian but may include small amounts of meat, poultry, or seafood.

In prospective studies of adults, compared to non-vegetarian eating patterns, vegetarian-style eating patterns have been associated with improved health outcomes—lower levels of obesity, a reduced risk of cardiovascular disease, and lower total mortality. Several clinical trials have documented that vegetarian eating patterns lower blood pressure.

On average, vegetarians consume a lower proportion of calories from fat (particularly saturated fatty acids); fewer overall calories; and more fiber, potassium, and vitamin C than do non-vegetarians. Vegetarians generally have a lower body mass index. These characteristics and other lifestyle factors associated with a vegetarian diet may contribute to the positive health outcomes that have been identified among vegetarians.

Common Elements Of Healthy Eating Patterns

Although healthy eating patterns around the world are diverse, some common threads exist. They are abundant in vegetables and fruits. Many emphasize whole grains. They include moderate amounts and a variety of foods high in protein (seafood, beans and peas, nuts, seeds, soy products, meat, poultry, and eggs). They include only limited amounts of foods high in added sugars and may include more oils than solid fats. Most are low in full-fat milk and milk products. However, some include substantial amounts of low-fat milk and milk products. Compared to typical American diets, these patterns tend to have a high unsaturated to saturated fatty acid ratio and a high dietary fiber and potassium content. In addition, some are relatively low in sodium compared to current American intake.

Although there is no single "American" or "Western" eating pattern, average American eating patterns currently bear little resemblance to dietary recommendations. Americans eat too many calories and too much solid fat, added sugars, refined grains, and sodium. Americans also consume too little potassium; dietary fiber; calcium; vitamin D; unsaturated fatty acids from oils, nuts, and seafood; and other important nutrients. These nutrients are mostly found in vegetables, fruits, whole grains, and low-fat milk and milk products.

Table 1.5. Eating Pattern Comparison: Usual U.S. Intake, Mediterranean, DASH, And USDA Food Patterns (average daily intake at or adjusted to a 2,000 calorie level).

Pattern	Usual U.S. Intake Adults[a]	Mediterranean Patterns[b] Greece (G) Spain (S)	DASH[b]	USDA Food Pattern
Food Groups				
Vegetables[1]: Total	1.6	1.2 (S) – 4.1 (G)	2.1	2.5
Dark-green	0.1	nd[c]	nd	0.2
Beans and peas	0.1	<0.1 (G) – 0.4 (S)	See protein foods	0.2
Red and orange	0.4	nd	nd	0.8
Other	0.5	nd	nd	0.6
Starchy	0.5	nd – 0.6 (G)	nd	0.7
Fruit And Juices[1]	1.0	1.4 (S) – 2.5 (G) (including nuts)	2.5	2.0
Grains: Total[2]	6.4	2.0 (S) – 5.4 (G)	7.3	6.0
Whole grains	0.6	nd	3.9	>=3.0
Milk and milk products dairy products)[1]	1.5	1.0 (G) – 2.1 (S)	2.6	3.0
Protein foods[2]:				
Meat	2.5	3.5 (G) – 3.6 (S) (including poultry)	1.4	1.8
Poultry	1.2	nd	1.7	1.5
Eggs	0.4	nd – 1.9 (S)	nd	0.4

Principles For Achieving A Healthy Eating Pattern

A healthy eating pattern focuses on nutrient-dense foods—vegetables, fruits, whole grains, fat-free or low-fat milk and milk products, lean meats and poultry, seafood, eggs, beans and peas, and nuts and seeds that are prepared without added solid fats, sugars, starches, and sodium. Combined into an eating pattern, these foods can provide the full range of essential nutrients and fiber, without excessive calories. The oils contained in seafood, nuts and seeds, and vegetable oils added to foods also contribute essential nutrients.

Most people's eating patterns can accommodate only a limited number of calories from solid fats and added sugars. These calories are best used to increase the palatability of nutrient-dense foods rather than to consume foods or beverages that are primarily solid fats, added sugars, or both. A few examples of nutrient-dense foods containing some solid fats or added

Table 1.5. continued

Pattern	Usual U.S. Intake Adults[a]	Mediterranean Patterns[b] Greece (G) Spain (S)	DASH[b]	USDA Food Pattern
Fish/seafood	0.5	0.8 (G) – 2.4 (S)	1.4	1.2
Beans and peas[2]	See vegetables	See vegetables	0.4	See vegetables
Nuts, seeds, and soy products	0.5	See fruits	0.9	0.6
Oils[3]	18.0	19 (S) – 40 (G)	25.0	27.0
Solid fats[3]	43.0	nd	nd	16[d]
Added Sugars[3]	79.0	nd – 24 (G)	12.0	32[d]
Alcohol[3,4]	9.9	7.1 (S) – 7.9 (G)	nd	nd[e]

[1]Cups, [2]Ounces, [3]Grams

[4]Anyone younger than the legal drinking age should not consume any alcohol. Besides being illegal, alcohol consumption increases the risk of drowning, car accidents, and traumatic injury, which are common causes of death in children and adolescents.

Other Notes:

a Source: U.S. Department of Agriculture, Agricultural Research Service and U.S. Department of Health and Human Services, Centers for Disease Control and Prevention. What We Eat In America, NHANES [National Health and Nutrition Examination Survey] 2001–2004, 1 day mean intakes for adult males and females, adjusted to 2,000 calories and aver-aged.

b See the *Dietary Guidelines for Americans* report for additional information and references at www.dietaryguidelines.gov.

c nd = Not determined.

d Amounts of solid fats and added sugars are examples only of how calories from solid fats and added sugars in the USDA Food Patterns could be divided.

e In the USDA Food Patterns, some of the calories assigned to limits for solid fats and added sugars may be used for alcohol consumption instead.

sugars include whole-grain breakfast cereals that contain small amounts of added sugars, cuts of meat that are marbled with fat, poultry baked with skin on, vegetables topped with butter or stick margarine, fruit sprinkled with sugar, and fat-free chocolate milk.

Vegetarian Adaptations Of The USDA Food Patterns

The USDA food patterns allow for additional flexibility in choices through their adaptations for vegetarians—a vegan pattern that contains only plant foods and a lacto-ovo vegetarian pattern that includes milk and milk products and eggs. The adaptations include changes in the protein foods group and, in the vegan adaptation, in the dairy group. Vegetarian variations represent healthy eating patterns, but rely on fortified foods for some nutrients. In the vegan patterns especially, fortified foods provide much of the calcium and vitamin B12, and either fortified foods or supplements should be selected to provide adequate intake of these nutrients.

Chapter 2

Understanding Calories

"That's loaded with calories!"

"Are you counting your calories?"

When people talk about the calories in food, what do they mean? A calorie is a unit of measurement—but it doesn't measure weight or length. A calorie is a unit of energy. When you hear something contains 100 calories, it's a way of describing how much energy your body could get from eating or drinking it.

Are Calories Bad For You?

Calories aren't bad for you. Your body needs calories for energy. But eating too many calories—and not burning enough of them off through activity—can lead to weight gain.

Most foods and drinks contain calories. Some foods, such as lettuce, contain few calories. (A cup of shredded lettuce has less than 10 calories.) Other foods, like peanuts, contain a lot of calories. (A half of a cup of peanuts has 427 calories.)

You can find out how many calories are in a food by looking at the nutrition facts label. The label also will describe the components of the food—how many grams of carbohydrate, protein, and fat it contains. Here's how many calories are in one gram of each:

- **Carbohydrate:** 4 calories
- **Protein:** 4 calories
- **Fat:** 9 calories

About This Chapter: "Learning About Calories," March 2007, reprinted with permission from www.kidshealth .org. Copyright © 2007 The Nemours Foundation. This information was provided by KidsHealth, one of the largest resources online for medically reviewed health information written for parents, kids, and teens. For more articles like this one, visit www.KidsHealth.org, or www.TeensHealth.org.

What's It Mean?

Calorie: Unit of (heat) energy available from the metabolism of food that is required to sustain the body's various functions, including metabolic processes and physical activity. Carbohydrate, fat, protein, and alcohol provide all of the energy supplied by foods and beverages.

Source: Excerpted from *Dietary Guidelines for Americans 2010*, U.S. Department of Agriculture, December 2010.

That means if you know how many grams of each one are in a food, you can calculate the total calories. You would multiply the number of grams by the number of calories in a gram of that food component. For example, if a serving of potato chips (about 20 chips) has 10 grams of fat, 90 calories are from fat. That's 10 grams times 9 calories per gram.

Some people watch their calories if they are trying to lose weight. Most kids don't need to do this, but all kids can benefit from eating a healthy, balanced diet that includes the right number of calories—not too many, not too few. But how do you know how many calories you need?

How Many Calories Do Kids Need?

Kids come in all sizes and each person's body burns energy (calories) at different rates, so there isn't one perfect number of calories that a kid should eat. But there is a recommended range for most school-age kids: 1,600 to 2,500 per day.

When they reach puberty, girls need more calories, but they tend to need fewer calories than boys. As boys enter puberty, they will need as many as 2,500 to 3,000 calories per day. But whether they are girls or boys, kids who are active and move around a lot will need more calories than kids who don't.

Most kids don't have to worry about not getting enough calories because the body—and feelings of hunger—help regulate how many calories a person eats. But kids with certain medical problems may need to make sure they eat enough calories. Kids with cystic fibrosis, for instance, have to eat high-calorie foods because their bodies have trouble absorbing the nutrients and energy from food.

Kids who are overweight might have to make sure they don't eat too many calories. (Only your doctor can say if you are overweight, so check with him or her if you're concerned. And never go on a diet without talking to your doctor.)

If you eat more calories than your body needs, the leftover calories are converted to fat. Too much fat can lead to health problems. Often, kids who are overweight can start by avoiding high-calorie foods, such as sugary sodas, candy, and fast food, and by eating a healthy, balanced diet. Exercising and playing are really important, too, because activity burns calories.

Calories Burned

A 154-pound man (5' 10") will use up about the number of calories listed doing each activity in Table 2.1. Those who weigh more will use more calories, and those who weigh less will use fewer. The calorie values listed include both calories used by the activity and the calories used for normal body functioning.

Table 2.1. Approximate Calories Used By A 154-Pound Man

Moderate Physical Activities	In 1 hour	In 30 minutes
Hiking	370	185
Light gardening/yard work	330	165
Dancing	330	165
Golf (walking and carrying clubs)	330	165
Bicycling (less than 10 miles per hour)	290	145
Walking (3½ miles per hour)	280	140
Weight training (general light workout)	220	110
Stretching	180	90
Vigorous physical activities:	**In 1 hour**	**In 30 minutes**
Running/jogging (5 miles per hour)	590	295
Bicycling (more than 10 miles per hour)	590	295
Swimming (slow freestyle laps)	510	255
Aerobics	480	240
Walking (4½ miles per hour)	460	230
Heavy yard work (chopping wood)	440	220
Weight lifting (vigorous effort)	440	220
Basketball (vigorous)	440	220

Excerpted from "How Many Calories Does Physical Activity Use?" U.S. Department of Agriculture, May 18, 2011.

How The Body Uses Calories

Some people mistakenly believe they have to burn off all the calories they eat or they will gain weight. This isn't true. Your body needs some calories just to operate—to keep your heart beating and your lungs breathing. As a kid, your body also needs calories from a variety of foods to grow and develop. And you burn off some calories without even thinking about it—by walking your dog or making your bed.

But it is a great idea to play and be active for at least one hour and up to several hours a day. That means time spent playing sports, just running around outside, or riding your bike. It all adds up. Being active every day keeps your body strong and can help you maintain a healthy weight.

Watching TV and playing video games doesn't burn many calories at all, which is why you should try to limit those activities to one to two hours per day. A person burns only about one calorie per minute while watching TV, about the same as sleeping.

Chapter 3

Understanding The Food Label

Benefits Of The Food Label

Health professionals agree that the relationship between diet and health is important. Our eating habits can help or hurt our overall health and wellbeing. Good eating habits include being a smart shopper and selecting foods that reflect the *Dietary Guidelines for Americans*.

The food label was designed to help people choose foods for a healthful diet. By using the food label, we can compare the nutrient content of similar foods, see how foods fit into our overall diets, and understand the relationship between certain nutrients and diseases.

The Dietary Guidelines For Americans

Developed by the United States Department of Agriculture (USDA) in 1980, and updated every five years, the *Dietary Guidelines for Americans* reflect the most recent scientific research about nutrition and health. Released in 2005, the latest version of the *Dietary Guidelines* contains key recommendations for the general population as well as recommendations for specific population groups. Information found on both the front and back of food packages can aid consumers in choosing foods that follow these recommendations. For more information about the *Dietary Guidelines for Americans* visit www.healthierus.gov/dietaryguidelines for the USDA's complete *Dietary Guidelines for Americans* report. [Ed. Note: See Chapter 1 for additional information about the newly released 2010 *Dietary Guidelines*.]

About This Chapter: This chapter begins with text under the heading "Benefits of the Food Label," from "Understanding the Food Label," by J. Anderson, L. Young and S. Perryman, December 2010. © Colorado State University Extension (www.ext.colostate.edu). Reprinted with permission. Text under the heading "How To Understand and Use the Nutrition Facts Label" is from the U.S. Food and Drug Administration (www.fda.gov), June 2009.

Remember

The food label provides:

- Nutrition labeling for most foods
- Standardized serving sizes
- Information on saturated fat, trans fat, cholesterol, dietary fiber, and other nutrients of major concern
- Nutrient reference values to help us understand how that food fits into a daily diet
- Uniform definitions for nutrient claims, such as "light," "low-fat," and "high-fiber"
- Health claims about the relationship between a nutrient and a disease

Source: December 2010. © Colorado State University Extension.

Nutrition Facts

Serving Size 1 cup (228g)
Servings Per Container 2

Amount Per Serving	
Calories 250	Calories from Fat 110

	% Daily Value*
Total Fat 12g	18%
Saturated Fat 3g	15%
Trans Fat 1.5g	
Cholesterol 30mg	10%
Sodium 470mg	20%
Total Carbohydrate 31g	10%
Dietary Fiber 0g	0%
Sugars 5g	
Protein 5g	

Vitamin A	4%
Vitamin C	2%
Calcium	20%
Iron	4%

* Percent Daily Values are based on a 2,000 calorie diet. Your Daily Values may be higher or lower depending on your calorie needs:

	Calories:	2,000	2,500
Total Fat	Less than	65g	80g
Sat Fat	Less than	20g	25g
Cholesterol	Less than	300mg	300mg
Sodium	Less than	2,400mg	2,400mg
Total Carbohydrate		300g	375g
Dietary Fiber		25g	30g

Figure 3.1. A sample nutrition facts panel.

The Front Of The Package

Nutrient Descriptors And Claims: The front of the package is designed to get your attention. Manufacturers use different packaging techniques to get us to buy their products. For many years, specific nutrient descriptors and claims appeared on packages with a loosely defined form of standardization. Today, descriptors such as "high fiber," "light," or "low fat," as well as specific nutrient claims, have standard definitions and requirements that consumers can use as a quick guide for making smart selections. By understanding what the nutrient descriptors and claims mean, you can more effectively and efficiently select foods and choose between products. Table 3.2 provides a glossary of nutrient descriptors and claims.

Health Claims: Health claims describe the relationship between a nutrient or a food and the risk of a disease. Products that make a health claim must contain a defined amount of the nutrient that is directly linked to the health-related condition.

For example, to make a claim about the relationship between sodium and hypertension, the product must contain 140 milligrams or less of sodium per serving. If the package states that the product "may reduce the risk of hypertension," we know that it is a low-sodium product, because low sodium also is defined as 140 milligrams or less sodium per serving.

Additionally, the claims must make it clear that other factors, such as exercise or heredity, may also influence the development of certain diseases. Health claims cannot state the degree of risk reduction and must use words such as "may" or "might" in discussing the food-disease relationship. Examples of health claims approved for food labels:

Calcium And Osteoporosis

- *Claim:* A diet adequate in calcium may help reduce the risk for osteoporosis, a degenerative bone disease.

- *Requirements:* At least 200 milligrams calcium, no more phosphorus than calcium per serving, and calcium must be in a form that can be readily absorbed by the body.

Fat And Cancer

- *Claim:* A low-fat diet may help the risk for developing some types of cancer.

- *Requirements:* 3 grams or less fat per serving or fish and game meats that are "extra-lean" (fewer than 5 grams fat, fewer than 2 grams saturated fat, and fewer than 95 milligrams cholesterol per serving).

Fiber-Containing Fruits, Vegetables, And Grain Products And Risk Of CHD

- *Claim:* Along with eating a diet low in fat, saturated fat, and cholesterol, fiber may help reduce blood cholesterol levels and the risk for developing heart disease.

- *Requirements:* Must be or contain a fruit, vegetable, or grain product, 3 grams or less fat per serving, fewer than 20 milligrams cholesterol per serving, 1 gram or less saturated fat per serving, and 15% or less calories from saturated fat, 0.6 grams or more dietary fiber per serving.

Folate or Folic Acid and Neural Birth Defects

- *Claim:* Healthful diets with adequate folate may reduce a woman's risk of having a child with a neural tube defect.

- *Requirements:* The food must meet or exceed the criteria for a good source: 40 micrograms folic acid per serving or at least 10% of Daily Value. A serving cannot contain more than 100% of the Daily Value for vitamins A or D because of potential risk to fetuses.

Omega-3 Fatty Acids

- *Claim:* Supportive but not conclusive research shows that consumption of EPA and DHA omega-3 fatty acids may reduce the risk of coronary heart disease.

- *Requirements:* With the exception of fish and dietary supplements, foods must be low in cholesterol and low in saturated fat.

A complete listing of health claims approved for food labels is available from the Center for Food Safety and Applied Nutrition at www.cfsan.fda.gov/label.html.

Organic Labeling

The Organic Foods Production Act and the National Organic Program (NOP) ensure that organic foods purchased in the United Sates are produced, processed, and certified to consistent national organic standards. On food labels, products that use the term "organic" must meet the following guidelines.

- Products labeled as "100% organic" must contain (excluding water and salt) only organically produced ingredients.

- Products labeled "organic" must consist of at least 95% organically produced ingredients (excluding water and salt). Any remaining product ingredients must consist of nonagricultural substances approved on the National List or non-organically produced agricultural products that are not commercially available in organic form.

- Processed products that contain at least 70% organic ingredients can use the phrase "made with organic ingredients" and list up to three of the organic ingredients or food groups on the principal display panel. For example, soup made with at least 70% organic ingredients and only organic vegetables may be labeled either "soup made with organic peas, potatoes, and carrots," or "soup made with organic vegetables."

The Back Of The Package

The "Nutrition Facts" section on the back of the food label allows you to make comparisons between the nutrient contents of similar foods and to see how the foods fit into your overall diet. The nutrition facts panel provides information on saturated fat, cholesterol, dietary fiber, and other nutrients that are of major health concern. As of 2006, the Food and Drug Administration (FDA) also requires that all manufacturers list trans fats on the nutrition facts panel. Scientific research shows that consumption of trans fat raises LDL ("bad") cholesterol levels and increases risk for developing heart disease.

The components of the nutrition panel include mandatory and voluntary dietary information. The mandatory components are listed on the nutrition facts panel in the order shown in Figure 3.1. Immediately to the right of each nutrient, the absolute amount of that nutrient (in grams or milligrams) is listed per serving.

Additionally, a column labeled "% Daily Value" helps us determine how each nutrient fits into an average daily diet. "Daily Value" is used to refer to two separate sets of reference values. The reference daily intakes (RDIs) are reference values for 19 vitamins and minerals, based on the dietary reference intakes (DRIs). Daily reference values (DRVs) also are provided for eight additional nutrients based on dietary guidelines. The RDI and DRV form the basis for the %DV.

Voluntary dietary components on the label include: calories from saturated fat, polyunsaturated fat, monounsaturated fat, potassium, soluble fiber, insoluble fiber, sugar alcohol, other carbohydrate, and other essential vitamins and minerals. The standard "Nutrition Facts" panel may be presented in different formats depending on the size of the package or the total nutrient content in the food.

Table 3.1. Nutrition Reference Amounts In Grams (g) For Different Calorie Levels*

	Calories					
Food Component	**1,600**	**2,000**	**2,200**	**2,500**	**2,800**	**3,200**
total fat (g)	53	65	73	80	93	107
saturated fat (g)	18	20	24	25	31	36
total carbohydrate (g)	240	300	330	375	420	480
dietary fiber (g)**	20	25	25	30	32	37
protein (g)***	46	50	55	65	70	80

* Numbers may be rounded.
** 20 grams is the minimum recommended by the National Cancer Institute.
*** 46 grams is the minimum recommended.

List Of Ingredients

Ingredients for all foods must be listed on the food label, including standardized foods. The label must also list the FDA-certified color additives by name. Ingredients are listed in descending order by weight. Specific ingredient information, such as the source of the protein, also is included. This allows people to avoid substances to which they are allergic or sensitive, or for religious or cultural reasons.

As of January 2006, food manufacturers also must disclose in plain language whether products contain any of the top eight food allergens. While numerous foods have been identified as sources of allergic reactions, 90% of the allergic reactions associated with foods are caused by one of eight foods: milk, eggs, fish, crustacean shellfish, peanuts, tree nuts, wheat, and soy.

Manufacturers have two options for declaring the presence of these food substances in foods. One option is to provide a "contains" statement next to the ingredient list that identifies the types of allergenic ingredients contained in the product; for example, "contains milk and wheat." The second option is to place the food source in parentheses next to ingredients derived from one of the eight potential offending foods classes, such as sodium caseinate (milk), albumin (egg).

However, the new law does not specifically address gluten. Gluten describes a group of proteins found in certain grains, such as wheat, barley, and rye, that cannot be tolerated by people with celiac disease. The new law requires the FDA to issue a proposed rule that allows voluntary use of the term "gluten free" as of August 2006 and to have a final rule on "gluten free" in place by August 2008. [Ed. Note: FDA did issue a proposed rule, but it resulted in the need for more study. As of early 2011, the final rule had not yet been published.]

Getting The Right Balance Of Each Nutrient

The % Daily Value allows us to determine the nutrient contribution of that particular food or beverage relative to a 2,000 calorie per day diet. Not everyone consumes exactly 2,000 calories each day. That number was established as the average reference intake of Americans. Factors that contribute to energy needs include gender, age and activity level. Therefore, it is important to establish your individual energy needs and make adjustments accordingly to fit your personal "% Daily Value."

Table 3.1 lists various calorie intake levels and corresponding nutrient recommendations. Remember that the reference amounts listed on the label are based on a 2,000 calorie diet. Some labels also may contain reference values for a 2,500 calorie diet. DVs are listed as the percent of a minimum or a maximum value. For example, DVs for some nutrients (total fat, saturated fat, cholesterol and sodium) represent the upper limit considered desirable.

By using the "% Daily Value," you can easily determine what amount of a nutrient a food provides and then choose the other foods you eat during the day according to your specific needs. For example, if you consume 2,000 calories per day, your total fat intake should not exceed 65 grams. If you eat 13 grams of fat at breakfast or 20% of your Daily Value (DV), and about 20 grams of fat at lunch (30% of your DV), then you should not consume more than about 32 grams of fat (or 50% of your daily fat intake) for the remainder of the day (snacks and dinner combined).

The Daily Value is not a rigid number, but rather a reference value to aim for in balancing your intake. Use it to compare different products. Keep in mind variety and moderation—the important fundamentals of good eating habits.

Serving Sizes

The serving size is the basis for reporting the nutrient content of each food. In the past the serving size was up to the discretion of the manufacturer. Now serving sizes must be consistent between similar products (for example, breakfast cereals) and reflective of typical consumption.

Serving sizes must be expressed in metric measures as well as common household units to make it easier for consumers to make quick comparisons. For example, if you are trying to decide between two breakfast cereals and want to purchase the one higher in dietary fiber, you can make an easier and more educated comparison because the serving sizes are the same.

Source: December 2010. © Colorado State University Extension.

Making Quick Comparisons Between Similar Products

Regardless of the format, the serving size is the basis for reporting the nutrient content of each food. However, unlike in the past, where the serving size was up to the discretion of the manufacturer, serving sizes now must be consistent between similar products (for example, breakfast cereals) and reflective of typical consumption.

Serving sizes must be expressed in metric measures as well as common household units to make it easier for consumers to make quick comparisons. For example, if you are trying to decide between two breakfast cereals and want to purchase the one higher in dietary fiber, you can make an easier and more educated comparison because the serving sizes are the same.

References

FDA Backgrounder: The New Food Label. BG 92-4 (December 10, 1992).

Smart Selections for Healthy Eating: Using the new food label. A project of Public Voice for Food and Health Policy in cooperation with Campbell Soup Company.

Browne, M.B. Label Facts for Healthful Eating. National Food Processors Association, 1993.

FDA Consumer. An FDA Consumer Special Report. Focus on Food Labeling. May 1993.

FDA Consumer. Focus on Food Labeling, Vol. 27:4, May 1993.

The National Organic Program. Labeling and Marketing Information. October 2002. Available at www.ams.usda.gov/nop/FactSheets/LabelingE.html.

Reviewed and revised by K. Topham and C. Fitzgerald. 12/10.

Table 3.2. Glossary Of Nutrient Claims And Descriptors

Term	Description
Calorie free	Less than 5 calories per serving.
Cholesterol free	Less than 2 mg cholesterol and 2 g or less saturated fat per serving.
Enriched or fortified	Has been nutritionally altered so that one serving provides at least 10% more of the Daily Value of a nutrient than the comparison food.
Extra lean	Less than 5 g fat, 2 g saturated fat, and 95 mg of cholesterol per serving and per 100 g.
Fat free	Less than 0.5 g of fat per serving.
Free	"Without," "no," or "zero" can all be used in place of "free."
Fresh	Generally used on food in its raw state. It cannot be used on food that has been frozen or cooked, or on food that contains preservatives.
Fresh-frozen	Foods that have been quickly frozen while still fresh.
Good source	One serving provides 10–19% of the Daily Value for a particular nutrient.
Good source of fiber	Contains 10 to 19% of the Daily Value for fiber (2.5–4.75 g) per serving. If a food is not "low fat," it must declare the level of total fat per serving and refer to the nutrition panel when a fiber claim is mentioned.
High	One serving provides at least 20% or more of the Daily Value for a particular nutrient.
High fiber	Contains 20% or more of the Daily Value for fiber (at least 5 g) per serving. If a food is not "low fat," it must declare the level of total fat per serving and refer to the nutrition panel when a fiber claim is made.
Lean	Less than 10 g fat, 4 g saturated fat, and 95 mg cholesterol per serving and per 100 g.
Light	1) At least one-third fewer calories per serving than a comparison food; or 2) contains no more than half the fat per serving of a comparison food. If a food derives 50% or more of its calories from fat, the reduction must be at least 50% of the fat; or 3) contains at least 50% less sodium per serving than a comparison food; or 4) can refer to texture and/or color, if clearly explained, for example, "light brown sugar."
Low	"Little," "few," or "low source of" may be used in place of "low."
Low calorie	40 calories or less per serving.
Low cholesterol	20 mg or less cholesterol and 2 g or less saturated fat per serving.
Low fat	3 g or less per serving.
Low saturated fat	1 g or less saturated fat per serving and 15% or less calories from fat.
Low sodium	140 mg or less per serving.
More	One serving contains at least 10% more of the Daily Value of a nutrient than the comparison food.
Percent fat free	A claim made on a "low fat" or "fat free" product which accurately reflects the amount of fat present in 100 g of food; a food with 3 g of fat per 100 g would be "97% fat free."
Reduced	A nutritionally altered product which must contain 25% less of a nutrient or of calories than the regular or reference product.
Salt or sodium free	Less than 5 mg per serving.
Sugar free	Less than 0.5 g of sugars per serving.
Unsalted	Has no salt added during processing. To use this term, the product it resembles must normally be processed with salt and the label must note that the food is not a sodium-free food if it does not meet the requirements for "sodium free."
Very low sodium	Less than 35 mg or less sodium per serving.

How To Understand And Use The Nutrition Facts Label

The following label-building skills are intended to make it easier for you to use nutrition labels to make quick, informed food choices that contribute to a healthy diet (refer to Figure 3.1 [on page 22] to see the components as they appear on a Nutrition Facts Label).

The Serving Size

The first place to start when you look at the Nutrition Facts label is the serving size and the number of servings in the package. Serving sizes are standardized to make it easier to compare similar foods; they are provided in familiar units, such as cups or pieces, followed by the metric amount, for example, the number of grams.

The size of the serving on the food package influences the number of calories and all of the nutrient amounts listed on the top part of the label. Pay attention to the serving size, especially how many servings there are in the food package. Then ask yourself, "How many servings am I consuming"? (for example, half serving, one serving, or more)

Calories And Calories From Fat

Calories provide a measure of how much energy you get from a serving of this food. Many Americans consume more calories than they need without meeting recommended intakes for a number of nutrients. The calorie section of the label can help you manage your weight (that is, gain, lose, or maintain.) Remember: The number of servings you consume determines the number of calories you actually eat (your portion amount).

General Guide To Calories: This general guide to calories provides a general reference for calories when you look at a Nutrition Facts label. This guide is based on a 2,000 calorie diet. Eating too many calories per day is linked to overweight and obesity.

- 40 calories is low

- 100 calories is moderate

- 400 calories or more is high

The Nutrients: How Much?

Look at the top of the nutrient section in the label. It shows you some key nutrients that impact on your health and separates them into two main groups.

The nutrients listed first are the ones Americans generally eat in adequate amounts, or even too much. Eating too much fat, saturated fat, trans fat, cholesterol, or sodium may increase your risk of certain chronic diseases, like heart disease, some cancers, or high blood pressure.

Health experts recommend that you keep your intake of saturated fat, trans fat and cholesterol as low as possible as part of a nutritionally balanced diet.

Get Enough Of These: Most Americans don't get enough dietary fiber, vitamin A, vitamin C, calcium, and iron in their diets. Eating enough of these nutrients can improve your health and help reduce the risk of some diseases and conditions. For example, getting enough calcium may reduce the risk of osteoporosis, a condition that results in brittle bones as one ages. Eating a diet high in dietary fiber promotes healthy bowel function. Additionally, a diet rich in fruits, vegetables, and grain products that contain dietary fiber, particularly soluble fiber, and low in saturated fat and cholesterol may reduce the risk of heart disease.

Quick Guide To Percent Daily Value

Comparisons: The %DV also makes it easy for you to make comparisons. You can compare one product or brand to a similar product. Just make sure the serving sizes are similar, especially the weight (for example, gram, milligram, or ounces) of each product. It's easy to see which foods are higher or lower in nutrients because the serving sizes are generally consistent for similar types of foods except in a few cases like cereals.

Nutrient Content Claims: Use the %DV to help you quickly distinguish one claim from another, such as "reduced fat" vs. "light" or "nonfat." Just compare the %DVs for Total Fat in each food product to see which one is higher or lower in that nutrient—there is no need to memorize definitions. This works when comparing all nutrient content claims, for example, less, light, low, free, more, high, etc.

Dietary Trade-Offs: You can use the %DV to help you make dietary trade-offs with other foods throughout the day. You don't have to give up a favorite food to eat a healthy diet. When a food you like is high in fat, balance it with foods that are low in fat at other times of the day. Also, pay attention to how much you eat so that the total amount of fat for the day stays below 100%DV.

Limit Or Increase Nutrients

You can use the Nutrition Facts label not only to help limit those nutrients you want to cut back on but also to increase those nutrients you need to consume in greater amounts.

Source: U.S. Food and Drug Administration, 2009.

Tip For Limiting Nutrients

To limit nutrients that have no %DV, like trans fat and sugars, compare the labels of similar products and choose the food with the lowest amount.

Source: U.S. Food and Drug Administration, 2009.

Calcium: Look at the %DV for calcium on food packages so you know how much one serving contributes to the total amount you need per day. Remember, a food with 20%DV or more contributes a lot of calcium to your daily total, while one with 5%DV or less contributes a little.

Experts advise adult consumers to consume adequate amounts of calcium, that is, 1,000 mg or 100%DV in a daily 2,000 calorie diet. This advice is often given in milligrams (mg), but the Nutrition Facts label only lists a %DV for calcium.

For certain populations, they advise that adolescents, especially girls, consume 1,300mg (130%DV) of calcium daily. The DV for calcium on food labels is 1,000 mg.

Nutrients Without A %DV: Trans Fats, Protein, And Sugars

Trans Fat: Experts could not provide a reference value for trans fat nor any other information that FDA believes is sufficient to establish a Daily Value or %DV. Scientific reports link trans fat (and saturated fat) with raising blood LDL ("bad") cholesterol levels, both of which increase your risk of coronary heart disease, a leading cause of death in the U.S.

Protein: A %DV is required to be listed if a claim is made for protein, such as "high in protein." Otherwise, unless the food is meant for use by infants and children under four-years-old, none is needed. Current scientific evidence indicates that protein intake is not a public health concern for adults and children over four years of age.

Sugars: No daily reference value has been established for sugars because no recommendations have been made for the total amount to eat in a day. Keep in mind, the sugars listed on the Nutrition Facts label include naturally occurring sugars (like those in fruit and milk) as well as those added to a food or drink.

If you are concerned about your intake of sugars, make sure that added sugars are not listed as one of the first few ingredients. Other names for added sugars include: corn syrup, high-fructose corn syrup, fruit juice concentrate, maltose, dextrose, sucrose, honey, and maple syrup.

Chapter 4

Grains

What foods are in the grains group?

Any food made from wheat, rice, oats, cornmeal, barley, or another cereal grain is a grain product. Bread, pasta, oatmeal, breakfast cereals, tortillas, and grits are examples of grain products.

Grains are divided into two subgroups, whole grains and refined grains. Whole grains contain the entire grain kernel—the bran, germ, and endosperm. Examples include whole-wheat flour, bulgur (cracked wheat), oatmeal, whole cornmeal, and brown rice.

Refined grains have been milled, a process that removes the bran and germ. This is done to give grains a finer texture and improve their shelf life, but it also removes dietary fiber, iron, and many B vitamins. Some examples of refined grain products are white flour, degermed cornmeal, white bread, and white rice.

Most refined grains are enriched. This means certain B vitamins (thiamin, riboflavin, niacin, folic acid) and iron are added back after processing. Fiber is not added back to enriched grains. Check the ingredient list on refined grain products to make sure that the word "enriched" is included in the grain name. Some food products are made from mixtures of whole grains and refined grains.

Commonly eaten grain products include the following:

- **Whole Grains:** Amaranth; brown rice; buckwheat; bulgur (cracked wheat); millet; oatmeal; popcorn; ready-to-eat breakfast cereals (whole wheat cereal flakes, muesli); rolled oats; quinoa; sorghum; triticale; whole grain barley; whole grain cornmeal; whole rye; whole wheat bread; whole wheat crackers; whole wheat pasta; whole wheat sandwich buns and rolls; whole wheat tortillas; wild rice

About This Chapter: From "Good Groups: Grains," U.S. Department of Agriculture (ChooseMyPlate.gov), May 31, 2011.

- **Refined Grains:** Cornbread*; corn tortillas*; couscous*; crackers*; flour tortillas*; grits; noodles*; pasta* (spaghetti, macaroni); pitas*; pretzels; ready-to-eat breakfast cereals (corn flakes); white bread; white sandwich buns and rolls; white rice. (*Most of these products are made from refined grains. Some are made from whole grains. Check the ingredient list for the words "whole grain" or "whole wheat" to decide if they are made from a whole grain. Some foods are made from a mixture of whole and refined grains.)

Some grain products contain significant amounts of bran. Bran provides fiber, which is important for health. However, products with added bran or bran alone (for example, oat bran) are not necessarily whole grain products.

How many grain foods are needed daily?

The amount of grains you need to eat depends on your age, sex, and level of physical activity. Recommended daily amounts are listed in Table 4.1. Most Americans consume enough grains, but few are whole grains. At least half of all the grains eaten should be whole grains.

> **Whole Grains**
>
> Make at least half your grains whole grains.

Table 4.1. Recommendations For Grain Foods

		Daily recommendation*	Daily minimum amount of whole grains*
Children	2–3 years old	3 ounce equivalents	1½ ounce equivalents
	4–8 years old	5 ounce equivalents	2½ ounce equivalents
Girls	9–13 years old	5 ounce equivalents	3 ounce equivalents
	14–18 years old	6 ounce equivalents	3 ounce equivalents
Boys	9–13 years old	6 ounce equivalents	3 ounce equivalents
	14–18 years old	8 ounce equivalents	4 ounce equivalents
Women	19–30 years old	6 ounce equivalents	3 ounce equivalents
	31–50 years old	6 ounce equivalents	3 ounce equivalents
	51+ years old	5 ounce equivalents	3 ounce equivalents
Men	19–30 years old	8 ounce equivalents	4 ounce equivalents
	31-50 years old	7 ounce equivalents	3½ ounce equivalents
	51+ years old	6 ounce equivalents	3 ounce equivalents

*These amounts are appropriate for individuals who get less than 30 minutes per day of moderate physical activity, beyond normal daily activities. Those who are more physically active may be able to consume more while staying within calorie needs. To see what counts as an ounce-equivalent of grains, see Table 4.2.

Check Food Labels To Identify Whole Grains

- Choose foods that name a whole-grain ingredient first on the label's ingredient list (see the lists of whole grains and refined grains in the chapter to help you identify which grains are whole grains).

- Foods labeled with the words "multi-grain," "stone-ground," "100% wheat," "cracked wheat," "seven-grain," or "bran" are usually not whole-grain products.

- Color is not an indication of a whole grain. Bread can be brown because of molasses or other added ingredients. Read the ingredient list to see if it is a whole grain.

- Use the Nutrition Facts label and choose whole grain products with a higher % Daily Value (%DV) for fiber. Many, but not all, whole grain products are good or excellent sources of fiber.

- Read the food label's ingredient list. Look for terms that indicate added sugars (such as sucrose, high-fructose corn syrup, honey, malt syrup, maple syrup, molasses, or raw sugar) that add extra calories. Choose foods with fewer added sugars.

- Most sodium in the food supply comes from packaged foods. Similar packaged foods can vary widely in sodium content, including breads. Use the Nutrition Facts label to choose foods with a lower % DV for sodium. Foods with less than 140 mg sodium per serving can be labeled as low sodium foods. Claims such as "low in sodium" or "very low in sodium" on the front of the food label can help you identify foods that contain less salt (or sodium).

What counts as an ounce equivalent of grains?

In general, one slice of bread, one cup of ready-to-eat cereal, or a half cup of cooked rice, cooked pasta, or cooked cereal can be considered as one ounce equivalent from the grains group. Table 4.2 lists specific amounts that count as one ounce equivalent of grains towards your daily recommended intake. In some cases the number of ounce-equivalents for common portions are also shown.

Why is it important to eat grains, especially whole grains?

Eating grains, especially whole grains, provides health benefits. People who eat whole grains as part of a healthy diet have a reduced risk of some chronic diseases. Grains provide many nutrients that are vital for the health and maintenance of our bodies.

Health Benefits

- Consuming whole grains as part of a healthy diet may reduce the risk of heart disease.

- Consuming foods containing fiber, such as whole grains, as part of a healthy diet, may reduce constipation.

Table 4.2. Grain Ounce Equivalents

Food		1 ounce equivalent*	ounce equivalents of common portions**
Bagels	WG: whole wheat RG: plain, egg	1 "mini" bagel	1 large bagel = 4 oz. equivalents
Biscuits	RG: baking powder/buttermilk	1 small (2" diameter)	1 large (3" diameter) = 2 oz. equivalents
Breads	WG: 100% whole wheat RG: white, wheat, French, sourdough	1 regular slice 1 small slice French 4 snack-size slices rye bread	2 regular slices = 2 oz. equivalents
Bulgur	WG: cracked wheat	½ cup cooked	
Cornbread	RG	1 small piece (2½" x 1¼" x 1¼")	1 medium piece (2½" x 2½" x 1¼") = 2 oz. equivalents
Crackers	WG: 100% whole wheat, rye RG: saltines, snack crackers	5 whole wheat crackers 2 rye crispbreads 7 square or round crackers	
English muffins	WG: whole wheat RG: plain, raisin	½ muffin	1 muffin = 2 oz. equivalents
Muffins	WG: whole wheat RG: bran, corn, plain	1 small (2½" diameter)	1 large (3½" diameter) = 3 oz. equivalents
Oatmeal	WG	½ cup cooked 1 packet instant 1 oz. (1/3 cup) dry (regular or quick)	
Pancakes	WG: whole wheat, buckwheat RG: buttermilk, plain	1 pancake (4½" diameter) 2 small pancakes (3" diameter)	3 pancakes (4½" diameter) = 3 oz. equivalents
Popcorn	WG	3 cups, popped	1 mini microwave bag or 100-calorie bag, popped = 2 oz. equivalents
Ready-to-eat breakfast cereal	WG: toasted oat, whole wheat flakes RG: corn flakes, puffed rice	1 cup flakes or rounds 1¼ cup puffed	
Rice	WG: brown, wild RG: enriched, white, polished	½ cup cooked 1 ounce dry	1 cup cooked = 2 oz. equivalents
Pasta (spaghetti, macaroni, noodles)	WG: whole wheat RG: enriched, durum	½ cup cooked 1 oz. dry	1 cup cooked = 2 oz. equivalents
Tortillas	WG: whole wheat, whole grain corn RG: Flour, corn	1 small flour tortilla (6" diameter) 1 corn tortilla (6" diameter)	1 large tortilla (12" diameter) = 4 ounce equivalents

WG = whole grains; RG = refined grains; oz. = ounce

*Amount of the food item that counts as being equivalent to 1 ounce of grains.

**Commonly consumed portions sometimes differ from standard serving sizes. The ounce equivalents here are for some common portions.

- Eating whole grains may help with weight management.

- Eating grain products fortified with folate before and during pregnancy helps prevent neural tube defects during fetal development.

Tips To Help You Eat Whole Grains

At Meals

To eat more whole grains, substitute a whole-grain product for a refined product—such as eating whole-wheat bread instead of white bread or brown rice instead of white rice. It's important to substitute the whole-grain product for the refined one, rather than adding the whole-grain product. Here are some more tips:

- For a change, try brown rice or whole-wheat pasta. Try brown rice stuffing in baked green peppers or tomatoes and whole-wheat macaroni in macaroni and cheese.

- Use whole grains in mixed dishes, such as barley in vegetable soup or stews and bulgur wheat in casserole or stir-fries.

- Create a whole grain pilaf with a mixture of barley, wild rice, brown rice, broth and spices. For a special touch, stir in toasted nuts or chopped dried fruit.

- Experiment by substituting whole wheat or oat flour for up to half of the flour in pancake, waffle, muffin or other flour-based recipes. They may need a bit more leavening.

- Use whole-grain bread or cracker crumbs in meatloaf.

- Try rolled oats or a crushed, unsweetened whole grain cereal as breading for baked chicken, fish, veal cutlets, or eggplant parmesan.

- Try an unsweetened, whole grain ready-to-eat cereal as croutons in salad or in place of crackers with soup.

- Freeze leftover cooked brown rice, bulgur, or barley. Heat and serve it later as a quick side dish.

Whole Grain Snacks

- Snack on ready-to-eat, whole grain cereals such as toasted oat cereal.

- Add whole-grain flour or oatmeal when making cookies or other baked treats.

- Try 100% whole-grain snack crackers.

- Popcorn, a whole grain, can be a healthy snack if made with little or no added salt and butter.

Nutrients

- Grains are important sources of many nutrients, including dietary fiber, several B vitamins (thiamin, riboflavin, niacin, and folate), and minerals (iron, magnesium, and selenium).

- Dietary fiber from whole grains or other foods, may help reduce blood cholesterol levels and may lower risk of heart disease, obesity, and type 2 diabetes. Fiber is important for proper bowel function. It helps reduce constipation and diverticulosis. Fiber-containing foods such as whole grains help provide a feeling of fullness with fewer calories.

- The B vitamins thiamin, riboflavin, and niacin play a key role in metabolism—they help the body release energy from protein, fat, and carbohydrates. B vitamins are also essential for a healthy nervous system. Many refined grains are enriched with these B vitamins.

- Folate (folic acid), another B vitamin, helps the body form red blood cells. Women of childbearing age who may become pregnant should consume adequate folate from foods, and in addition 400 mcg of synthetic folic acid from fortified foods or supplements. This reduces the risk of neural tube defects, spina bifida, and anencephaly during fetal development.

- Iron is used to carry oxygen in the blood. Many teenage girls and women in their childbearing years have iron-deficiency anemia. They should eat foods high in heme-iron (meats) or eat other iron containing foods along with foods rich in vitamin C, which can improve absorption of non-heme iron. Whole and enriched refined grain products are major sources of non-heme iron in American diets.

- Whole grains are sources of magnesium and selenium. Magnesium is a mineral used in building bones and releasing energy from muscles. Selenium protects cells from oxidation. It is also important for a healthy immune system.

Chapter 5

Vegetables

What foods are in the vegetable group?

Any vegetable or 100% vegetable juice counts as a member of the vegetable group. Vegetables may be raw or cooked; fresh, frozen, canned, or dried/dehydrated; and may be whole, cut-up, or mashed.

Vegetables are organized into five subgroups, based on their nutrient content. Some commonly eaten vegetables in each subgroup include the following:

- Dark green vegetables: Bok choy; broccoli; collard greens; dark green leafy lettuce; kale; mesclun; mustard greens; romaine lettuce; spinach; turnip greens; watercress

- Red and orange vegetables: Acorn squash; butternut squash; carrots; hubbard squash; pumpkin; red peppers; sweet potatoes; tomatoes; tomato juice

- Beans and peas: Black beans; black-eyed peas (mature, dry); garbanzo beans (chickpeas); kidney beans; lentils; navy beans; pinto beans; soy beans; split peas; white beans

- Starchy vegetables: Cassava; corn; fresh cowpeas, field peas, or black-eyed peas (not dry); green bananas; green peas; green lima beans; plantains; potatoes; taro; water chestnuts

- Other vegetables: Artichokes; asparagus; avocado; bean sprouts; beets; brussels sprouts; cabbage; cauliflower; celery; cucumbers; eggplant; green beans; green peppers; iceberg (head) lettuce; mushrooms; okra; onions; parsnips; turnips; wax beans; zucchini

About This Chapter: From "Good Groups: Vegetables," U.S. Department of Agriculture (ChooseMyPlate.gov), June 8, 2011.

Beans And Peas Are Unique Foods

Beans and peas include kidney beans, pinto beans, black beans, garbanzo beans (chickpeas), lima beans, black-eyed peas, split peas, and lentils. They are excellent sources of protein. They also provide other nutrients, such as iron and zinc, similar to seafood, meat, and poultry. They are excellent sources of dietary fiber and nutrients such as potassium and folate, which are also found in other vegetables.

Because of their high nutrient content, beans and peas may be considered both as a vegetable and as a protein food. Individuals have flexibility in counting beans and peas as either a vegetable or a protein food.

Green peas and green (string) beans are not considered to be "Beans and Peas." Green peas are similar to other starchy vegetables and are grouped with them. Green beans are grouped with other vegetables such as onions, lettuce, celery, and cabbage because their nutrient content is similar to those foods.

Table 5.1. Vegetable Consumption Recommendations

		Daily recommendation*
Children	2–3 years old	1 cup
	4–8 years old	1½ cups
Girls	9–13 years old	2 cups
	14–18 years old	2½ cups
Boys	9–13 years old	2½ cups
	14–18 years old	3 cups
Women	19–30 years old	2½ cups
	31–50 years old	2½ cups
	51+ years old	2 cups
Men	19–30 years old	3 cups
	31–50 years old	3 cups
	51+ years old	2½ cups

*These amounts are appropriate for individuals who get less than 30 minutes per day of moderate physical activity, beyond normal daily activities. Those who are more physically active may be able to consume more while staying within calorie needs. For information about what counts as a cup of vegetables, see Table 5.2.

How many vegetables are needed daily or weekly?

The amount of vegetables you need to eat depends on your age, sex, and level of physical activity. Recommended total daily amounts are shown in Table 5.1.

Vegetable subgroup recommendations are given as amounts to eat weekly. It is not necessary to eat vegetables from each subgroup daily. However, over a week, try to consume the amounts listed from each subgroup as a way to reach your daily intake recommendation. Recommended weekly amounts from each vegetable subgroup are shown in Table 5.2.

Table 5.2. Weekly Vegetable Subgroup Recommendations

	Dark green vegetables	Red and orange vegetables	Beans and peas	Starchy vegetables	Other vegetables
Children					
2–3 yrs old	½ cup	2½ cups	½ cup	2 cups	1½ cups
4–8 yrs old	1 cup	3 cups	½ cup	3½ cups	2½ cups
Girls					
9–13 yrs old	1½ cups	4 cups	1 cup	4 cups	3½ cups
14–18 yrs old	1½ cups	5½ cups	1½ cups	5 cups	4 cups
Boys					
9–13 yrs old	1½ cups	5½ cups	1½ cups	5 cups	4 cups
14–18 yrs old	2 cups	6 cups	2 cups	6 cups	5 cups
Women					
19–30 yrs old	1½ cups	5½ cups	1½ cups	5 cups	4 cups
31–50 yrs old	1½ cups	5½ cups	1½ cups	5 cups	4 cups
51+ yrs old	1½ cups	4 cups	1 cup	4 cups	3½ cups
Men					
19–30 yrs old	2 cups	6 cups	2 cups	6 cups	5 cups
31–50 yrs old	2 cups	6 cups	2 cups	6 cups	5 cups
51+ yrs old	1½ cups	5½ cups	1½ cups	5 cups	4 cups

What counts as a cup of vegetables?

In general, one cup of raw or cooked vegetables or vegetable juice, or two cups of raw leafy greens can be considered as one cup from the Vegetable Group. Table 5.3 lists specific amounts that count as one cup of vegetables (in some cases equivalents for ½ cup are also shown) towards your recommended intake.

Table 5.3. Vegetables: Common Cup Equivalents

	Amount that counts as 1 cup of vegetables	Amount that counts as ½ cup of vegetables
Dark Green Vegetables		
Broccoli	1 cup chopped or florets 3 spears 5" long raw or cooked	
Greens (collards, mustard greens, turnip greens, kale)	1 cup cooked	
Spinach	1 cup, cooked 2 cups raw is equivalent to 1 cup of vegetables	1 cup raw is equivalent to ½ cup of vegetables
Raw leafy greens (spinach, romaine, watercress, dark green leafy lettuce, endive, escarole)	2 cups raw is equivalent to 1 cup of vegetables	1 cup raw is equivalent to ½ cup of vegetables
Red And Orange Vegetables		
Carrots	1 cup, strips, slices, or chopped, raw or cooked 2 medium carrot 1 cup baby carrots (about 12)	1 medium carrot About 6 baby carrots
Pumpkin	1 cup mashed, cooked	
Red peppers	1 cup chopped, raw, or cooked 1 large pepper (3" diameter, 3¾" long)	1 small pepper
Tomatoes	1 large raw whole (3") 1 cup chopped or sliced, raw, canned, or cooked	1 small raw whole (2¼" diameter) 1 medium canned
Tomato juice	1 cup	½ cup
Sweet potato	1 large baked (2¼" or more diameter) 1 cup sliced or mashed, cooked	
Winter squash (acorn, butternut, hubbard)	1 cup cubed, cooked	½ acorn squash, baked = ¾ cup
Beans And Peas		
Dry beans and peas (such as black, garbanzo, kidney, pinto, or soy beans, or black eyed peas or split peas)	1 cup whole or mashed, cooked	

Why is it important to eat vegetables?

Eating vegetables provides health benefits—people who eat more vegetables and fruits as part of an overall healthy diet are likely to have a reduced risk of some chronic diseases. Vegetables provide nutrients vital for health and maintenance of your body.

Table 5.3. Vegetables: Common Cup Equivalents (continued)

	Amount that counts as 1 cup of vegetables	Amount that counts as ½ cup of vegetables
Starchy Vegetables		
Corn, yellow or white	1 cup 1 large ear (8" to 9" long)	1 small ear (about 6" long)
Green peas	1 cup	
White potatoes	1 cup diced, mashed 1 medium boiled or baked potato (2½" to 3" diameter) French fried: 20 medium to long strips (2½" to 4" long) (Contains added calories from solid fats.)	
Other Vegetables		
Bean sprouts	1 cup cooked	
Cabbage, green	1 cup, chopped or shredded raw or cooked	
Cauliflower	1 cup pieces or florets raw or cooked	
Celery	1 cup, diced or sliced, raw or cooked 2 large stalks (11" to 12" long)	1 large stalk (11" to 12" long)
Cucumbers	1 cup raw, sliced or chopped	
Green or wax beans	1 cup cooked	
Green peppers	1 cup chopped, raw or cooked 1 large pepper (3" diameter, 3¾" long)	1 small pepper
Lettuce, iceberg or head	2 cups raw, shredded or chopped = equivalent to 1 cup of vegetables	1 cup raw, shredded or chopped = equivalent to ½ cup of vegetables
Mushrooms	1 cup raw or cooked	
Onions	1 cup chopped, raw or cooked	
Summer squash or zucchini	1 cup cooked, sliced or diced	

Health Benefits

- Eating a diet rich in vegetables and fruits as part of an overall healthy diet may reduce risk for heart disease, including heart attack and stroke.

- Eating a diet rich in some vegetables and fruits as part of an overall healthy diet may protect against certain types of cancers.

- Diets rich in foods containing fiber, such as some vegetables and fruits, may reduce the risk of heart disease, obesity, and type 2 diabetes.

- Eating vegetables and fruits rich in potassium as part of an overall healthy diet may lower blood pressure and may also reduce the risk of developing kidney stones and help to decrease bone loss.

- Eating foods such as vegetables that are lower in calories per cup instead of some other higher-calorie food may be useful in helping to lower calorie intake.

Nutrients

- Most vegetables are naturally low in fat and calories. None have cholesterol. (Sauces or seasonings may add fat, calories, or cholesterol.)

- Vegetables are important sources of many nutrients, including potassium, dietary fiber, folate (folic acid), vitamin A, and vitamin C.

- Diets rich in potassium may help to maintain healthy blood pressure. Vegetable sources of potassium include sweet potatoes, white potatoes, white beans, tomato products (paste, sauce, and juice), beet greens, soybeans, lima beans, spinach, lentils, and kidney beans.

- Dietary fiber from vegetables, as part of an overall healthy diet, helps reduce blood cholesterol levels and may lower risk of heart disease. Fiber is important for proper bowel function. It helps reduce constipation and diverticulosis. Fiber-containing foods such as vegetables help provide a feeling of fullness with fewer calories.

For The Best Nutritional Value From Vegetables

- Select vegetables with more potassium often, such as sweet potatoes, white potatoes, white beans, tomato products (paste, sauce, and juice), beet greens, soybeans, lima beans, spinach, lentils, and kidney beans.

- Sauces or seasonings can add calories, saturated fat, and sodium to vegetables. Use the Nutrition Facts label to compare the calories and % Daily Value for saturated fat and sodium in plain and seasoned vegetables.

- Prepare more foods from fresh ingredients to lower sodium intake. Most sodium in the food supply comes from packaged or processed foods.

- Buy canned vegetables labeled "reduced sodium," "low sodium," or "no salt added." If you want to add a little salt it will likely be less than the amount in the regular canned product.

- Folate (folic acid) helps the body form red blood cells. Women of childbearing age who may become pregnant should consume adequate folate from foods, and in addition 400 mcg of synthetic folic acid from fortified foods or supplements. This reduces the risk of neural tube defects, spina bifida, and anencephaly during fetal development.

- Vitamin A keeps eyes and skin healthy and helps to protect against infections.

- Vitamin C helps heal cuts and wounds and keeps teeth and gums healthy. Vitamin C aids in iron absorption.

How can I add more vegetables to my diet?

- Buy fresh vegetables in season. They cost less and are likely to be at their peak flavor.

- Stock up on frozen vegetables for quick and easy cooking in the microwave.

- Buy vegetables that are easy to prepare. Pick up pre-washed bags of salad greens and add baby carrots or grape tomatoes for a salad in minutes. Buy packages of veggies such as baby carrots or celery sticks for quick snacks.

- Use a microwave to quickly "zap" vegetables. White or sweet potatoes can be baked quickly this way.

- Vary your veggie choices to keep meals interesting.

- Try crunchy vegetables, raw or lightly steamed.

- Plan some meals around a vegetable main dish, such as a vegetable stir-fry or soup. Then add other foods to complement it.

- Try a main dish salad for lunch. Go light on the salad dressing.

- Include a green salad with your dinner every night.

- Shred carrots or zucchini into meatloaf, casseroles, quick breads, and muffins.

- Include chopped vegetables in pasta sauce or lasagna.

- Order a veggie pizza with toppings like mushrooms, green peppers, and onions, and ask for extra veggies.

- Use pureed, cooked vegetables such as potatoes to thicken stews, soups and gravies. These add flavor, nutrients, and texture.

- Grill vegetable kabobs as part of a barbecue meal. Try tomatoes, mushrooms, green peppers, and onions.

- Many vegetables taste great with a dip or dressing. Try a low-fat salad dressing with raw broccoli, red and green peppers, celery sticks or cauliflower.

- Add color to salads by adding baby carrots, shredded red cabbage, or spinach leaves. Include in-season vegetables for variety through the year.

- Include beans or peas in flavorful mixed dishes, such as chili or minestrone soup.

- Decorate plates or serving dishes with vegetable slices.

- Keep a bowl of cut-up vegetables in a see-through container in the refrigerator. Carrot and celery sticks are traditional, but consider red or green pepper strips, broccoli florets, or cucumber slices.

Vegetables—Keep It Safe

Rinse vegetables before preparing or eating them. Under clean, running water, rub vegetables briskly with your hands to remove dirt and surface microorganisms. Dry with a clean cloth towel or paper towel after rinsing. Remember to keep vegetables separate from raw meat, poultry and seafood while shopping, preparing, or storing.

Chapter 6

Fruits

What foods are in the fruit group?

Any fruit or 100% fruit juice counts as part of the fruit group. Fruits may be fresh, canned, frozen, or dried, and may be whole, cut-up, or pureed. Some commonly eaten fruits include apples; apricots; bananas; berries (strawberries, blueberries, raspberries); cherries; grapefruit; grapes; kiwi fruit; lemons; limes; mangoes; melons (cantaloupe, honeydew, watermelon); mixed fruits (fruit cocktail); nectarines; oranges; peaches; pears; papaya; pineapple; plums; prunes; raisins; tangerines.

Some commonly consumed 100% fruit juices include orange, apple, grape, and grapefruit.

How much fruit is needed daily?

The amount of fruit you need to eat depends on age, sex, and level of physical activity. Recommended daily amounts are shown in Table 6.1.

What counts as a cup of fruit?

In general, one cup of fruit or 100% fruit juice, or ½ cup of dried fruit can be considered as one cup from the fruit group. The amounts listed in Table 6.2 count as one cup of fruit (in some cases equivalents for ½ cup are also shown) towards your daily recommended intake.

Why is it important to eat fruit?

Eating fruit provides health benefits—people who eat more fruits and vegetables as part of an overall healthy diet are likely to have a reduced risk of some chronic diseases. Fruits provide nutrients vital for health and maintenance of your body.

About This Chapter: From "Good Groups: Fruits," U.S. Department of Agriculture (ChooseMyPlate.gov), May 31, 2011.

Table 6.1. Fruit Recommendations

		Daily recommendation*
Children	2–3 years old	1 cup
	4–8 years old	1 to 1½ cups
Girls	9–13 years old	1½ cups
	14–18 years old	1½ cups
Boys	9–13 years old	1½ cups
	14–18 years old	2 cups
Women	19–30 years old	2 cups
	31–50 years old	1½ cups
	51+ years old	1½ cups
Men	19–30 years old	2 cups
	31–50 years old	2 cups
	51+ years old	2 cups

*These amounts are appropriate for individuals who get less than 30 minutes per day of moderate physical activity, beyond normal daily activities. Those who are more physically active may be able to consume more while staying within calorie needs. For information about what counts as a cup equivalent for fruit, see Table 6.2.

Health Benefits

- Eating a diet rich in vegetables and fruits as part of an overall healthy diet may reduce risk for heart disease, including heart attack and stroke.

- Eating a diet rich in some vegetables and fruits as part of an overall healthy diet may protect against certain types of cancers.

- Diets rich in foods containing fiber, such as some vegetables and fruits, may reduce the risk of heart disease, obesity, and type 2 diabetes.

- Eating vegetables and fruits rich in potassium as part of an overall healthy diet may lower blood pressure, and may also reduce the risk of developing kidney stones and help to decrease bone loss.

- Eating foods such as fruits that are lower in calories per cup instead of some other higher-calorie food may be useful in helping to lower calorie intake.

Table 6.2. Common Fruit Equivalents

	Amount that counts as 1 cup of fruit	Amount that counts as ½ cup of fruit
Apple	½ large (3.25" diameter) 1 small (2.5" diameter) 1 cup sliced or chopped, raw or cooked	½ cup sliced or chopped, raw or cooked
Applesauce	1 cup	1 snack container (4 oz)
Banana	1 cup sliced 1 large (8" to 9" long)	1 small (less than 6" long)
Cantaloupe	1 cup diced or melon balls	1 medium wedge (1/8 of a med. melon)
Grapes	1 cup whole or cut-up 32 seedless grapes	16 seedless grapes
Grapefruit	1 medium (4" diameter) 1 cup sections	½ medium (4" diameter)
Mixed fruit (fruit cocktail)	1 cup diced or sliced, raw or canned, drained	1 snack container (4 oz) drained = 3/8 cup
Orange	1 large (3 1/16" diameter) 1 cup sections	1 small (2 3/8" diameter)
Orange, mandarin	1 cup canned, drained	
Peach	1 large (2¾" diameter) 1 cup sliced or diced, raw, cooked, or canned, drained 2 halves, canned	1 small (2" diameter) 1 snack container (4 oz) drained = 3/8 cup
Pear	1 medium pear (2.5 per lb)	
	1 cup sliced or diced, raw, cooked, or canned, drained	1 snack container (4 oz) drained – 3/8 cup
Pineapple	1 cup chunks, sliced or crushed, raw, cooked or canned, drained	1 snack container (4 oz) drained = 3/8 cup
Plum	1 cup sliced raw or cooked 3 medium or 2 large plums	1 large plum
Strawberries	About 8 large berries 1 cup whole, halved, or sliced, fresh or frozen	½ cup whole, halved, or sliced
Watermelon	1 small wedge (1" thick) 1 cup diced or balls	6 melon balls
Dried fruit (raisins, prunes, apricots, etc.)	½ cup dried fruit is equivalent to 1 cup fruit: ½ cup raisins ½ cup prunes ½ cup dried apricots	¼ cup dried fruit is equivalent to ½ cup fruit 1 small box raisins (1.5 oz)
100% fruit juice (orange, apple, grape, grapefruit, etc.)	1 cup	½ cup

Nutrients

- Most fruits are naturally low in fat, sodium, and calories. None have cholesterol.

- Fruits are sources of many essential nutrients that are under-consumed, including potassium, dietary fiber, vitamin C, and folate (folic acid).

- Diets rich in potassium may help to maintain healthy blood pressure. Fruit sources of potassium include bananas, prunes and prune juice, dried peaches and apricots, cantaloupe, honeydew melon, and orange juice.

- Dietary fiber from fruits, as part of an overall healthy diet, helps reduce blood cholesterol levels and may lower risk of heart disease. Fiber is important for proper bowel function. It helps reduce constipation and diverticulosis. Fiber-containing foods such as fruits help provide a feeling of fullness with fewer calories. Whole or cut-up fruits are sources of dietary fiber; fruit juices contain little or no fiber.

- Vitamin C is important for growth and repair of all body tissues, helps heal cuts and wounds, and keeps teeth and gums healthy.

- Folate (folic acid) helps the body form red blood cells. Women of childbearing age who may become pregnant should consume adequate folate from foods, and in addition 400 mcg of synthetic folic acid from fortified foods or supplements. This reduces the risk of neural tube defects, spina bifida, and anencephaly during fetal development.

How can I add more fruit to my diet?

Some general tips for adding fruit to your diet include keeping a bowl of whole fruit on the table, counter, or in the refrigerator. You can also refrigerate cut-up fruit to store for later.

Consider convenience when shopping. Try pre-cut packages of fruit (such as melon or pineapple chunks) for a healthy snack in seconds. Choose packaged fruits that do not have added sugars.

Buy fresh fruits in season when they may be less expensive and at their peak flavor, and buy fruits that are dried, frozen, and canned (in water or 100% juice) as well as fresh, so that you always have a supply on hand.

For the best nutritional value from fruit, make most of your choices whole or cut-up fruit rather than juice, for the benefits dietary fiber provides. Select fruits with more potassium often, such as bananas, prunes and prune juice, dried peaches and apricots, and orange juice. When choosing canned fruits, select fruit canned in 100% fruit juice or water rather than syrup. Also remember to vary your fruit choices. Fruits differ in nutrient content.

Tips For Eating More Fruit

At Meals

- At breakfast, top your cereal with bananas or peaches; add blueberries to pancakes; drink 100% orange or grapefruit juice. Or, mix fresh fruit with plain fat-free or low-fat yogurt.
- At lunch, pack a tangerine, banana, or grapes to eat, or choose fruits from a salad bar. Individual containers of fruits like peaches or applesauce are easy and convenient.
- At dinner, add crushed pineapple to coleslaw, or include orange sections or grapes in a tossed salad.
- Make a Waldorf salad, with apples, celery, walnuts, and a low-calorie salad dressing.
- Try meat dishes that incorporate fruit, such as chicken with apricots or mangoes.
- Add fruit like pineapple or peaches to kabobs as part of a barbecue meal.
- For dessert, have baked apples, pears, or a fruit salad.

As Snacks

- Cut-up fruit makes a great snack. Either cut them yourself, or buy pre-cut packages of fruit pieces like pineapples or melons. Or, try whole fresh berries or grapes.
- Dried fruits also make a great snack. They are easy to carry and store well. Because they are dried, ¼ cup is equivalent to ½ cup of other fruits.
- Keep a package of dried fruit in your bag or backpack. Some fruits that are available dried include apricots, apples, pineapple, bananas, cherries, figs, dates, cranberries, blueberries, prunes (dried plums), and raisins (dried grapes).
- As a snack, spread peanut butter on apple slices or top plain fat-free or low-fat yogurt with berries or slices of kiwi fruit.
- Frozen juice bars (100% juice) make healthy alternatives to high-fat snacks.

Here are some tips to help make fruit more appealing:

- Many fruits taste great with a dip or dressing. Try fat-free or low-fat yogurt as a dip for fruits like strawberries or melons.

- Make a fruit smoothie by blending fat-free or low-fat milk or yogurt with fresh or frozen fruit. Try bananas, peaches, strawberries, or other berries.

- Try unsweetened applesauce as a lower calorie substitute for some of the oil when baking cakes.

- Try different textures of fruits. For example, apples are crunchy, bananas are smooth and creamy, and oranges are juicy.

- For fresh fruit salads, mix apples, bananas, or pears with acidic fruits like oranges, pineapple, or lemon juice to keep them from turning brown.

Fruit: Keep It Safe

Rinse fruits before preparing or eating them. Under clean, running water, rub fruits briskly with your hands to remove dirt and surface microorganisms. Dry with a clean cloth towel or paper towel after rinsing. Keep fruits separate from raw meat, poultry and seafood while shopping, preparing, or storing.

Chapter 7

The Dairy Group

What foods are included in the dairy group?

All fluid milk products and many foods made from milk are considered part of this food group. Most dairy group choices should be fat-free or low fat. Foods made from milk that retain their calcium content are part of the group. Foods made from milk that have little to no calcium, such as cream cheese, cream, and butter, are not. Calcium-fortified soymilk (soy beverage) is also part of the dairy group.

Some commonly eaten choices in the dairy group are:

- Milk*: All fluid milk: fat-free (skim); low fat (1%); reduced fat (2%); whole milk; flavored milks (chocolate, strawberry); lactose-reduced milks; lactose-free milks

- Milk-based desserts*: Puddings; ice milk; frozen yogurt; ice cream

- Calcium-fortified soymilk (soy beverage)

- Cheese*: Hard natural cheeses (cheddar, mozzarella); Swiss; Parmesan; soft cheeses (ricotta, cottage cheese); processed cheeses (American)

- Yogurt*: All yogurt: fat-free; low fat; reduced fat; whole milk yogurt

*For items marked with an asterisk (*), refer to the following selection tips:

Choose fat-free or low-fat milk, yogurt, and cheese. If you choose milk or yogurt that is not fat-free, or cheese that is not low-fat, the fat in the product counts against your maximum limit for "empty calories" (calories from solid fats and added sugars).

About This Chapter: From "Good Groups: Dairy," U.S. Department of Agriculture (ChooseMyPlate.gov), June 14, 2011.

If sweetened milk products are chosen (flavored milk, yogurt, drinkable yogurt, desserts), the added sugars also count against your maximum limit for "empty calories" (calories from solid fats and added sugars).

For those who are lactose intolerant, smaller portions (such as 4 fluid ounces of milk) may be well tolerated. Lactose-free and lower-lactose products are available. These include lactose-reduced or lactose-free milk, yogurt, and cheese, and calcium-fortified soymilk (soy beverage). Also, enzyme preparations can be added to milk to lower the lactose content. Calcium-fortified foods and beverages such as cereals, orange juice, or rice or almond beverages may provide calcium, but may not provide the other nutrients found in dairy products.

How much food from the dairy group is needed daily?

The amount of food from the dairy group you need to eat depends on age. Recommended daily amounts are shown in Table 7.1.

Fat-Free Milk

Switch to fat-free or low-fat (1%) milk.

What counts as a cup in the dairy group?

In general, 1 cup of milk, yogurt, or soymilk (soy beverage), 1½ ounces of natural cheese, or 2 ounces of processed cheese can be considered as 1 cup from the dairy group. Table 7.2 lists specific amounts that count as one cup in the dairy group towards your daily recommended intake.

Table 7.1. Dairy Group Daily Recommendations

Children	2–3 years old	2 cups
	4-8 years old	2½ cups
Girls	9–13 years old	3 cups
	14–18 years old	3 cups
Boys	9–13 years old	3 cups
	14-18 years old	3 cups
Women	19–30 years old	3 cups
	31-50 years old	3 cups
	51+ years old	3 cups
Men	19–30 years old	3 cups
	31–50 years old	3 cups
	51+ years old	3 cups

Table 7.2. Dairy Group Cup Equivalents

	Amount that counts as a cup in the Dairy Group	Common portions and cup equivalents
Milk (choose fat-free or low-fat milk)	1 cup milk 1 half-pint container milk ½ cup evaporated milk	
Yogurt (choose fat-free or low-fat yogurt)	1 regular container (8 fluid ounces) 1 cup yogurt	1 small container (6 ounces) = ¾ cup 1 snack size container (4 ounces) = ½ cup
Cheese (choose reduced-fat or low-fat cheeses)	1½ ounces hard cheese (cheddar, mozzarella, Swiss, Parmesan) 1/3 cup shredded cheese 2 ounces processed cheese (American) ½ cup ricotta cheese 2 cups cottage cheese	1 slice of hard cheese is equivalent to ½ cup milk 1 slice of processed cheese is equivalent to 1/3 cup milk ½ cup cottage cheese is equivalent to ¼ cup milk
Milk-based desserts (choose fat-free or low-fat types)	1 cup pudding made with milk 1 cup frozen yogurt 1½ cups ice cream	1 scoop ice cream is equivalent to 1/3 cup milk
Soymilk (soy beverage)	1 cup calcium-fortified soymilk 1 half-pint container calcium-fortified soymilk	

What health benefits and nutrients do dairy products provide?

Consuming dairy products provides health benefits—especially improved bone health. Foods in the dairy group provide nutrients that are vital for health and maintenance of your body. These nutrients include calcium, potassium, vitamin D, and protein.

Health Benefits

- Intake of dairy products is linked to improved bone health, and may reduce the risk of osteoporosis.

- The intake of dairy products is especially important to bone health during childhood and adolescence, when bone mass is being built.

- Intake of dairy products is also associated with a reduced risk of cardiovascular disease and type 2 diabetes, and with lower blood pressure in adults.

Nutrients

- Calcium is used for building bones and teeth and in maintaining bone mass. Dairy products are the primary source of calcium in American diets. Diets that provide 3 cups or the equivalent of dairy products per day can improve bone mass.

- Diets rich in potassium may help to maintain healthy blood pressure. Dairy products, especially yogurt, fluid milk, and soymilk (soy beverage), provide potassium.

- Vitamin D functions in the body to maintain proper levels of calcium and phosphorous, thereby helping to build and maintain bones. Milk and soymilk (soy beverage) that are fortified with vitamin D are good sources of this nutrient. Other sources include vitamin D-fortified yogurt and vitamin D-fortified ready-to-eat breakfast cereals.

- Milk products that are consumed in their low-fat or fat-free forms provide little or no solid fat.

Why is it important to make fat-free or low-fat choices from the dairy group?

Choosing foods from the dairy group that are high in saturated fats and cholesterol can have health implications. Diets high in saturated fats raise "bad" cholesterol levels in the blood. The "bad" cholesterol is called LDL (low-density lipoprotein) cholesterol. High LDL cholesterol, in turn, increases the risk for coronary heart disease. Many cheeses, whole milk, and products made from them are high in saturated fat. To help keep blood cholesterol levels healthy, limit the amount of these foods you eat. In addition, a high intake of fats makes it difficult to avoid consuming more calories than are needed.

How can I make wise choices in the dairy group?

- Include milk or calcium-fortified soymilk (soy beverage) as a beverage at meals. Choose fat-free or low-fat milk.

- If you usually drink whole milk, switch gradually to fat-free milk, to lower saturated fat and calories. Try reduced fat (2%), then low-fat (1%), and finally fat-free (skim).

- If you drink cappuccinos or lattes—ask for them with fat-free (skim) milk.

- Add fat-free or low-fat milk instead of water to oatmeal and hot cereals.

- Use fat-free or low-fat milk when making condensed cream soups (such as cream of tomato).

- Have fat-free or low-fat yogurt as a snack.

- Make a dip for fruits or vegetables from yogurt.

- Make fruit-yogurt smoothies in the blender.

- For dessert, make chocolate or butterscotch pudding with fat-free or low-fat milk.

- Top cut-up fruit with flavored yogurt for a quick dessert.

- Top casseroles, soups, stews, or vegetables with shredded reduced-fat or low-fat cheese.

- Top a baked potato with fat-free or low-fat yogurt.

How can I meet nutrient recommendations if I choose not to consume milk products?

If you avoid milk because of lactose intolerance, the most reliable way to get the health benefits of dairy products is to choose lactose-free alternatives within the dairy group, such as cheese, yogurt, lactose-free milk, or calcium-fortified soymilk (soy beverage) or to consume the enzyme lactase before consuming milk.

Calcium choices for those who do not consume dairy products include the following:

- Calcium fortified juices, cereals, breads, rice milk, or almond milk.

- Canned fish (sardines, salmon with bones) soybeans and other soy products (tofu made with calcium sulfate, soy yogurt, tempeh), some other beans, and some leafy greens (collard and turnip greens, kale, bok choy). The amount of calcium that can be absorbed from these foods varies.

Keep It Safe To Eat

- Avoid raw (unpasteurized) milk or any products made from unpasteurized milk.

- Chill (refrigerate) perishable food promptly and defrost foods properly. Refrigerate or freeze perishables, prepared food, and leftovers as soon as possible. If food has been left at temperatures between 40° and 140° F for more than two hours, discard it, even though it may look and smell good.

- Separate raw, cooked and ready-to-eat foods.

Chapter 8

The Protein Group

What foods are in the protein foods group?

All foods made from meat, poultry, seafood, beans and peas, eggs, processed soy products, nuts, and seeds are considered part of the protein foods group. Beans and peas are also part of the vegetable group.

Select a variety of protein foods to improve nutrient intake and health benefits, including at least eight ounces of cooked seafood per week. Young children need less, depending on their age and calories needs. The advice to consume seafood does not apply to vegetarians. Vegetarian options in the protein foods group include beans and peas, processed soy products, and nuts and seeds. Meat and poultry choices should be lean or low-fat.

Some commonly eaten choices in the protein foods group include the following:

- Meats*: Lean cuts of beef, ham, lamb, pork, veal; Game meats: bison; rabbit; venison. Lean ground meats: beef; pork; lamb. Lean luncheon or deli meats. Organ meats: liver; giblets

- Poultry*: Chicken; duck; goose; turkey; ground chicken and turkey

- Eggs*: Chicken eggs; duck eggs

- Beans and peas: Black beans; black-eyed peas; chickpeas (garbanzo beans); falafel; kidney beans; lentils; lima beans (mature); navy beans; pinto beans; soy beans; split peas; processed soy products; tofu (bean curd made from soybeans); white beans; bean burgers; veggie burgers; tempeh; texturized vegetable protein (TVP)

About This Chapter: From "Food Groups: Protein Foods," U.S. Department of Agriculture (ChooseMyPlate.gov), June 8, 2011.

- Nuts and seeds*: Almonds; cashews; hazelnuts (filberts); mixed nuts; peanuts; peanut butter; pecans; pistachios; pumpkin seeds; sesame seeds; sunflower seeds; walnuts

- Seafood*: Finfish such as catfish, cod, flounder, haddock, halibut, herring, mackerel, pollock, porgy, salmon, sea bass, snapper, swordfish, trout, tuna. Shellfish such as clams, crab, crayfish, lobster, mussels, octopus, oysters, scallops, squid (calamari), shrimp. Canned fish such as anchovies, clams, tuna, sardines

For items marked with an asterisk (*), refer to the following selection tips:

Choose lean or low-fat meat and poultry. If higher fat choices are made, such as regular ground beef (75 to 80% lean) or chicken with skin, the fat counts against your maximum limit for empty calories (calories from solid fats or added sugars).

If solid fat is added in cooking, such as frying chicken in shortening or frying eggs in butter or stick margarine, this also counts against your maximum limit for empty calories (calories from solid fats and added sugars).

Select some seafood that is rich in omega-3 fatty acids, such as salmon, trout, sardines, anchovies, herring, Pacific oysters, and Atlantic and Pacific mackerel.

Processed meats such as ham, sausage, frankfurters, and luncheon or deli meats have added sodium. Check the Nutrition Facts label to help limit sodium intake. Fresh chicken, turkey, and pork that have been enhanced with a salt-containing solution also have added sodium. Check the product label for statements such as "self-basting" or "contains up to __% of __", which mean that a sodium-containing solution has been added to the product.

Choose unsalted nuts and seeds to keep sodium intake low.

How much food from the protein foods group is needed daily?

The amount of food from the protein foods group you need to eat depends on age, sex, and level of physical activity. Most Americans eat enough food from this group, but need to make leaner and more varied selections of these foods. Recommended daily amounts are shown in Table 8.1.

What counts as an ounce equivalent in the protein foods group?

In general, 1 ounce of meat, poultry, or fish, ¼ cup cooked beans, one egg, 1 tablespoon of peanut butter, or ½ ounce of nuts or seeds can be considered as one ounce equivalent from the protein foods group.

Table 8.2 lists specific amounts that count as one ounce equivalent in the protein foods group towards your daily recommended intake.

What are the types of protein?

Proteins are made up of amino acids. Think of amino acids as the building blocks. There are 20 different amino acids that join together to make all types of protein. Some of these amino acids can't be made by our bodies, so these are known as essential amino acids. It's essential that our diet provide these.

In the diet, protein sources are labeled according to how many of the essential amino acids they provide:

- A complete protein source is one that provides all of the essential amino acids. You may also hear these sources called high quality proteins. Animal-based foods; for example, meat, poultry, fish, milk, eggs, and cheese are considered complete protein sources.

- An incomplete protein source is one that is low in one or more of the essential amino acids. Complementary proteins are two or more incomplete protein sources that together provide adequate amounts of all the essential amino acids.

For example, rice contains low amounts of certain essential amino acids; however, these same essential amino acids are found in greater amounts in dry beans. Similarly, dry beans contain lower amounts of other essential amino acids that can be found in larger amounts in rice. Together, these two foods can provide adequate amounts of all the essential amino acids the body needs.

Source: Excerpted from "Protein," Centers for Disease Control and Prevention (www.cdc.gov), February 23, 2011.

Why is it important to make lean or low-fat choices from the protein foods group?

Foods in the meat, poultry, fish, eggs, nuts, and seed group provide nutrients that are vital for health and maintenance of your body. However, choosing foods from this group that are high in saturated fat and cholesterol may have health implications.

Nutrients

- Meat, poultry, fish, dry beans and peas, eggs, nuts, and seeds supply many nutrients. These include protein, B vitamins (niacin, thiamin, riboflavin, and B6), vitamin E, iron, zinc, and magnesium.

- Proteins function as building blocks for bones, muscles, cartilage, skin, and blood. They are also building blocks for enzymes, hormones, and vitamins. Proteins are one of three nutrients that provide calories (the others are fat and carbohydrates).

- B vitamins found in this food group serve a variety of functions in the body. They help the body release energy, play a vital role in the function of the nervous system, aid in the formation of red blood cells, and help build tissues.

- Iron is used to carry oxygen in the blood. Many teenage girls and women in their child-bearing years have iron-deficiency anemia. They should eat foods high in heme-iron (meats) or eat other non-heme iron containing foods along with a food rich in vitamin C, which can improve absorption of non-heme iron.

- Magnesium is used in building bones and in releasing energy from muscles.

- Zinc is necessary for biochemical reactions and helps the immune system function properly.

- EPA (eicosapentaenoic acid) and DHA (docosahexaenoic acid) are omega-3 fatty acids found in varying amounts in seafood. Eating eight ounces per week of seafood may help reduce the risk for heart disease.

Health Implications

- Diets that are high in saturated fats raise "bad" cholesterol levels in the blood. The "bad" cholesterol is called LDL (low-density lipoprotein) cholesterol. High LDL cholesterol, in turn, increases the risk for coronary heart disease. Some food choices in this group

Table 8.1. Daily Recommendations* For Protein Foods

Children	2–3 years old	2 ounce equivalents**
	4–8 years old	4 ounce equivalents**
Girls	9–13 years old	5 ounce equivalents**
	14–18 years old	5 ounce equivalents**
Boys	9–13 years old	5 ounce equivalents**
	14–18 years old	6½ ounce equivalents**
Women	19–30 years old	5½ ounce equivalents**
	31–50 years old	5 ounce equivalents**
	51+ years old	5 ounce equivalents**
Men	19–30 years old	6½ ounce equivalents**
	31–50 years old	6 ounce equivalents**
	51+ years old	5½ ounce equivalents**

*These amounts are appropriate for individuals who get less than 30 minutes per day of moderate physical activity, beyond normal daily activities. Those who are more physically active may be able to consume more while staying within calorie needs.

**See Table 8.2 for information about what counts as one ounce equivalent in the protein foods group.

are high in saturated fat. These include fatty cuts of beef, pork, and lamb; regular ground beef; regular sausages, hot dogs, and bacon; some luncheon meats such as regular bologna and salami; and some poultry such as duck. To help keep blood cholesterol levels healthy, limit the amount of these foods you eat.

- Diets that are high in cholesterol can raise LDL cholesterol levels in the blood. Cholesterol is only found in foods from animal sources. Some foods from this group are high in cholesterol. These include egg yolks (egg whites are cholesterol-free) and organ meats such as liver and giblets. To help keep blood cholesterol levels healthy, limit the amount of these foods you eat.

- A high intake of fats makes it difficult to avoid consuming more calories than are needed.

Table 8.2. Protein Foods Group Ounce Equivalents

	Amount that counts as 1 ounce equivalent in the protein foods group	Common portions and ounce equivalents
Meats	1 ounce cooked lean beef	1 small steak (eye of round, filet) = 3½ to 4 ounce equivalents
	1 ounce cooked lean pork or ham	1 small lean hamburger = 2 to 3 ounce equivalents
Poultry	1 ounce cooked chicken or turkey, without skin 1 sandwich slice of turkey (4½ x 2½ x 1/8")	1 small chicken breast half = 3 ounce equivalents ½ Cornish game hen = 4 ounce equivalents
Seafood	1 ounce cooked fish or shell fish	1 can of tuna, drained = 3 to 4 ounce equivalents 1 salmon steak = 4 to 6 ounce equivalents 1 small trout = 3 ounce equivalents
Eggs	1 egg	3 egg whites = 2 ounce equivalents 3 egg yolks = 1 ounce equivalent
Nuts and seeds	½ ounce of nuts (12 almonds, 24 pistachios, 7 walnut halves) ½ ounce of seeds (pumpkin, sunflower or squash seeds, hulled, roasted) 1 Tablespoon of peanut butter or almond butter	1 ounce of nuts or seeds = 2 ounce equivalents
Beans and peas	¼ cup of cooked beans (such as black, kidney, pinto, or white beans) ¼ cup of cooked peas (such as chickpeas, cowpeas, lentils, or split peas) ¼ cup of baked beans, refried beans ¼ cup (about 2 ounces) of tofu 1 oz. tempeh, cooked ¼ cup roasted soybeans 1 falafel patty (2¼", 4 oz) 2 Tablespoons hummus	1 cup split pea soup = 2 ounce equivalents 1 cup lentil soup = 2 ounce equivalents 1 cup bean soup = 2 ounce equivalents 1 soy or bean burger patty = 2 ounce equivalents

Why is it important to eat eight ounces of seafood per week?

Seafood contains a range of nutrients, notably the omega-3 fatty acids, EPA and DHA. Eating about eight ounces per week of a variety of seafood contributes to the prevention of heart disease. Smaller amounts of seafood are recommended for young children.

Seafood varieties that are commonly consumed in the United States that are higher in EPA and DHA and lower in mercury include salmon, anchovies, herring, sardines, Pacific oysters, trout, and Atlantic and Pacific mackerel (not king mackerel, which is high in mercury). The health benefits from consuming seafood outweigh the health risk associated with mercury, a heavy metal found in seafood in varying levels.

What are the benefits of eating nuts and seeds?

Eating peanuts and certain tree nuts (walnuts, almonds, and pistachios) may reduce the risk of heart disease when consumed as part of a diet that is nutritionally adequate and within calorie needs. Because nuts and seeds are high in calories, eat them in small portions and use them to replace other protein foods, like some meat or poultry, rather than adding them to what you already eat. In addition, choose unsalted nuts and seeds to help reduce sodium intakes.

How can I make wise choices from the protein foods group?

Go lean with protein. Start with a lean choice and keep it lean when you prepare foods:

- Trim away all of the visible fat from meats and poultry before cooking.

- Broil, grill, roast, poach, or boil meat, poultry, or fish instead of frying.

- Drain off any fat that appears during cooking.

- Skip or limit the breading on meat, poultry, or fish. Breading adds calories. It will also cause the food to soak up more fat during frying.

- Prepare beans and peas without added fats.

- Choose and prepare foods without high fat sauces or gravies.

Vary your protein choices. Choose seafood at least twice a week as the main protein food. Look for seafood rich in omega-3 fatty acids, such as salmon, trout, and herring. Some ideas are salmon steak or filet, salmon loaf, and grilled or baked trout.

Choose beans, peas, or soy products as a main dish or part of a meal often. Some choices are chili with kidney or pinto beans, stir-fried tofu, split pea, lentil, minestrone, or white bean soups, baked beans, black bean enchiladas, garbanzo or kidney beans on a chef's salad, rice and beans, veggie burgers, and hummus (chickpeas) spread on pita bread.

Choose unsalted nuts as a snack, on salads, or in main dishes. Use nuts to replace meat or poultry, not in addition to these items. Some other tips for using nuts include the following:

- Use pine nuts in pesto sauce for pasta.

- Add slivered almonds to steamed vegetables.

- Add toasted peanuts or cashews to a vegetable stir fry instead of meat.

- Sprinkle a few nuts on top of low-fat ice cream or frozen yogurt.

- Add walnuts or pecans to a green salad instead of cheese or meat.

Keep Protein Foods Safe To Eat

- Separate raw, cooked and ready-to-eat foods.
- Do not wash or rinse meat or poultry.
- Wash cutting boards, knives, utensils, and counter tops in hot soapy water after preparing each food item and before going on to the next one.
- Store raw meat, poultry, and seafood on the bottom shelf of the refrigerator so juices don't drip onto other foods.
- Cook foods to a safe temperature to kill microorganisms. Use a meat thermometer, which measures the internal temperature of cooked meat and poultry, to make sure that the meat is cooked all the way through.
- Chill (refrigerate) perishable food promptly and defrost foods properly. Refrigerate or freeze perishables, prepared food and leftovers within two hours.
- Plan ahead to defrost foods. Never defrost food on the kitchen counter at room temperature. Thaw food by placing it in the refrigerator, submerging air-tight packaged food in cold tap water (change water every 30 minutes), or defrosting on a plate in the microwave.
- Avoid raw or partially cooked eggs or foods containing raw eggs and raw or undercooked meat and poultry.
- Women who may become pregnant, pregnant women, nursing mothers, and young children should avoid some types of fish and eat types lower in mercury. See www.cfsan.fda .gov/~dms/admehg3.html or call 888-SAFEFOOD for more information.

Source: U.S. Department of Agriculture (ChooseMyPlate.gov), June 8, 2011.

What are vegetarian choices in the protein foods group?

Vegetarians get enough protein from this group as long as the variety and amounts of foods selected are adequate. Protein sources from the protein foods group for vegetarians include eggs (for ovo-vegetarians), beans and peas, nuts, nut butters, and soy products (tofu, tempeh, veggie burgers). [For more information about vegetarian and vegan food choices, see Chapter 35.]

Chapter 9

Oils

What are oils?

Oils are fats that are liquid at room temperature, like the vegetable oils used in cooking. Oils come from many different plants and from fish. Oils are NOT a food group, but they provide essential nutrients. Therefore, oils are included in USDA food patterns. Some common oils are canola oil, corn oil, cottonseed oil, olive oil, safflower oil, soybean oil, and sunflower oil.

Some oils are used mainly as flavorings, such as walnut oil and sesame oil. A number of foods are naturally high in oils, like nuts, olives, some fish, and avocados.

Foods that are mainly oil include mayonnaise, certain salad dressings, and soft (tub or squeeze) margarine with no trans fats. Check the nutrition facts label to find margarines with 0 grams of trans fat. Amounts of trans fat are required to be listed on labels.

Most oils are high in monounsaturated or polyunsaturated fats, and low in saturated fats. Oils from plant sources (vegetable and nut oils) do not contain any cholesterol. In fact, no plant foods contain cholesterol.

A few plant oils, however, including coconut oil, palm oil, and palm kernel oil, are high in saturated fats, and for nutritional purposes they should be considered to be solid fats.

Solid fats are fats that are solid at room temperature, like butter and shortening. Solid fats come from many animal foods and can be made from vegetable oils through a process called hydrogenation. Some common solid fats are butter, milk fat, beef fat (tallow, suet), chicken fat, pork fat (lard), stick margarine, shortening, and partially hydrogenated oil.

About This Chapter: From "What Are Oils?" U.S. Department of Agriculture (ChooseMyPlate.gov), June 4, 2011.

Oils Instead Of Solid Fats

Oils are not a food group, but are emphasized because they contribute essential fatty acids and vitamin E to the diet. Replacing some saturated fatty acids with unsaturated fatty acids lowers both total and low-density lipoprotein (LDL) blood cholesterol levels.

Oils are naturally present in foods such as olives, nuts, avocados, and seafood. Many common oils are extracted from plants, such as canola, corn, olive, peanut, safflower, soybean, and sunflower oils. Foods that are mainly oil include mayonnaise, oil-based salad dressings, and soft (tub or squeeze) margarine with no trans fatty acids. Coconut oil, palm kernel oil, and palm oil are high in saturated fatty acids and partially hydrogenated oils contain trans fatty acids. For nutritional purposes, they should be considered solid fats.

Americans consume more solid fats but less oil than is desirable. Because oils are a concentrated source of calories, Americans should replace solid fats with oils, rather than add oil to the diet, and should use oils in small amounts. For example, individuals can use soft margarine instead of stick margarine, replace some meats and poultry with seafood or unsalted nuts, and use vegetable oils instead of solid fats, such as butter, in cooking.

Source: Excerpted from *Dietary Guidelines for Americans 2010*, U.S. Department of Agriculture, December 2010.

How are oils different from solid fats?

All fats and oils are a mixture of saturated fatty acids and unsaturated fatty acids. Solid fats contain more saturated fats and/or trans fats than oils. Oils contain more monounsaturated (MUFA) and polyunsaturated (PUFA) fats. Saturated fats, trans fats, and cholesterol tend to raise "bad" (LDL) cholesterol levels in the blood, which in turn increases the risk for heart disease. To lower risk for heart disease, cut back on foods containing saturated fats, trans fats, and cholesterol.

Why is it important to consume oils?

Oils are not a food group, but they do provide essential nutrients and are therefore included in USDA recommendations for what to eat. Note that only small amounts of oils are recommended.

Most of the fats you eat should be polyunsaturated (PUFA) or monounsaturated (MUFA) fats. Oils are the major source of MUFAs and PUFAs in the diet. PUFAs contain some fatty acids that are necessary for health—called "essential fatty acids."

Because oils contain these essential fatty acids, there is an allowance for oils in the food guide.

The MUFAs and PUFAs found in fish, nuts, and vegetable oils do not raise LDL ("bad") cholesterol levels in the blood. In addition to the essential fatty acids they contain, oils are the major source of vitamin E in typical American diets.

While consuming some oil is needed for health, oils still contain calories. In fact, oils and solid fats both contain about 120 calories per tablespoon. Therefore, the amount of oil consumed needs to be limited to balance total calorie intake. The nutrition facts label provides information to help you make smart choices.

How much is my allowance for oils?

Some Americans consume enough oil in the foods they eat, such as nuts, fish, cooking oil, and salad dressings, Others could easily consume the recommended allowance by substituting oils for some solid fats they eat. A person's allowance for oils depends on age, sex, and level of physical activity. Daily allowances are shown in Table 9.1.

How do I count the oils I eat?

Table 9.2 gives a quick guide to the amount of oils in some common foods.

Table 9.1. Daily Allowance For Oils*

Children	2-3 years old	3 teaspoons
	4-8 years old	4 teaspoons
Girls	9-13 years old	5 teaspoons
	14-18 years old	5 teaspoons
Boys	9-13 years old	5 teaspoons
	14-18 years old	6 teaspoons
Women	19-30 years old	6 teaspoons
	31-50 years old	5 teaspoons
	51+ years old	5 teaspoons
Men	19-30 years old	7 teaspoons
	31-50 years old	6 teaspoons
	51+ years old	6 teaspoons

*These amounts are appropriate for individuals who get less than 30 minutes per day of moderate physical activity, beyond normal daily activities. Those who are more physically active may be able to consume more while staying within calorie needs.

Table 9.2. Oils In Common Foods.

	Amount of food	Amount of oil	Calories from oil	Total calories
		Teaspoons/ grams	Approximate calories	Approximate calories
Vegetable oils (such as canola, corn, cottonseed, olive, peanut, safflower, soybean, and sunflower)	1 Tbsp	3 tsp/14 g	120	120
Foods rich in oils:				
Margarine, soft (trans fat free)	1 Tbsp	2½ tsp/11 g	100	100
Mayonnaise	1 Tbsp	2½ tsp/11 g	100	100
Mayonnaise-type salad dressing	1 Tbsp	1 tsp/5 g	45	55
Italian dressing	2 Tbsp	2 tsp/8 g	75	85
Thousand Island dressing	2 Tbsp	2½ tsp/11 g	100	120
Olives*, ripe, canned	4 large	½ tsp/2 g	15	20
Avocado*	½ med	3 tsp/15 g	130	160
Peanut butter*	2 T	4 tsp/16 g	140	190
Peanuts, dry roasted*	1 oz	3 tsp/14 g	120	165
Mixed nuts, dry roasted*	1 oz	3 tsp/15 g	130	170
Cashews, dry roasted*	1 oz	3 tsp/13 g	115	165
Almonds, dry roasted*	1 oz	3 tsp/15 g	130	170
Hazelnuts*	1 oz	4 tsp/18 g	160	185
Sunflower seeds*	1 oz	3 tsp/14 g	120	165

*Avocados and olives are part of the vegetable group; nuts and seeds are part of the protein foods group. These foods are also high in oils. Soft margarine, mayonnaise, and salad dressings are mainly oil and are not considered to be part of any food group.

Chapter 10

Empty Calories

What are "empty calories"?

Currently, many of the foods and beverages Americans eat and drink contain empty calories—calories from solid fats and/or added sugars. Solid fats and added sugars add calories to the food but few or no nutrients. For this reason, the calories from solid fats and added sugars in a food are often called empty calories. Learning more about solid fats and added sugars can help you make better food and drink choices.

Solid fats are fats that are solid at room temperature, like butter, beef fat, and shortening. Some solid fats are found naturally in foods. They can also be added when foods are processed by food companies or when they are prepared.

Added sugars are sugars and syrups that are added when foods or beverages are processed or prepared.

Solid fats and added sugars can make a food or beverage more appealing, but they also can add a lot of calories. The following foods and beverages provide the most empty calories for Americans:

- Cakes, cookies, pastries, and donuts (contain both solid fat and added sugars)
- Sodas, energy drinks, sports drinks, and fruit drinks (contain added sugars)
- Cheese (contains solid fat)
- Pizza (contains solid fat)
- Ice cream (contains both solid fat and added sugars)
- Sausages, hot dogs, bacon, and ribs (contain solid fat)

About This Chapter: From "Empty Calories," U.S. Department of Agriculture (ChooseMyPlate.gov), June 4, 2011.

These foods and beverages are the major sources of empty calories, but many can be found in forms with less or no solid fat or added sugars. For example, low-fat cheese and low-fat hot dogs can be purchased. You can choose water, milk, or sugar-free soda instead of drinks with sugar. Check that the calories in these products are less than in the regular product.

In some foods, like most candies and sodas, all the calories are empty calories. These foods are often called "empty calorie foods." However, empty calories from solid fats and added sugars can also be found in some other foods that contain important nutrients. Some examples of foods that provide nutrients, shown in forms with and without empty calories are listed in Table 10.1. Making better choices, like unsweetened applesauce or extra lean ground beef, can help keep your intake of added sugars and solid fats low.

Table 10.1. Foods With And Without Empty Calories

Food with some empty calories	Food with few or no empty calories
Sweetened applesauce (contains added sugars)	Unsweetened applesauce
Regular ground beef (75% lean) (contains solid fats)	Extra lean ground beef (90% or more lean)
Fried chicken (contains solid fats from frying and skin)	Baked chicken breast without skin
Sugar-sweetened cereals (contain added sugars)	Unsweetened cereals
Whole milk (contains solid fats)	Fat-free milk

A small amount of empty calories is okay, but most people eat far more than is healthy. It is important to limit empty calories to the amount that fits your calorie and nutrient needs. You can lower your intake by eating and drinking foods and beverages containing empty calories less often or by decreasing the amount you eat or drink.

How many empty calories can I have?

The limit for empty calories is based on estimated calorie needs by age/gender group. Physical activity increases calorie needs, so those who are more physically active need more total calories and have a larger limit for empty calories. Table 10.2 gives a general guide.

What are solid fats?

Solid fats are fats that are solid at room temperature. Solid fats mainly come from animal foods and can also be made from vegetable oils through a process called hydrogenation. Some common solid fats are butter, milk fat, beef fat (tallow, suet), chicken fat, cream, pork fat (lard), stick margarine, shortening, hydrogenated and partially hydrogenated oils*, coconut oil*, and palm and palm kernel oils*.

Table 10.2. Estimated Empty Calorie Allowances

Age and gender	Total daily calorie needs*	Daily limit for empty calories
Children 2–3 yrs	1000 cals	135**
Children 4–8 yrs	1200–1400 cals	120
Girls 9–13 yrs	1600 cals	120
Boys 9–13 yrs	1800 cals	160
Girls 14–18 yrs	1800 cals	160
Boys 14–18 yrs	2200 cals	265
Females 19–30 yrs	2000 cals	260
Males 19–30 yrs	2400 cals	330
Females 31–50 yrs	1800 cals	160
Males 31–50 yrs	2200 cals	265
Females 51+ yrs	1600 cals	120
Males 51+ yrs	2000 cals	260

*These amounts are appropriate for individuals who get less than 30 minutes of moderate physical activity most days. Those who are more active need more total calories, and have a higher limit for empty calories.

** The limit for empty calories is higher for children 2 and 3 years old than it is for some older children because younger children have lower nutrient needs and smaller recommended intakes from the basic food groups.

The starred items (*) are called "oils" because they come from plant sources. Even though they are called "oils," they are considered to be solid fats because they are high in saturated or trans fatty acids.

Most solid fats are high in saturated fats and/or trans fats and have less monounsaturated or polyunsaturated fats. Animal products containing solid fats also contain cholesterol. Saturated fats and trans fats tend to raise "bad" (LDL) cholesterol levels in the blood. This, in turn increases the risk for heart disease. To lower risk for heart disease, cut back on foods containing saturated fats and trans fats.

Some foods that contain solid fats include many desserts and baked goods, such as cakes, cookies, donuts, pastries, and croissants; many cheeses and foods containing cheese, such as pizza; sausages, hot dogs, bacon, and ribs; ice cream and other dairy desserts; fried potatoes (French fries)—if fried in a solid fat or hydrogenated oil, regular ground beef and cuts of meat with marbling or visible fat, and fried chicken and other chicken dishes with the skin.

Table 10.3. Empty Calories In Common Foods (calories from solid fats and added sugars)

Food	Amount	Estimated Total Calories	Estimated Empty Calories
Dairy Group			
Fat-free milk (skim)	1 cup	83	0
1% milk (low fat)	1 cup	102	18
2% milk (reduced fat)	1 cup	122	37
Whole milk	1 cup	149	63
Low-fat chocolate milk	1 cup	158	64
Cheddar cheese	1½ ounces	172	113
Nonfat mozzarella cheese	1½ ounces	59	0
Whole milk mozzarella cheese	1½ ounces	128	76
Fruit flavored low-fat yogurt	1 cup (8 fl oz.)	250	152
Frozen yogurt	1 cup	224	119
Ice cream, vanilla	1 cup	275	210
Cheese sauce	¼ cup	120	64
Protein Foods Group			
Extra lean ground beef, 95% lean	3 oz., cooked	146	0
Regular ground beef, 80% lean	3 oz., cooked	229	64
Turkey roll, light meat	3 slices (1 oz. each)	165	0
Roasted chicken breast (skinless)	3 oz., cooked	138	0
Roasted chicken thigh with skin	3 oz., cooked	209	47
Fried chicken with skin and batter	3 medium wings	478	382
Beef sausage, pre-cooked	3 oz., cooked	345	172
Pork sausage	2 patties (2 oz.)	204	96
Beef bologna	3 slices (1 oz. each)	261	150
Grains Group			
Whole wheat bread	1 slice (1 oz.)	69	0
White bread	1 slice (1 oz.)	69	0
English muffin	1 muffin	132	0
Blueberry muffin	1 small muffin (2 oz.)	259	69
Croissant	1 medium (2 oz.)	231	111

Table 10.3. continued

Food	Amount	Estimated Total Calories	Estimated Empty Calories
Grains Group, *continued*			
Biscuit, plain	1 medium (2.5" diameter)	186	71
Cornbread	1 piece (2 ½" x 2 ½" x 1 ¼")	167	52
Corn flakes cereal	1 cup	90	8
Frosted corn flakes cereal	1 cup	147	56
Graham crackers	2 large pieces	118	54
Whole wheat crackers	5 crackers	85	25
Round snack crackers	7 crackers	106	42
Chocolate chip cookies	2 large	161	109
Chocolate cake	1 slice of two-layer cake	408	315
Glazed doughnut, yeast type	1 medium, 3¾" diameter	255	170
Cinnamon sweet roll	1 medium roll	223	137
Vegetable Group			
Baked potato	1 medium	159	0
French fries	1 medium order	431	185
Onion rings	1 order (8 to 9 rings)	275	160
Fruit Group			
Unsweetened applesauce	1 cup	105	0
Sweetened applesauce	1 cup	173	68
Other			
Pepperoni pizza	1 slice of a 14" pizza, regular crust	340	139
Regular soda	1 can (12 fluid oz.)	136	136
Regular soda	1 bottle (19.9 fluid oz.)	192	192
Fruit-flavored drink	1 cup	128	128
Butter	1 teaspoon	36	33
Stick margarine	1 teaspoon	36	32
Cream cheese	1 Tablespoon	41	36
Heavy (whipping) cream	1 Tablespoon	51	45
Frozen whipped topping (non dairy)	¼ cup	60	55

Watch Serving Sizes

The calories per serving are listed on the nutrition facts label on food packages. Be sure to compare the stated serving size to the amount actually eaten. If you eat twice the stated serving size, you will have twice the calories.

In some cases, the fat in foods is not visible. For example, the fat in fluid milk is a solid fat. Milk fat (butter) is solid at room temperature but it is suspended in the fluid milk by the process of homogenization.

In contrast to solid fats, oils are fats that are liquid at room temperature, like the vegetable oils used in cooking. Oils come from many different plants—such as corn and peanuts—and from fish. [See Chapter 9 for more information about oils.]

Solid fats and oils provide the same number of calories per gram. However, oils are generally better for your health than solid fats because they contain less saturated fats and/or trans fats. Foods containing partially hydrogenated vegetable oils usually contain trans fats. Trans fats can be found in many cakes, cookies, crackers, icings, margarines, and microwave popcorns.

What are added sugars?

Added sugars are sugars and syrups that are added to foods or beverages when they are processed or prepared. This does not include naturally occurring sugars such as those in milk and fruits.

The major food and beverage sources of added sugars for Americans are regular soft drinks, energy drinks, and sports drinks; candy, cakes, cookies, pies, and cobblers; sweet rolls, pastries, and donuts; fruit drinks, such as fruitades and fruit punch; and dairy desserts, such as ice cream,

Reading the ingredient label on processed foods can help to identify added sugars. Names for added sugars on food labels include the following:

- Anhydrous dextrose
- Confectioner's powdered sugar
- Corn syrup solids
- Fructose
- Honey
- Lactose

- Brown sugar
- Corn syrup
- Dextrose
- High-fructose corn syrup (HFCS)
- Invert sugar
- Malt syrup

- Maltose
- Molasses
- Pancake syrup
- Sucrose
- White granulated sugar
- Maple syrup
- Nectars (for example, peach nectar, pear nectar)
- Raw sugar
- Sugar

You may also see other names used for added sugars, but these are not recognized by the U.S. Food and Drug Administration (FD)A as an ingredient name. These include cane juice, evaporated corn sweetener, fruit juice concentrate, crystal dextrose, glucose, liquid fructose, sugar cane juice, and fruit nectar.

How do I count the empty calories I eat?

Fats are concentrated sources of calories. Eating even small amounts of foods high in solid fats can send you over your empty calorie limit. Some foods and beverages with added sugars, like sodas, are often served in large portions. These large portions can also send you over your empty calorie limit.

You can lower your intake of empty calories by eating and drinking foods with empty calories less often. You can also cut down on empty calories by choosing a smaller amount to eat or drink. Or, you can choose foods and beverages with fewer solid fats and added sugars.

Table 10.3 provides a quick guide to the number of empty calories in some common foods.

Chapter 11

Water: Meeting Your Daily Fluid Needs

Ever notice how lifeless a houseplant looks when you forget to water it? Just a little water and it seems to perk back up. Water is just as essential for our bodies because it is in every cell, tissue, and organ in your body. That is why getting enough water every day is important for your health.

Healthy people meet their fluid needs by drinking when thirsty and drinking fluids with meals. But, if you're outside in hot weather for most of the day or doing vigorous physical activity, you'll need to make an effort to drink more fluids.

Where do I get the water I need?

Most of your water needs are met through the water and beverages you drink.

You can get some fluid through the foods you eat. For example, broth soups and other foods that are 85 percent to 95 percent water such as celery, tomatoes, oranges, and melons.

What does water do in my body?

Water helps your body with the following:

- Keeps its temperature normal
- Lubricates and cushions your joints
- Protects your spinal cord and other sensitive tissues
- Gets rid of wastes through urination, perspiration, and bowel movements

About This Chapter: Excerpted from "Water: Meeting Your Daily Fluid Needs," Centers for Disease Control and Prevention, December 2008.

Other Beverages

Beverages contribute substantially to overall dietary and calorie intake for most Americans. Although they provide needed water, many beverages add calories to the diet without providing essential nutrients. Their consumption should be planned in the context of total calorie intake and how they can fit into the eating pattern of each individual. Currently, American adults ages 19 years and older consume an average of about 400 calories per day as beverages. The major types of beverages consumed by adults, in descending order by average calorie intake, are: regular soda, energy, and sports drinks; alcoholic beverages; milk (including whole, 2%, 1%, and fat-free); 100% fruit juice; and fruit drinks. Children ages 2 to 18 years also consume an average of 400 calories per day as beverages. The major beverages for children are somewhat different and, in order by average calorie intake, are: milk (including whole, 2%, 1%, and fat-free); regular soda, energy, and sports drinks; fruit drinks; and 100% fruit juice. Among children and adolescents, milk and 100% fruit juice intake is higher for younger children, and soda intake is higher for adolescents.

The calorie content of beverages varies widely, and some of the beverages with the highest intake, including regular sodas, fruit drinks, and alcoholic beverages, contain calories but provide few or no essential nutrients. Other beverages, however, such as fat-free or low-fat milk and 100% fruit juice, provide a substantial amount of nutrients along with the calories they contain. Water and unsweetened beverages, such as coffee and tea, contribute to total water intake without adding calories. To limit excess calories and maintain healthy weight, individuals are encouraged to drink water and other beverages with few or no calories, in addition to recommended amounts of low-fat or fat-free milk and 100% fruit juices.

Source: Excerpted from *Dietary Guidelines for Americans 2010*, U.S. Department of Agriculture, December 2010.

Why do I need to drink enough water each day?

You need water to replace what your body loses through normal everyday functions. Of course, you lose water when you go to the bathroom or sweat, but you even lose small amounts of water when you exhale. You need to replace this lost water to prevent dehydration.

Your body also needs more water when you are in hot climates, more physically active, running a fever, or having diarrhea or vomiting.

To help you stay hydrated during prolonged physical activity or when it is hot outside, the *Dietary Guidelines for Americans* recommend these two steps:

- Drink fluid while doing the activity.
- Drink several glasses of water or other fluid after the physical activity is completed.

Also, when you are participating in vigorous physical activity, it's important to drink before you even feel thirsty. Thirst is a signal that your body is on the way to dehydration.

Some people may have fluid restrictions because of a health problem, such as kidney disease. If your healthcare provider has told you to restrict your fluid intake, be sure to follow that advice.

Do sugar-sweetened beverages count?

Although beverages that are sweetened with sugars do provide water, they usually have more calories than unsweetened beverages. To help with weight control, you should consume beverages and foods that don't have added sugars.

Examples of beverages with added sugars include fruit drinks, some sports drinks, and soft drinks and sodas (non-diet).

How can I increase fluid intake by drinking more water?

Under normal conditions, most people can drink enough fluids to meet their water needs. If you are outside in hot weather for most of the day or doing vigorous activity, you may need to increase your fluid intake.

If you think you're not getting enough water each day, the following tips may help:

- Carry a water bottle for easy access when you are at work or running errands.

- Freeze some freezer-safe water bottles. Take one with you for ice-cold water all day long.

- Choose water instead of sugar-sweetened beverages. This tip can also help with weight management. Substituting water for one 20-ounce sugar-sweetened soda will save you about 240 calories.

- Choose water instead of other beverages when eating out. Generally, you will save money and reduce calories.

- Give your water a little pizzazz by adding a wedge of lime or lemon. This may improve the taste, and you just might drink more water than you usually do.

Fluoride And Dental Health

Drinking fluoridated water and/or using fluoride-containing dental products helps reduce the risk of dental caries (cavities). Most bottled water is not fluoridated. With the increase in consumption of bottled water, Americans may not be getting enough fluoride to maintain oral health.

During the time that sugars and starches are in contact with teeth, they also contribute to dental caries. A combined approach of reducing the amount of time sugars and starches are in the mouth, drinking fluoridated water, and brushing and flossing teeth, is the most effective way to reduce dental caries.

Source: Excerpted from *Dietary Guidelines for Americans 2010*, U.S. Department of Agriculture, December 2010.

Part Two
Vitamins And Minerals

Chapter 12

Vitamin A And Carotenoids

Vitamin A: What is it?

Vitamin A is a group of compounds that play an important role in vision, bone growth, reproduction, cell division, and cell differentiation (in which a cell becomes part of the brain, muscle, lungs, blood, or other specialized tissue.) Vitamin A helps regulate the immune system, which helps prevent or fight off infections by making white blood cells that destroy harmful bacteria and viruses. Vitamin A also may help lymphocytes (a type of white blood cell) fight infections more effectively.

Vitamin A promotes healthy surface linings of the eyes and the respiratory, urinary, and intestinal tracts. When those linings break down, it becomes easier for bacteria to enter the body and cause infection. Vitamin A also helps the skin and mucous membranes function as a barrier to bacteria and viruses.

In general, there are two categories of vitamin A, depending on whether the food source is an animal or a plant.

Vitamin A found in foods that come from animals is called preformed vitamin A. It is absorbed in the form of retinol, one of the most usable (active) forms of vitamin A. Sources include liver, whole milk, and some fortified food products. Retinol can be made into retinal and retinoic acid (other active forms of vitamin A) in the body.

Vitamin A that is found in colorful fruits and vegetables is called provitamin A carotenoid. They can be made into retinol in the body. In the United States, approximately 26% of vitamin A consumed by men and 34% of vitamin A consumed by women is in the form of provitamin

About This Chapter: Excerpted from "Vitamin A and Carotenoids," Office of Dietary Supplements, April 2006.

A carotenoids. Common provitamin A carotenoids found in foods that come from plants are beta-carotene, alpha-carotene, and beta-cryptoxanthin. Among these, beta-carotene is most efficiently made into retinol. Alpha-carotene and beta-cryptoxanthin are also converted to vitamin A, but only half as efficiently as beta-carotene.

Of the 563 identified carotenoids, fewer than 10% can be made into vitamin A in the body. Lycopene, lutein, and zeaxanthin are carotenoids that do not have vitamin A activity but have other health promoting properties. The Institute of Medicine (IOM) encourages consumption of all carotenoid-rich fruits and vegetables for their health-promoting benefits.

Some provitamin A carotenoids have been shown to function as antioxidants in laboratory studies; however, this role has not been consistently demonstrated in humans. Antioxidants protect cells from free radicals, which are potentially damaging by-products of oxygen metabolism that may contribute to the development of some chronic diseases.

What foods provide vitamin A?

Retinol is found in foods that come from animals such as whole eggs, milk, and liver. Most fat-free milk and dried nonfat milk solids sold in the United States are fortified with vitamin A to replace the amount lost when the fat is removed. Fortified foods such as fortified breakfast cereals also provide vitamin A. Provitamin A carotenoids are abundant in darkly colored fruits and vegetables. The 2000 National Health and Nutrition Examination Survey (NHANES) indicated that major dietary contributors of retinol are milk, margarine, eggs, beef liver and fortified breakfast cereals, whereas major contributors of provitamin A carotenoids are carrots, cantaloupes, sweet potatoes, and spinach.

Vitamin A in foods that come from animals is well absorbed and used efficiently by the body. Vitamin A in foods that come from plants is not as well absorbed as animal sources of vitamin A. Tables 12.1 and 12.2 suggest many sources of vitamin A and provitamin A carotenoids.

What are recommended intakes of vitamin A?

Recommendations for vitamin A are provided in the dietary reference intakes (DRIs) developed by the Institute of Medicine (IOM). DRI is the general term for a set of reference values used for planning and assessing nutrient intake in healthy people. Three important types of reference values included in the DRIs are recommended dietary allowances (RDA), adequate intakes (AI), and tolerable upper intake levels (UL). The RDA recommends the average daily dietary intake level that is sufficient to meet the nutrient requirements of nearly all (97% to 98%) healthy individuals in each age and gender group. An AI is set when there

Table 12.1. Selected Animal Sources Of Vitamin A

Food	Vitamin A (IU)*	percent DV**
Liver, beef, cooked, 3 ounces	27,185	545
Liver, chicken, cooked, 3 ounces	12,325	245
Milk, fortified skim, 1 cup	500	10
Cheese, cheddar, 1 ounce	284	6
Milk, whole (3.25% fat), 1 cup	249	5
Egg substitute, ¼ cup	226	5

Table 12.2. Selected Plant Sources Of Vitamin A (From Beta-Carotene)

Food	Vitamin A (IU)*	percent DV**
Carrot juice, canned, ½ cup	22,567	450
Carrots, boiled, ½ cup slices	13,418	270
Spinach, frozen, boiled, ½ cup	11,458	230
Kale, frozen, boiled, ½ cup	9,558	190
Carrots, 1 raw (7½ inches)	8,666	175
Vegetable soup, canned, chunky, ready-to-serve, 1 cup	5,820	115
Cantaloupe, 1 cup cubes	5,411	110
Spinach, raw, 1 cup	2,813	55
Apricots with skin, juice pack, ½ cup	2,063	40
Apricot nectar, canned, ½ cup	1,651	35
Papaya, 1 cup cubes	1,532	30
Mango, 1 cup sliced	1,262	25
Oatmeal, instant, fortified, plain, prepared with water, 1 cup	1,252	25
Peas, frozen, boiled, ½ cup	1,050	20
Tomato juice, canned, 6 ounces	819	15
Peaches, canned, juice pack, ½ cup halves or slices	473	10
Peach, 1 medium	319	6
Pepper, sweet, red, raw, 1 ring (3 inches diameter by ¼ inch thick)	313	6

* IU = International Units

** DV = Daily Value. DVs are reference numbers based on the Recommended Dietary Allowances (RDAs). They were developed to help consumers determine if a food contains a lot or a little of a nutrient. The DV for vitamin A is 5,000 IU. Most food labels do not list vitamin A content. The percent DV (% DV) column in the table above indicates the percentage of the DV provided in one serving. A food providing 5% or less of the DV is a low source while a food that provides 10% to 19% of the DV is a good source. A food that provides 20% or more of the DV is high in that nutrient. It is important to remember that foods that provide lower percentages of the DV also contribute to a healthful diet. For foods not listed in this table, refer to the U.S. Department of Agriculture's Nutrient Database Web site: http://www.nal.usda.gov/fnic/cgi-bin/nut_search.pl.

are insufficient scientific data to establish an RDA. AIs meet or exceed the amount needed to maintain nutritional adequacy in nearly all people. The UL, on the other hand, is the maximum daily intake unlikely to result in adverse health effects.

In Table 12.3, RDAs for vitamin A are listed as micrograms (mcg) of retinol activity equivalents (RAE) to account for the different biological activities of retinol and provitamin A carotenoids. Table 12.3 also lists RDAs for vitamin A in international units (IU), which are used on food and supplement labels (1 RAE = 3.3 IU).

The NHANES III survey (1988–1994) found that most Americans consume recommended amounts of vitamin A. More recent NHANES data (1999–2000) show average adult intakes to be about 3,300 IU per day, which also suggests that most Americans get enough vitamin A.

There is no RDA for beta-carotene or other provitamin A carotenoids. The IOM states that consuming three mg to six mg of beta-carotene daily (equivalent to 833 IU to 1,667 IU vitamin A) will maintain blood levels of beta-carotene in the range associated with a lower risk of chronic diseases. A diet that provides five or more servings of fruits and vegetables per day and includes some dark green and leafy vegetables and deep yellow or orange fruits should provide sufficient beta-carotene and other carotenoids.

When can vitamin A deficiency occur?

Vitamin A deficiency is common in developing countries but rarely seen in the United States. Approximately 250,000 to 500,000 malnourished children in the developing world become blind each year from a deficiency of vitamin A. In the United States, vitamin A deficiency is most often associated with strict dietary restrictions and excess alcohol intake. Severe zinc deficiency, which is also associated with strict dietary limitations, often accompanies vitamin A deficiency. Zinc is required to make retinol binding protein (RBP) which transports vitamin A. Therefore, a deficiency in zinc limits the body's ability to move vitamin A stores from the liver to body tissues.

Table 12.3. Recommended Dietary Allowances (RDAs) For Vitamin A

Age (years)	Children (mcg RAE)	Males (mcg RAE)	Females (mcg RAE)	Pregnancy (mcg RAE)	Lactation (mcg RAE)
1–3	300 (1,000 IU)				
4–8	400 (1,320 IU)				
9–13	600 (2,000 IU)				
14–18		900 (3,000 IU)	700 (2,310 IU)	750 (2,500 IU)	1,200 (4,000 IU)
19+		900 (3,000 IU)	700 (2,310 IU)	770 (2,565 IU)	1,300 (4,300 IU)

Night Blindness And Vitamin A Deficiency

Night blindness is one of the first signs of vitamin A deficiency. In ancient Egypt, it was known that night blindness could be cured by eating liver, which was later found to be a rich source of the vitamin. Vitamin A deficiency contributes to blindness by making the cornea very dry and damaging the retina and cornea.

Vitamin A deficiency diminishes the ability to fight infections. In countries where such deficiency is common and immunization programs are limited, millions of children die each year from complications of infectious diseases such as measles. In vitamin A-deficient individuals, cells lining the lungs lose their ability to remove disease-causing microorganisms. This may contribute to the pneumonia associated with vitamin A deficiency.

There is increased interest in early forms of vitamin A deficiency, described as low storage levels of vitamin A that do not cause obvious deficiency symptoms. This mild degree of vitamin A deficiency may increase children's risk of developing respiratory and diarrheal infections, decrease growth rate, slow bone development, and decrease likelihood of survival from serious illness. Children in the United States who are considered to be at increased risk for subclinical vitamin A deficiency include the following:

- Toddlers and preschool age children

- Children living at or below the poverty level

- Children with inadequate health care or immunizations

- Children living in areas with known nutritional deficiencies

- Recent immigrants or refugees from developing countries with high incidence of vitamin A deficiency or measles

- Children with diseases of the pancreas, liver, or intestines, or with inadequate fat digestion or absorption

A deficiency can occur when vitamin A is lost through chronic diarrhea and through an overall inadequate intake, as is often seen with protein-energy malnutrition. Low blood retinol concentrations indicate depleted levels of vitamin A. This occurs with vitamin A deficiency but also can result from an inadequate intake of protein, calories, and zinc, since these nutrients are needed to make RBP. Iron deficiency can also affect vitamin A metabolism, and iron supplements provided to iron-deficient individuals may improve body stores of vitamin A and iron.

Excess alcohol intake depletes vitamin A stores. Also, diets high in alcohol often do not provide recommended amounts of vitamin A. It is very important for people who consume excessive amounts of alcohol to include good sources of vitamin A in their diets. Vitamin A supplements may not be recommended for individuals who abuse alcohol, however, because their livers may be more susceptible to potential toxicity from high doses of vitamin A. A medical doctor will need to evaluate this situation and determine the need for vitamin A supplements.

Who may need extra vitamin A to prevent a deficiency?

Vitamin A deficiency rarely occurs in the United States, but the World Health Organization (WHO) and the United Nations Children's Fund (UNICEF) recommend vitamin A administration for all children diagnosed with measles in communities where vitamin A deficiency is a serious problem and where death from measles is greater than 1%. In 1994, the American Academy of Pediatrics recommended vitamin A supplements for two subgroups of children likely to be at high risk for subclinical vitamin A deficiency: children aged six months to 24 months who are hospitalized with measles, and hospitalized children older than six months.

Fat malabsorption can result in diarrhea and prevent normal absorption of vitamin A. Over time this may result in vitamin A deficiency. Those conditions include the following:

- **Celiac Disease:** Often referred to as sprue, celiac disease is a genetic disorder. People with celiac disease become sick when they eat a protein called gluten found in wheat and some other grains. In celiac disease, gluten can trigger damage to the small intestine, where most nutrient absorption occurs. Approximately 30% to 60% of people with celiac disease have gastrointestinal-motility disorders such as diarrhea. They must follow a gluten-free diet to avoid malabsorption and other symptoms.

- **Crohn Disease:** This inflammatory bowel disease affects the small intestine. People with Crohn disease often experience diarrhea, fat malabsorption, and malnutrition.

- **Pancreatic Disorders:** Because the pancreas secretes enzymes that are important for fat absorption, pancreatic disorders often result in fat malabsorption. Without these enzymes, it is difficult to absorb fat. Many people with pancreatic disease take pancreatic enzymes in pill form to prevent fat malabsorption and diarrhea.

Healthy adults usually have a reserve of vitamin A stored in their livers and should not be at risk of deficiency during periods of temporary or short-term fat malabsorption. Long-term problems absorbing fat, however, may result in deficiency. In these instances physicians may recommend additional vitamin A.

Vitamin A For Vegetarians

Vegetarians who do not consume eggs and dairy foods need provitamin A carotenoids to meet their need for vitamin A. They should include a minimum of five servings of fruits and vegetables in their daily diet and regularly choose dark green leafy vegetables and orange and yellow fruits to consume recommended amounts of vitamin A.

What are the health risks of too much vitamin A?

Hypervitaminosis A refers to high storage levels of vitamin A in the body that can lead to toxic symptoms. There are four major adverse effects of hypervitaminosis A: birth defects, liver abnormalities, reduced bone mineral density that may result in osteoporosis (see the previous section), and central nervous system disorders.

Toxic symptoms can also arise after consuming very large amounts of preformed vitamin A over a short period of time. Signs of acute toxicity include nausea and vomiting, headache, dizziness, blurred vision, and muscular uncoordination. Although hypervitaminosis A can occur when large amounts of liver are regularly consumed, most cases result from taking excess amounts of the nutrient in supplements.

The IOM has established tolerable upper intake levels (ULs) for vitamin A that apply to healthy populations. The UL was established to help prevent the risk of vitamin A toxicity. The risk of adverse health effects increases at intakes greater than the UL. The UL does not apply to malnourished individuals receiving vitamin A either periodically or through fortification programs as a means of preventing vitamin A deficiency. It also does not apply to individuals being treated with vitamin A by medical doctors for diseases such as retinitis pigmentosa.

What are the health risks of too many carotenoids?

Provitamin A carotenoids such as beta-carotene are generally considered safe because they are not associated with specific adverse health effects. Their conversion to vitamin A decreases when body stores are full. A high intake of provitamin A carotenoids can turn the skin yellow, but this is not considered dangerous to health.

Chapter 13

B Vitamins

Vitamin B6

What is it?

Vitamin B6 is a water-soluble vitamin that exists in three major chemical forms: pyridoxine, pyridoxal, and pyridoxamine. It performs a wide variety of functions in your body and is essential for your good health. For example, vitamin B6 is needed for more than 100 enzymes involved in protein metabolism. It is also essential for red blood cell metabolism. The nervous and immune systems need vitamin B6 to function efficiently, and it is also needed for the conversion of tryptophan (an amino acid) to niacin (a vitamin).

Hemoglobin within red blood cells carries oxygen to tissues. Your body needs vitamin B6 to make hemoglobin. Vitamin B6 also helps increase the amount of oxygen carried by hemoglobin. A vitamin B6 deficiency can result in a form of anemia that is similar to iron deficiency anemia.

An immune response is a broad term that describes a variety of biochemical changes that occur in an effort to fight off infections. Calories, protein, vitamins, and minerals are important to your immune defenses because they promote the growth of white blood cells that directly fight infections. Vitamin B6, through its involvement in protein metabolism and cellular growth, is important to the immune system. It helps maintain the health of lymphoid organs (thymus, spleen, and lymph nodes) that make your white blood cells. Animal studies show that a vitamin B6 deficiency can decrease your antibody production and suppress your immune response.

About This Chapter: Excepted from "Vitamin B6," August 2007, and "Vitamin B12," July 2010, both produced by the Office of Dietary Supplements.

Vitamin B6 And Blood Glucose

Vitamin B6 helps maintain your blood glucose (sugar) within a normal range. When caloric intake is low your body needs vitamin B6 to help convert stored carbohydrate or other nutrients to glucose to maintain normal blood sugar levels. While a shortage of vitamin B6 will limit these functions, supplements of this vitamin do not enhance them in well-nourished individuals.

Table 13.1. Food Sources Of Vitamin B6

Food	Milligrams (mg) per serving	% DV*
Ready-to-eat cereal (100% fortified, ¾ C)	2.00	100
Potato (Baked, flesh and skin, 1 medium)	0.70	35
Banana (raw, 1 medium)	0.68	34
Garbanzo beans (canned, ½ C)	0.57	30
Chicken breast (meat only, cooked, ½ breast)	0.52	25
Ready-to-eat cereal (25% fortified, ¾ C)	0.50	25
Oatmeal (instant, fortified, 1 packet)	0.42	20
Pork loin (lean only, cooked, 3 oz)	0.42	20
Roast beef (eye of round, lean only, cooked, 3 oz)	0.32	15
Trout (rainbow, cooked, 3 oz)	0.29	15
Sunflower seeds (kernels, dry roasted, 1 oz)	0.23	10
Spinach (frozen, cooked, ½ C)	0.14	8
Tomato juice (canned, 6 oz)	0.20	10
Avocado (raw, sliced, ½ cup)	0.20	10
Salmon (Sockeye, cooked, 3 oz)	0.19	10
Tuna (canned in water, drained solids, 3 oz)	0.18	10
Wheat bran (crude or unprocessed, ¼ C)	0.18	10
Peanut butter (smooth, 2 Tbs.)	0.15	8
Walnuts (English/Persian, 1 oz)	0.15	8
Soybeans (green, boiled, drained, ½ C)	0.05	2
Lima beans (frozen, cooked, drained, ½ C)	0.10	6

* DV = Daily Value. DVs are reference numbers based on the Recommended Dietary Allowance (RDA). They were developed to help consumers determine if a food contains a lot or a little of a specific nutrient. The DV for vitamin B6 is 2.0 milligrams (mg). The% DV (%DV) listed on the nutrition facts panel of food labels tells you what percentage of the DV is provided in one serving. Percent DVs are based on a 2,000 calorie diet. Your Daily Values may be higher or lower depending on your calorie needs. Foods that provide lower percentages of the DV also contribute to a healthful diet.

What foods provide vitamin B6?

Vitamin B6 is found in a wide variety of foods including fortified cereals, beans, meat, poultry, fish, and some fruits and vegetables. Table 13.1 shows selected food sources of vitamin B6 and suggests many dietary sources of B6.

What is the recommended dietary allowance for vitamin B6 for adults?

The recommended dietary allowance (RDA) is the average daily dietary intake level that is sufficient to meet the nutrient requirements of nearly all (97 to 98%) healthy individuals in each life-stage and gender group.

Table 13.2 shows the RDAs for vitamin B6 for adults in 1998.

Table 13.2. 1998 RDAs For Vitamin B6 For Adults, In Milligrams (mg)

Life-Stage	Men	Women	Pregnancy	Lactation
Ages 19-50	1.3 mg	1.3 mg		
Ages 51+	1.7 mg	1.5 mg		
All Ages			1.9 mg	2.0 mg

Results of two national surveys, the National Health and Nutrition Examination Survey (NHANES III 1988-94) and the Continuing Survey of Food Intakes by Individuals (1994-96 CSFII), indicated that diets of most Americans meet current intake recommendations for vitamin B6.

When can a vitamin B6 deficiency occur?

Clinical signs of vitamin B6 deficiency are rarely seen in the United States. Many older Americans, however, have low blood levels of vitamin B6, which may suggest a marginal or sub-optimal vitamin B6 nutritional status. Vitamin B6 deficiency can occur in individuals with poor quality diets that are deficient in many nutrients. Symptoms occur during later stages of deficiency, when intake has been very low for an extended time. Signs of vitamin B6 deficiency include dermatitis (skin inflammation), glossitis (a sore tongue), depression, confusion, and convulsions. Vitamin B6 deficiency also can cause anemia. Some of these symptoms can also result from a variety of medical conditions other than vitamin B6 deficiency. It is important to have a physician evaluate these symptoms so that appropriate medical care can be given.

Who may need extra vitamin B6 to prevent a deficiency?

Individuals with a poor quality diet or an inadequate B6 intake for an extended period may benefit from taking a vitamin B6 supplement if they are unable to increase their dietary intake of vitamin B6. Alcoholics and older adults are more likely to have inadequate vitamin B6 intakes than other segments of the population because they may have limited variety in their diet. Alcohol also promotes the destruction and loss of vitamin B6 from the body.

Asthmatic children treated with the medicine theophylline may need to take a vitamin B6 supplement. Theophylline decreases body stores of vitamin B6, and theophylline-induced seizures have been linked to low body stores of the vitamin. A physician should be consulted about the need for a vitamin B6 supplement when theophylline is prescribed.

What are some current issues and controversies about vitamin B6?

Vitamin B6 And The Nervous System: Vitamin B6 is needed for the synthesis of neurotransmitters such as serotonin and dopamine. These neurotransmitters are required for normal nerve cell communication. Researchers have been investigating the relationship between vitamin B6 status and a wide variety of neurologic conditions such as seizures, chronic pain, depression, headache, and Parkinson disease.

Lower levels of serotonin have been found in individuals suffering from depression and migraine headaches. So far, however, vitamin B6 supplements have not proved effective for relieving these symptoms. One study found that a sugar pill was just as likely as vitamin B6 to relieve headaches and depression associated with low dose oral contraceptives.

Vitamin B6 And Carpal Tunnel Syndrome: Vitamin B6 was first recommended for carpal tunnel syndrome almost 30 years ago. Several popular books still recommend taking 100 to 200 milligrams (mg) of vitamin B6 daily to treat carpal tunnel syndrome, even though scientific studies do not indicate it is effective. Anyone taking large doses of vitamin B6 supplements for carpal tunnel syndrome needs to be aware that the Institute of Medicine recently established an upper tolerable limit of 100 mg per day for adults. There are documented cases in the literature of neuropathy caused by excessive vitamin B6 taken for treatment of carpal tunnel syndrome.

Vitamin B6 And Premenstrual Syndrome: Vitamin B6 has become a popular remedy for treating the discomforts associated with premenstrual syndrome (PMS). Unfortunately, clinical trials have failed to support any significant benefit. One recent study indicated that a sugar pill was as likely to relieve symptoms of PMS as vitamin B6. In addition, vitamin B6 toxicity has been seen in increasing numbers of women taking vitamin B6 supplements for PMS. One review indicated that neuropathy was present in 23 of 58 women taking daily vitamin B6 supplements for PMS whose blood levels of B6 were above normal. There is no convincing scientific evidence to support recommending vitamin B6 supplements for PMS.

What is the relationship between vitamin B6, homocysteine, and heart disease?

A deficiency of vitamin B6, folic acid, or vitamin B12 may increase your level of homocysteine, an amino acid normally found in your blood. There is evidence that an elevated homocysteine level is an independent risk factor for heart disease and stroke. The evidence suggests that high levels of homocysteine may damage coronary arteries or make it easier for blood clotting cells called platelets to clump together and form a clot. However, there is currently no evidence available to suggest that lowering homocysteine level with vitamins will reduce your risk of heart disease. Clinical intervention trials are needed to determine whether supplementation with vitamin B6, folic acid, or vitamin B12 can help protect you against developing coronary heart disease.

What is the health risk of too much vitamin B6?

Too much vitamin B6 can result in nerve damage to the arms and legs. This neuropathy is usually related to high intake of vitamin B6 from supplements, and is reversible when supplementation is stopped. According to the Institute of Medicine, "Several reports show sensory neuropathy at doses lower than 500 mg per day."

As previously mentioned, the Food and Nutrition Board of the Institute of Medicine has established an upper tolerable intake level (UL) for vitamin B6 of 100 mg per day for all adults. "As intake increases above the UL, the risk of adverse effects increases."

Is vitamin B6 found in healthy diets?

Vitamin B6 is found in a wide variety of foods. Foods such as fortified breakfast cereals, fish including salmon and tuna fish, meats such as pork and chicken, bananas, beans and peanut butter, and many vegetables will contribute to your vitamin B6 intake. According to the *Dietary Guidelines for Americans*, "Nutrient needs should be met primarily through consuming foods. Foods provide an array of nutrients and other compounds that may have beneficial effects on health. In certain cases, fortified foods and dietary supplements may be useful sources of one or more nutrients that otherwise might be consumed in less than recommended amounts. However, dietary supplements, while recommended in some cases, cannot replace a healthful diet."

Vitamin B12

What is vitamin B12 and what does it do?

Vitamin B12 is a nutrient that helps keep the body's nerve and blood cells healthy. It also helps prevent a type of anemia that makes people tired and weak.

How much vitamin B12 do I need?

It depends on your age. Table 13.3 shows the amounts of vitamin B12 people of different ages should get on average each day.

Table 13.3. Average Daily Amounts Of Vitamin B12 For Different Ages In Micrograms (mcg)

Birth to 6 months	0.4 mcg
Infants 7-12 months	0.5 mcg
Children 1–3 years	0.9 mcg
Children 4–8 years	1.2 mcg
Children 9–13 years	1.8 mcg
Teens 14-18 years	2.4 mcg
Adults	2.4 mcg
Pregnant teens and women	2.6 mcg
Breastfeeding teens and women	2.8 mcg

What is a healthy diet?

The *Dietary Guidelines for Americans* describes a healthy diet as one that does the following:

- Emphasizes a variety of fruits, vegetables, whole grains, and fat-free or low-fat milk and milk products
- Includes lean meats, poultry, fish, beans, eggs, and nuts
- Is low in saturated fats, trans fats, cholesterol, salt (sodium), and added sugars
- Stays within your daily calorie needs

What foods provide vitamin B12?

Foods from animals, but not plants, naturally have vitamin B12. You can get enough vitamin B12 by eating a variety of foods including beef liver, clams, fish, meat, poultry, eggs, milk, and other dairy products. Vitamin B12 is added to some breakfast cereals and other food products (check the product labels).

What kinds of vitamin B12 dietary supplements are available?

Almost all multivitamins have vitamin B12. Some dietary supplements have vitamin B12 only. Others have vitamin B12 with folic acid, vitamin B6, and other nutrients.

You can also get vitamin B12 from a shot or a nasal gel with a doctor's prescription. These forms are usually used to treat vitamin B12 deficiency.

Am I getting enough vitamin B12?

Most people get enough vitamin B12 from the foods they eat. But some people have trouble absorbing vitamin B12 and might have a deficiency, even if they get enough vitamin B12.

Many older adults, for example, have trouble absorbing the vitamin B12 found naturally in food. However, most older adults can absorb the vitamin B12 that is added to fortified foods, such as some breakfast cereals, and dietary supplements. People over age 50 should get most of their vitamin B12 from these sources.

People with pernicious anemia have trouble absorbing vitamin B12 from all foods and dietary supplements. Others who might have trouble getting enough vitamin B12 include people who eat little or no animal foods such as strict vegetarians and vegans; people who have had weight loss surgery; and people with digestive disorders, such as celiac disease or Crohn disease. Your doctor can test your vitamin B12 level to see if you have a deficiency.

What happens if I don't get enough vitamin B12?

People who don't get enough vitamin B12 can have many symptoms. Some of these are tiredness, weakness, memory loss, constipation, loss of appetite, weight loss, and anemia. Nerve problems such as numbness and tingling in the hands and feet can also occur.

What are some effects of vitamin B12 on health?

Scientists are studying vitamin B12 to see how it affects health. Here are a few examples of what this research has shown:

Heart Disease: Research on vitamin B12, usually combined with folic acid and vitamin B6, shows that taking vitamin B12 does not reduce the risk of having a heart attack or stroke.

Dementia: As they get older, some people develop dementia or confusion. Scientists don't know yet whether vitamin B12 helps prevent or treat dementia.

Energy And Athletic Performance: Vitamin B12 supplements do not appear to improve energy or athletic performance, except in people with a vitamin B12 deficiency.

Can vitamin B12 be harmful?

Vitamin B12 has not been shown to cause any harm.

Are there any interactions with vitamin B12 that I should know about?

Yes. For example, metformin for diabetes as well as some medicines that people take for acid reflux and peptic ulcer disease can affect how well the body absorbs vitamin B12.

Tell your doctor, pharmacist, and other health care providers about any dietary supplements and medicines you take. They can tell you if those dietary supplements might interact or interfere with your prescription or over-the-counter medicines or if the medicines might affect how your body uses vitamin B12.

Chapter 14

Vitamin C

What is vitamin C and what does it do?

Vitamin C is a nutrient in food that people need to stay healthy. It helps heal wounds and protects the body from infections, viruses, and damage that naturally occurs when the body turns food into energy.

How much vitamin C do I need?

It depends on your age. Table 14.1 shows the amounts of vitamin C people of different ages should get on average each day.

What foods provide vitamin C?

Fruits and vegetables are the best sources of vitamin C. You can get enough vitamin C by eating a variety of foods including citrus fruits (such as oranges and grapefruit) and their juices, as well as red and green pepper, kiwifruit, broccoli, strawberries, baked potatoes, and tomatoes. Vitamin C is added to some foods and beverages (check the product labels).

What kinds of vitamin C dietary supplements are available?

Most multivitamins have vitamin C. Vitamin C is also available alone as a dietary supplement or combined with other nutrients.

About This Chapter: Excerpted from "Vitamin C," Office of Dietary Supplements, July 2010.

Table 14.1. Average Daily Amounts Of Vitamin C For Different Ages In Milligrams (mg)*

Birth to 6 months	40 mg
Infants 7–12 months	50 mg
Children 1–3 years	15 mg
Children 4–8 years	25 mg
Children 9–13 years	45 mg
Teens 14–18 years (boys)	75 mg
Teens 14–18 years (girls)	65 mg
Adults (men)	90 mg
Adults (women)	75 mg
Pregnant teens	80 mg
Pregnant women	85 mg
Breastfeeding teens	115 mg
Breastfeeding women	120 mg

*If you smoke, add 35 mg to the numbers listed above to get the amount you need each day.

Am I getting enough vitamin C?

Most people get enough vitamin C. However, people who don't eat a variety of foods might not get as much vitamin C as they need. People who smoke might also have trouble getting enough vitamin C because they need higher amounts. Some people with cancer and people with kidney disease on dialysis might also not get enough vitamin C.

What happens if I don't get enough vitamin C?

Vitamin C deficiency is rare in the United States and Canada. People who get very little vitamin C for many weeks can get a disease called scurvy. Scurvy causes tiredness, swollen gums, small red or purple spots on the skin, joint pain, poor wound healing, and corkscrew hairs. Scurvy can also cause depression, bleeding gums, loose teeth, and anemia. People can die from scurvy if it is not treated.

What are some effects of vitamin C on health?

Scientists are studying vitamin C to see how it affects health. Here are a few examples of what this research has shown.

Cancer: People who get a lot of vitamin C from eating fruits and vegetables might have a lower risk of getting some types of cancer. However, taking vitamin C dietary supplements doesn't seem to help prevent cancer.

It is not clear whether taking high doses of vitamin C helps treat cancer. Vitamin C dietary supplements might interact with chemotherapy and radiation therapy. If you are being treated for cancer, talk with your health care provider before taking vitamin C or other dietary supplements, especially in high doses.

Heart Disease: Eating lots of fruits and vegetables might lower your risk of getting heart disease. However, scientists aren't sure whether vitamin C, either from food or supplements, helps protect people from heart disease. It is also not clear whether vitamin C helps keep heart disease from getting worse in people who already have it.

Age-Related Macular Degeneration (AMD) And Cataracts: Over time, people with AMD lose the ability to see. In people who have early-stage AMD, a specific supplement with vitamin C and other ingredients might slow down the loss of vision.

Cataracts also cause vision loss. However, it is not clear whether vitamin C, either from food or dietary supplements, affects the risk of getting cataracts.

Table 14.2. Safe Upper Limits For Vitamin C

Birth to 12 months	Not established
Children 1–3 years	400 mg
Children 4–8 years	650 mg
Children 9–13 years	1,200 mg
Teens 14–18 years	1,800 mg
Adults	2,000 mg

Can vitamin C be harmful?

Too much vitamin C might cause diarrhea, nausea and stomach cramps. The safe upper limits for vitamin C are listed in Table 14.2.

Are there any interactions with vitamin C that I should know about?

Yes. For example, taking vitamin C supplements might affect how well some medicines work, such as niacin and statins for high cholesterol. Vitamin C supplements might also interact with chemotherapy or radiation therapy for cancer.

The Common Cold

When taken regularly before getting a cold, vitamin C supplements might slightly shorten the length of a cold and reduce symptoms somewhat. However, for most people, taking vitamin C supplements does not seem to lessen the chance of getting colds. Taking vitamin C supplements also doesn't appear to be helpful after someone actually comes down with a cold.

Tell your doctor, pharmacist, and other health care providers about any dietary supplements and medicines you take. They can tell you if those dietary supplements might interact or interfere with your prescription or over-the-counter medicines or if the medicines might affect how your body uses vitamin C.

Chapter 15

Vitamin D

What is vitamin D and what does it do?

Vitamin D is a nutrient found in some foods that is needed for health and to maintain strong bones. It does so by helping the body absorb calcium (one of bone's main building blocks) from food and supplements. People who get too little vitamin D may develop soft, thin, and brittle bones, a condition known as rickets in children and osteomalacia in adults.

Vitamin D is important to the body in many other ways as well. Muscles need it to move, for example, nerves need it to carry messages between the brain and every body part, and the immune system needs vitamin D to fight off invading bacteria and viruses. Together with calcium, vitamin D also helps protect older adults from osteoporosis. Vitamin D is found in cells throughout the body.

How much vitamin D do I need?

The amount of vitamin D you need each day depends on your age. Average daily recommended amounts from the Food and Nutrition Board (a national group of experts) for different ages are listed in Table 15.1.

What foods provide vitamin D?

Very few foods naturally have vitamin D. Fortified foods provide most of the vitamin D in American diets.

- Fatty fish such as salmon, tuna, and mackerel are among the best sources.

About This Chapter: Excerpted from "Vitamin D," Office of Dietary Supplements, National Institutes of Health, February 4, 2011.

Table 15.1. Vitamin D Requirements In International Units (IU)

Birth to 12 months	400 IU
Children 1–13 years	600 IU
Teens 14–18 years	600 IU
Adults 19–70 years	600 IU
Adults 71 years and older	800 IU
Pregnant and breastfeeding women	600 IU

- Beef liver, cheese, and egg yolks provide small amounts.

- Mushrooms provide some vitamin D. In some mushrooms that are newly available in stores, the vitamin D content is being boosted by exposing these mushrooms to ultraviolet light.

- Almost all of the U.S. milk supply is fortified with 400 IU of vitamin D per quart. But foods made from milk, like cheese and ice cream, are usually not fortified.

- Vitamin D is added to many breakfast cereals and to some brands of orange juice, yogurt, margarine, and soy beverages; check the labels.

Can I get vitamin D from the sun?

The body makes vitamin D when skin is directly exposed to the sun, and most people meet at least some of their vitamin D needs this way. Skin exposed to sunshine indoors through a window will not produce vitamin D. Cloudy days, shade, and having dark-colored skin also cut down on the amount of vitamin D the skin makes.

However, despite the importance of the sun to vitamin D synthesis, it is prudent to limit exposure of skin to sunlight in order to lower the risk for skin cancer. When out in the sun for more than a few minutes, wear protective clothing and apply sunscreen with an SPF (sun protection factor) of 8 or more. Tanning beds also cause the skin to make vitamin D, but pose similar risks for skin cancer.

People who avoid the sun or who cover their bodies with sunscreen or clothing should include good sources of vitamin D in their diets or take a supplement. Recommended intakes of vitamin D are set on the assumption of little sun exposure.

What kinds of vitamin D dietary supplements are available?

Vitamin D is found in supplements (and fortified foods) in two different forms: D2 (ergocalciferol) and D3 (cholecalciferol). Both increase vitamin D in the blood.

Am I getting enough vitamin D?

Because vitamin D can come from sun, food, and supplements, the best measure of one's vitamin D status is blood levels of a form known as 25-hydroxyvitamin D. Levels are described in either nanomoles per liter (nmol/L) or nanograms per milliliter (ng/mL), where 1 nmol/L = 0.4 ng/mL.

In general, levels below 30 nmol/L (12 ng/mL) are too low for bone or overall health, and levels above 125 nmol/L (50 ng/mL) are probably too high. Levels greater than or equal to 50 nmol/L (greater than or equal to 20 ng/mL) are sufficient for most people.

By these measures, some Americans are vitamin D deficient and almost no one has levels that are too high. In general, young people have higher blood levels of 25-hydroxyvitamin D than older people and males have higher levels than females. By race, non-Hispanic blacks tend to have the lowest levels and non-Hispanic whites the highest. The majority of Americans have blood levels lower than 75 nmol/L (30 ng/mL).

What happens if I don't get enough vitamin D?

People can become deficient in vitamin D because they don't consume enough or absorb enough from food, their exposure to sunlight is limited, or their kidneys cannot convert vitamin D to its active form in the body. In children, vitamin D deficiency causes rickets, where the bones become soft and bend. It's a rare disease but still occurs, especially among African American infants and children. In adults, vitamin D deficiency leads to osteomalacia, causing bone pain and muscle weakness.

What are some effects of vitamin D on health?

Vitamin D is being studied for its possible connections to several diseases and medical problems, including diabetes, hypertension, and autoimmune conditions such as multiple sclerosis. Two of them discussed below are bone disorders and some types of cancer.

Certain Groups May Not Get Enough Vitamin D

- Breastfed infants, since human milk is a poor source of the nutrient. Breastfed infants should be given a supplement of 400 IU of vitamin D each day.
- Older adults, since their skin doesn't make vitamin D when exposed to sunlight as efficiently as when they were young, and their kidneys are less able to convert vitamin D to its active form.
- People with dark skin, because their skin has less ability to produce vitamin D from the sun.
- People with disorders such as Crohn disease or celiac disease who don't handle fat properly, because vitamin D needs fat to be absorbed.
- Obese people, because their body fat binds to some vitamin D and prevents it from getting into the blood.

Bone Disorders: As they get older, millions of people (mostly women, but men too) develop, or are at risk of, osteoporosis, where bones become fragile and may fracture if one falls. It is one consequence of not getting enough calcium and vitamin D over the long term. Supplements of both vitamin D3 (at 700–800 IU/day) and calcium (500–1,200 mg/day) have been shown to reduce the risk of bone loss and fractures in elderly people aged 62–85 years. Men and women should talk with their health care providers about their needs for vitamin D (and calcium) as part of an overall plan to prevent or treat osteoporosis.

Cancer: Some studies suggest that vitamin D may protect against colon cancer and perhaps even cancers of the prostate and breast. But higher levels of vitamin D in the blood have also been linked to higher rates of pancreatic cancer. At this time, it's too early to say whether low vitamin D status increases cancer risk and whether higher levels protect or even increase risk in some people.

Can vitamin D be harmful?

Yes, when amounts in the blood become too high. Signs of toxicity include nausea, vomiting, poor appetite, constipation, weakness, and weight loss. And by raising blood levels of calcium, too much vitamin D can cause confusion, disorientation, and problems with heart rhythm. Excess vitamin D can also damage the kidneys.

The safe upper limit for vitamin D is 1,000 to 1,500 IU/day for infants, 2,500 to 3,000 IU/day for children 1–8 years, and 4,000 IU/day for children 9 years and older, adults, and pregnant and lactating teens and women. Vitamin D toxicity almost always occurs from overuse of supplements. Excessive sun exposure doesn't cause vitamin D poisoning because the body limits the amount of this vitamin it produces.

Are there any interactions with vitamin D that I should know about?

Like most dietary supplements, vitamin D may interact or interfere with other medicines or supplements you might be taking. Here are several examples:

- Prednisone and other corticosteroid medicines to reduce inflammation impairs how the body handles vitamin D, which leads to lower calcium absorption and loss of bone over time.

- Both the weight-loss drug orlistat (brand names Xenical® and Alli®) and the cholesterol-lowering drug cholestyramine (brand names Questran®, LoCHOLEST®, and Prevalite®) can reduce the absorption of vitamin D and other fat-soluble vitamins (A, E, and K).

- Both phenobarbital and phenytoin (brand name Dilantin®), used to prevent and control epileptic seizures, increase the breakdown of vitamin D and reduce calcium absorption.

Tell your doctor, pharmacist, and other health care providers about any dietary supplements and medicines you take. They can tell you if those dietary supplements might interact or interfere with your prescription or over-the-counter medicines, or if the medicines might interfere with how your body absorbs, uses, or breaks down nutrients.

Chapter 16

Vitamin E

What is vitamin E and what does it do?

Vitamin E is a nutrient in food that people need to stay healthy. The body uses vitamin E, for example, to protect itself from infections and to keep blood flowing through the blood vessels.

How much vitamin E do I need?

It depends on your age. Table 16.1 shows the amounts people should get on average each day.

What foods provide vitamin E?

You can get enough vitamin E by eating a variety of foods that includes vegetable oils (such as wheat germ, sunflower, and safflower oils), nuts (such as almonds), seeds (such as sunflower seeds), and green vegetables (such as spinach and broccoli).

Vitamin E is added to some breakfast cereals, fruit juices, margarines and spreads, and other foods (check the product labels).

What kinds of vitamin E dietary supplements are available?

Most multivitamin-mineral supplements have vitamin E. It is also available alone as a dietary supplement or combined with other nutrients. The doses of vitamin E in these products are often much higher than the recommended amounts.

A chemical name for vitamin E is alpha-tocopherol. Vitamin E from natural (food) sources is listed on food and supplement labels as "d-alpha-tocopherol." Synthetic (laboratory-made) vitamin E is listed on labels as "dl-alpha-tocopherol." The natural form is stronger. For example, 100 IU of natural vitamin E is equal to about 150 IU of the synthetic form.

About This Chapter: Excepted from "Vitamin E," Office of Dietary Supplements, July 2010.

Other kinds of vitamin E supplements are named "gamma-tocopherol," "tocotrienols," and "mixed tocopherols." These supplements are often more expensive than alpha-tocopherol. For most people, alpha-tocopherol (natural or synthetic) is fine.

Table 16.1. Average Daily Amounts Of Vitamin E For Different Ages In Milligrams (mg) and International Units (IU).

Birth to 6 months	4 mg (6.0 IU)
Infants 7-12 months	5 mg (7.5 IU)
Children 1–3 years	6 mg (9.0 IU)
Children 4–8 years	7 mg (10.4 IU)
Children 9–13 years	11 mg (16.4 IU)
Teens 14–18 years	15 mg (22.4 IU)
Adults	15 mg (22.4 IU)
Pregnant teens and women	15 mg (22.4 IU)
Breastfeeding teens and women	19 mg (28.4 IU)

People At Risk

Many people do not get recommended amounts of vitamin E from food. But only people with certain diseases become deficient. These include people who have trouble digesting or absorbing fat, such as those with Crohn disease, cystic fibrosis, and certain rare inherited conditions.

What happens if I don't get enough vitamin E?

Usually, nothing obvious happens in the short run if you don't get enough vitamin E. But over time, not getting enough vitamin E can cause nerve and muscle damage and make your body less able to fight off infections.

What are some effects of vitamin E on health?

Scientists are studying vitamin E to see how it affects health. Here are a few examples of what this research has shown.

Heart Disease: Vitamin E does not seem to help prevent heart disease in middle-aged or older people or affect the risk of death from this disease. We do not know whether high intakes of vitamin E protect heart health in young, healthy people.

Cancer: It's not clear whether vitamin E prevents cancer. Vitamin E supplements might interact with chemotherapy and radiation therapy. If you are undergoing cancer treatment, talk with your health care provider before taking vitamin E or other dietary supplements, especially in high doses.

Eye Disorders: Age-related macular degeneration (AMD, the loss of straight-ahead vision) and cataracts (clouding of the surface of the eye) cause vision loss in older people. It is not clear whether taking extra vitamin E might help prevent these conditions. In people who have early-stage AMD, a supplement containing vitamin E and other ingredients might help slow vision loss.

Mental Function: Vitamin E supplements probably do not help healthy older people stay mentally active and alert. Vitamin E supplements cannot prevent or slow the decline in mental function, or prevent or treat Alzheimer disease.

Can vitamin E be harmful?

In healthy adults, up to 1,500 IU/day of natural vitamin E supplements or up to 1,100 IU/day of the synthetic form is safe. Higher doses can increase the time it takes blood to clot from a cut or injury. Very high doses can increase the risk of serious bleeding in the brain (stroke).

Are there any interactions with vitamin E that I should know about?

Vitamin E can increase the risk of bleeding in people taking anti-clotting drugs, such as warfarin (Coumadin). It might also interact with chemotherapy or radiation therapy. Also, vitamin E might lessen the effectiveness of medicines to lower cholesterol.

Tell your doctor, pharmacist, and other health care providers about any dietary supplements and medicines you take. They can tell you if those supplements might interact or interfere with your prescription or over-the-counter medicines or if the medicines might affect how your body uses vitamin E.

Chapter 17

Calcium

You probably heard "drink your milk" all the time from your parents when you were a kid, and you knew it was good for you. But now you may opt for sodas or sports drinks, and other than adding a splash to your morning Wheaties, you don't give much thought to milk.

But your parents were right to make you drink milk when you were little. It's loaded with calcium, a mineral vital for building strong bones and teeth.

Why Do I Need Calcium?

Bones grow rapidly during adolescence, and teens need enough calcium to build strong bones and fight bone loss later in life. But many don't get the recommended daily amount of calcium. In addition, people who smoke or drink soda, caffeinated beverages, or alcohol may get even less calcium because those substances interfere with the way the body absorbs and uses calcium.

Bone calcium begins to decrease in young adulthood and people gradually lose bone density as they age—particularly women. Teens, especially girls, whose diets don't provide the nutrients to build bones to their maximum potential are at greater risk of developing the bone disease osteoporosis, which increases the risk of fractures from weakened bones.

Calcium also plays an important role in muscle contraction, transmitting messages through the nerves, and the release of hormones. If people aren't getting enough calcium in their diet, the body takes calcium from the bones to ensure normal cell function, which can lead to weakened bones.

About This Chapter: "Calcium," June 2007, reprinted with permission from www.kidshealth.org. Copyright © 2007 The Nemours Foundation. This information was provided by KidsHealth, one of the largest resources online for medically reviewed health information written for parents, kids, and teens. For more articles like this one, visit www.KidsHealth.org, or www.TeensHealth.org.

If you got enough calcium and physical activity when you were a kid and continue to do so as a teen, you'll enter your adult years with the strongest bones possible.

How Much Do I Need And Where Can I Get It?

Teen guys and girls need 1,300 mg (milligrams) of calcium each day. Get it from:

- **Dairy Products:** Low-fat milk, yogurt, cheese, and cottage cheese are good sources of calcium.

- **Veggies:** You'll also find calcium in broccoli and dark green, leafy vegetables (especially collard and turnip greens, kale, and bok choy).

- **Soy Foods:** Turn to calcium-fortified (or "calcium-set") tofu, soy milk, tempeh, soy yogurt, and cooked soybeans (edamame).

- **Calcium-Fortified Foods:** Look for calcium-fortified orange juice, soy or rice milk, breads, and cereal.

- **Beans:** You can get decent amounts of calcium from baked beans, navy beans, white beans, and others.

- **Canned Fish:** You're in luck if you like sardines and canned salmon with bones.

If You're Lactose Intolerant

Teens who are lactose intolerant don't have enough of the intestinal enzyme lactase that helps digest the sugar (lactose) in dairy products, and may have gas, bloating, cramps, or diarrhea after drinking milk or eating dairy products.

Fortunately, there are low-lactose and lactose-free dairy products available, as well as lactase drops that can be added to dairy products and tablets that can be taken to make dairy products tolerable. Hard, aged cheeses (such as cheddar) are also lower in lactose, and yogurts that contain active cultures are easier to digest and much less likely to cause lactose problems.

If You're A Vegetarian

It can be a challenge to get enough calcium in a vegetarian diet that does not include dairy, but you can enjoy good sources of calcium such as dark green, leafy vegetables, broccoli, chickpeas, and calcium-fortified products, including orange juice, soy and rice drinks, and cereals.

Working Calcium Into Your Diet

Looking for ways to up your dietary calcium intake? Here are some easy ones:

- Put some cheddar in your omelet
- Pack a yogurt in your lunch
- Add white beans to your favorite soups
- Add a slice of American, Swiss, or provolone to sandwiches
- Use whole-grain soft-taco shells or tortillas to make burritos or wraps (fill them with eggs and cheese for breakfast; turkey, cheese, lettuce, tomato, and light dressing for lunch; and beans, salsa, taco sauce, and cheese for dinner)
- Create mini-pizzas by topping whole-wheat English muffins or bagels with pizza sauce and low-fat mozzarella or soy cheese
- Try whole-grain crackers with low-fat cheese as an afternoon treat
- Dig into chili with red beans and cheese
- Eat low-fat or fat-free frozen yogurt topped with fruit
- Create parfaits with layers of plain yogurt, fruit, and whole-grain cereal
- You're never too old to enjoy a glass of ice-cold milk with a couple of cookies or graham crackers

Other Considerations For Building Bones

Vitamin D is essential for calcium absorption, so it's important to get enough of this nutrient too. Made by the body when the skin is exposed to sunlight, vitamin D is also found in fortified dairy and other products, fish, and egg yolks.

Exercise is very important to bone health. Weight-bearing exercises—such as jumping rope, jogging, and walking—can help develop and maintain strong bones. In fact, current scientific evidence suggests that for teens, exercise may be even more strongly linked to better bone health than calcium intake.

Although it's best to get the calcium you need through a calcium-rich diet, sometimes it may not be possible. Discuss calcium supplements with your doctor if you're concerned that you're not getting enough.

Chapter 18

Other Important Minerals

Chromium

The Body Needs Chromium

Chromium is a mineral that humans require in trace amounts, although its mechanisms of action in the body and the amounts needed for optimal health are not well defined. It is found primarily in two forms: trivalent (chromium 3+, which is biologically active and found in food), and hexavalent (chromium 6+, a toxic form that results from industrial pollution). This chapter focuses exclusively on trivalent (3+) chromium.

Chromium is known to enhance the action of insulin, a hormone critical to the metabolism and storage of carbohydrate, fat, and protein in the body. In 1957, a compound in brewers' yeast was found to prevent an age-related decline in the ability of rats to maintain normal levels of sugar (glucose) in their blood. Chromium was identified as the active ingredient in this so-called "glucose tolerance factor" in 1959.

Chromium also appears to be directly involved in carbohydrate, fat, and protein metabolism, but more research is needed to determine the full range of its roles in the body. The challenges to meeting this goal include the following:

- Defining the types of individuals who respond to chromium supplementation

- Evaluating the chromium content of foods and its bioavailability

About This Chapter: Excepted from "Chromium," August 2005; "Folate," April 15, 2009; "Iron," August 24, 2007; "Magnesium," July 13, 2009; "Selenium," November 12, 2009; and "Zinc," June 24, 2011; all produced by the National Institutes of Health's Office of Dietary Substances (http://ods.od.nih.gov).

- Determining if a clinically relevant chromium-deficiency state exists in humans due to inadequate dietary intakes

- Developing valid and reliable measures of chromium status

Foods That Provide Chromium

Chromium is widely distributed in the food supply, but most foods provide only small amounts (less than two micrograms [mcg] per serving). Meat and whole-grain products, as well as some fruits, vegetables, and spices are relatively good sources. In contrast, foods high in simple sugars (like sucrose and fructose) are low in chromium.

Dietary intakes of chromium cannot be reliably determined because the content of the mineral in foods is substantially affected by agricultural and manufacturing processes and perhaps by contamination with chromium when the foods are analyzed.

Recommended Intakes Of Chromium

In 1989, the National Academy of Sciences established an "estimated safe and adequate daily dietary intake" range for chromium. For adults and adolescents that range was 50 to 200 mcg. In 2001, DRIs (daily reference intakes) for chromium were established. The research base was insufficient to establish RDAs (recommended dietary allowances), so AIs (adequate intakes) were developed based on average intakes of chromium from food as found in several studies. Chromium AIs are provided in Table 18.1.

About Intake Recommendations

Recommended intakes are provided in dietary reference intakes (DRIs) developed by the Institute of Medicine of the National Academy of Sciences. Dietary reference intakes is the general term for a set of reference values to plan and assess the nutrient intakes of healthy people. These values include the recommended dietary allowance (RDA) and the adequate intake (AI). The RDA is the average daily intake that meets a nutrient requirement of nearly all (97% to 98%) healthy individuals. An AI is established when there is insufficient research to establish an RDA. AIs meet or exceed the amount needed to maintain a nutritional state of adequacy in nearly all members of a specific age and gender group. The UL (upper level), on the other hand, is the maximum daily intake unlikely to result in adverse health effects.

Source: Office of Dietary Substances.

Table 18.1. Adequate Intakes (AIs) For Chromium In Micrograms (mcg)

Age	Infants and children (mcg/day)	Males (mcg/day)	Females (mcg/day)	Pregnancy (mcg/day)	Lactation (mcg/day)
0–6 months	0.2				
7–12 months	5.5				
1–3 years	11				
4–8 years	15				
9–13 years		25	21		
14–18 years		35	24	29	44
19–50 years		35	25	30	45
>50 years		30	20		

Supplemental Sources Of Chromium

Chromium is a widely used supplement. Estimated sales to consumers were $85 million in 2002, representing 5.6% of the total mineral-supplement market. Chromium is sold as a single-ingredient supplement as well as in combination formulas, particularly those marketed for weight loss and performance enhancement. Supplement doses typically range from 50 to 200 mcg.

The safety and efficacy of chromium supplements need more investigation. Please consult with a doctor or other trained healthcare professional before taking any dietary supplements.

Chromium supplements are available as chromium chloride, chromium nicotinate, chromium picolinate, high-chromium yeast, and chromium citrate. Chromium chloride in particular appears to have poor bioavailability. However, given the limited data on chromium absorption in humans, it is not clear which forms are best to take.

Meeting The Need For Chromium

Adult women in the United States consume about 23 to 29 mcg of chromium per day from food, which meets their AIs (adequate intakes) unless they're pregnant or lactating. In contrast, adult men average 39 to 54 mcg per day, which exceeds their AIs.

Source: Office of Dietary Substances, August 2005.

Folate

The Body Needs Folate

Folate is a water-soluble B vitamin that occurs naturally in food. Folic acid is the synthetic form of folate that is found in supplements and added to fortified foods.

Folate gets its name from the Latin word "folium" for leaf. A key observation of researcher Lucy Wills nearly 70 years ago led to the identification of folate as the nutrient needed to prevent the anemia of pregnancy. Dr. Wills demonstrated that the anemia could be corrected by a yeast extract. Folate was identified as the corrective substance in yeast extract in the late 1930s and was extracted from spinach leaves in 1941.

Folate helps produce and maintain new cells. This is especially important during periods of rapid cell division and growth such as infancy and pregnancy. Folate is needed to make DNA and RNA, the building blocks of cells. It also helps prevent changes to DNA that may lead to cancer. Both adults and children need folate to make normal red blood cells and prevent anemia. Folate is also essential for the metabolism of homocysteine, and helps maintain normal levels of this amino acid.

Foods That Provide Folate

Leafy green vegetables (like spinach and turnip greens), fruits (like citrus fruits and juices), and dried beans and peas are all natural sources of folate.

In 1996, the Food and Drug Administration (FDA) published regulations requiring the addition of folic acid to enriched breads, cereals, flours, corn meals, pastas, rice, and other grain products. Since cereals and grains are widely consumed in the U.S., these products have become a very important contributor of folic acid to the American diet.

Dietary Reference Intakes For Folate

The RDAs for folate are expressed in a term called the dietary folate equivalent (DFE). The DFE was developed to help account for the differences in absorption of naturally occurring dietary folate and the more bioavailable synthetic folic acid. Table 18.2 lists the RDAs for folate, expressed in micrograms of DFE, for children and adults.

The National Health and Nutrition Examination Survey (NHANES III 1988-94) and the Continuing Survey of Food Intakes by Individuals (1994-96 CSFII) indicated that most individuals surveyed did not consume adequate folate. However, the folic acid fortification program, which was initiated in 1998, has increased folic acid content of commonly eaten foods such as cereals and grains, and as a result most diets in the United States now provide recommended amounts of folate equivalents.

Caution About Folic Acid Supplements

Beware of the interaction between vitamin B12 and folic acid. Intake of supplemental folic acid should not exceed 1,000 micrograms (mcg) per day to prevent folic acid from triggering symptoms of vitamin B12 deficiency. Folic acid supplements can correct the anemia associated with vitamin B12 deficiency. Unfortunately, folic acid will not correct changes in the nervous system that result from vitamin B12 deficiency. Permanent nerve damage can occur if vitamin B12 deficiency is not treated.

Table 18.2. Recommended Dietary Allowances for Folate for Children and Adults in Micrograms (mcg) Of DFE*

Age (years)	Males and Females (mcg/day)	Pregnancy (mcg/day)	Lactation (mcg/day)
1–3	150		
4–8	200		
9–13	300		
14–18	400	600	500
19+	400	600	500

*1 DFE (Dietary Folate Equivalent) = 1 mcg food folate = 0.6 mcg folic acid from supplements and fortified foods

Folate intake from food is not associated with any health risk. The risk of toxicity from folic acid intake from supplements and/or fortified foods is also low. It is a water soluble vitamin, so any excess intake is usually lost in the urine. There is some evidence that high levels of folic acid can provoke seizures in patients taking anti-convulsant medications. Anyone taking such medications should consult with a medical doctor before taking a folic acid supplement.

Iron

The Body Needs Iron

Iron, one of the most abundant metals on Earth, is essential to most life forms and to normal human physiology. Iron is an integral part of many proteins and enzymes that maintain good health. In humans, iron is an essential component of proteins involved in oxygen transport. It is also essential for the regulation of cell growth and differentiation. A deficiency of iron limits oxygen delivery to cells, resulting in fatigue, poor work performance, and decreased immunity. On the other hand, excess amounts of iron can result in toxicity and even death.

Foods That Provide Iron

There are two forms of dietary iron: heme and nonheme. Heme iron is derived from hemoglobin, the protein in red blood cells that delivers oxygen to cells. Heme iron is found in animal

Iron In The Body

Almost two-thirds of iron in the body is found in hemoglobin, the protein in red blood cells that carries oxygen to tissues. Smaller amounts of iron are found in myoglobin, a protein that helps supply oxygen to muscle, and in enzymes that assist biochemical reactions. Iron is also found in proteins that store iron for future needs and that transport iron in blood. Iron stores are regulated by intestinal iron absorption.

Source: Office of Dietary Substances, August 2007.

foods that originally contained hemoglobin, such as red meats, fish, and poultry. Iron in plant foods such as lentils and beans is arranged in a chemical structure called nonheme iron. This is the form of iron added to iron-enriched and iron-fortified foods. Heme iron is absorbed better than nonheme iron, but most dietary iron is nonheme iron.

Recommended Intake For Iron

Table 18.3 lists the RDAs for iron for infants, children and adults.

Iron Deficiency

The World Health Organization considers iron deficiency the number one nutritional disorder in the world. As many as 80% of the world's population may be iron deficient, while 30% may have iron deficiency anemia.

Iron deficiency develops gradually and usually begins with a negative iron balance, when iron intake does not meet the daily need for dietary iron. This negative balance initially depletes the storage form of iron while the blood hemoglobin level, a marker of iron status, remains normal. Iron deficiency anemia is an advanced stage of iron depletion. It occurs when storage sites of iron are deficient and blood levels of iron cannot meet daily needs. Blood hemoglobin levels are below normal with iron deficiency anemia.

Iron deficiency anemia can be associated with low dietary intake of iron, inadequate absorption of iron, or excessive blood loss. Women of childbearing age, pregnant women, preterm and low birth weight infants, older infants and toddlers, and teenage girls are at greatest risk of developing iron deficiency anemia because they have the greatest need for iron. Women with heavy menstrual losses can lose a significant amount of iron and are at considerable risk for iron deficiency. Adult men and post-menopausal women lose very little iron, and have a low risk of iron deficiency.

Table 18.3. Recommended Dietary Allowances for Iron for Infants (7 to 12 months), Children, and Adults In Milligrams (mg)

Age	Males (mg/day)	Females (mg/day)	Pregnancy (mg/day)	Lactation (mg/day)
7–12 months	11	11		
1–3 years	7	7		
4–8 years	10	10		
9–13 years	8	8		
14–18 years	11	15	27	10
19–50 years	8	18	27	9
51+ years	8	8		

Signs of iron deficiency anemia include the following:

- Feeling tired and weak

- Decreased work and school performance

- Slow cognitive and social development during childhood

- Difficulty maintaining body temperature

- Decreased immune function, which increases susceptibility to infection

- Glossitis (an inflamed tongue)

Some Facts About Iron Supplements

Iron supplementation is indicated when diet alone cannot restore deficient iron levels to normal within an acceptable timeframe. Supplements are especially important when an individual is experiencing clinical symptoms of iron deficiency anemia. The goals of providing oral iron supplements are to supply sufficient iron to restore normal storage levels of iron and to replenish hemoglobin deficits. When hemoglobin levels are below normal, physicians often measure serum ferritin, the storage form of iron. A serum ferritin level less than or equal to 15 micrograms per liter confirms iron deficiency anemia in women, and suggests a possible need for iron supplementation.

Supplemental iron is available in two forms: ferrous and ferric. Ferrous iron salts (ferrous fumarate, ferrous sulfate, and ferrous gluconate) are the best absorbed forms of iron supplements. Elemental iron is the amount of iron in a supplement that is available for absorption.

The Risk Of Iron Toxicity

There is considerable potential for iron toxicity because very little iron is excreted from the body. Thus, iron can accumulate in body tissues and organs when normal storage sites are full. For example, people with hemochromatosis are at risk of developing iron toxicity because of their high iron stores.

In children, death has occurred from ingesting 200 mg of iron. It is important to keep iron supplements tightly capped and away from children's reach. Any time excessive iron intake is suspected, immediately call your physician or Poison Control Center, or visit your local emergency room. Doses of iron prescribed for iron deficiency anemia in adults are associated with constipation, nausea, vomiting, and diarrhea, especially when the supplements are taken on an empty stomach.

Iron Intakes And Healthful Diets

Iron is found in both animal and plant foods, but in different forms. Beef and turkey are good sources of heme iron while beans and lentils are high in nonheme iron. In addition, many foods, such as ready-to-eat cereals, are fortified with iron. It is important for anyone who is considering taking an iron supplement to first consider whether their needs are being met by natural dietary sources of heme and nonheme iron and foods fortified with iron, and to discuss their potential need for iron supplements with their physician.

Magnesium

The Body Needs Magnesium

Magnesium is the fourth most abundant mineral in the body and is essential to good health. Approximately 50% of total body magnesium is found in bone. The other half is found predominantly inside cells of body tissues and organs. Only 1% of magnesium is found in blood, but the body works very hard to keep blood levels of magnesium constant.

Magnesium is needed for more than 300 biochemical reactions in the body. It helps maintain normal muscle and nerve function, keeps heart rhythm steady, supports a healthy immune system, and keeps bones strong. Magnesium also helps regulate blood sugar levels, promotes normal blood pressure, and is known to be involved in energy metabolism and protein synthesis. There is an increased interest in the role of magnesium in preventing and managing disorders such as hypertension, cardiovascular disease, and diabetes. Dietary magnesium is absorbed in the small intestines. Magnesium is excreted through the kidneys.

Foods That Provide Magnesium

Green vegetables such as spinach are good sources of magnesium because the center of the chlorophyll molecule (which gives green vegetables their color) contains magnesium. Some legumes (beans and peas), nuts and seeds, and whole, unrefined grains are also good sources of magnesium. Refined grains are generally low in magnesium. When white flour is refined and processed, the magnesium-rich germ and bran are removed. Bread made from whole grain wheat flour provides more magnesium than bread made from white refined flour. Tap water can be a source of magnesium, but the amount varies according to the water supply. Water that naturally contains more minerals is described as "hard." "Hard" water contains more magnesium than "soft" water.

Eating a wide variety of legumes, nuts, whole grains, and vegetables will help you meet your daily dietary need for magnesium.

Dietary Reference Intakes For Magnesium

Table 18.4 lists the RDAs for magnesium, in milligrams, for children and adults.

Table 18.4. Recommended Dietary Allowances For Magnesium For Children And Adults In Milligrams (mg)

Age (years)	Male (mg/day)	Female (mg/day)	Pregnancy (mg/day)	Lactation (mg/day)
1–3	80	80		
4–8	130	130		
9–13	240	240		
14–18	410	360	400	360
19–30	400	310	350	310
31+	420	320	360	320

The Best Way To Get Extra Magnesium

Eating a variety of whole grains, legumes, and vegetables (especially dark-green, leafy vegetables) every day will help provide recommended intakes of magnesium and maintain normal storage levels of this mineral. Increasing dietary intake of magnesium can often restore mildly depleted magnesium levels. However, increasing dietary intake of magnesium may not be enough to restore very low magnesium levels to normal.

Oral magnesium supplements combine magnesium with another substance such as a salt. Examples of magnesium supplements include magnesium oxide, magnesium sulfate, and magnesium carbonate. Elemental magnesium refers to the amount of magnesium in each compound. The amount of elemental magnesium in a compound and its bioavailability influence the effectiveness of the magnesium supplement. Bioavailability refers to the amount of magnesium in food, medications, and supplements that is absorbed in the intestines and ultimately available for biological activity in your cells and tissues. Enteric coating (the outer layer of a tablet or capsule that allows it to pass through the stomach and be dissolved in the small intestine) of a magnesium compound can decrease bioavailability. In a study that compared four forms of magnesium preparations, results suggested lower bioavailability of magnesium oxide, with significantly higher and equal absorption and bioavailability of magnesium chloride and magnesium lactate. This supports the belief that both the magnesium content of a dietary supplement and its bioavailability contribute to its ability to restore deficient levels of magnesium.

The Health Risk Of Too Much Magnesium

Dietary magnesium does not pose a health risk, however pharmacologic doses of magnesium in supplements can promote adverse effects such as diarrhea and abdominal cramping. Risk of magnesium toxicity increases with kidney failure, when the kidney loses the ability to remove excess magnesium. Very large doses of magnesium-containing laxatives and antacids also have been associated with magnesium toxicity. For example, a case of hypermagnesemia after unsupervised intake of aluminum magnesia oral suspension occurred after a 16-year-old girl decided to take the antacid every two hours rather than four times per day, as prescribed. Three days later, she became unresponsive and demonstrated loss of deep tendon reflex. Doctors were unable to determine her exact magnesium intake, but the young lady presented with blood levels of magnesium five times higher than normal. Therefore, it is important for medical professionals to be aware of the use of any magnesium-containing laxatives or antacids. Signs of excess magnesium can be similar to magnesium deficiency and include changes in mental status, nausea, diarrhea, appetite loss, muscle weakness, difficulty breathing, extremely low blood pressure, and irregular heartbeat.

Selenium

The Body Needs Selenium

Selenium is a trace mineral that is essential to good health but required only in small amounts. Selenium is incorporated into proteins to make selenoproteins, which are important antioxidant enzymes. The antioxidant properties of selenoproteins help prevent cellular damage from free radicals. Free radicals are natural by-products of oxygen metabolism that may contribute to the development of chronic diseases such as cancer and heart disease. Other selenoproteins help regulate thyroid function and play a role in the immune system.

Foods That Provide Selenium

Plant foods are the major dietary sources of selenium in most countries throughout the world. The content of selenium in food depends on the selenium content of the soil where plants are grown or animals are raised. For example, researchers know that soils in the high plains of northern Nebraska and the Dakotas have very high levels of selenium. People living in those regions generally have the highest selenium intakes in the United States. In the United States, food distribution patterns across the country help prevent people living in low-selenium geographic areas from having low dietary selenium intakes. Soils in some parts of China and Russia have very low amounts of selenium. Selenium deficiency is often reported in those regions because most food in those areas is grown and eaten locally.

Selenium also can be found in some meats and seafood. Animals that eat grains or plants that were grown in selenium-rich soil have higher levels of selenium in their muscle. In the U.S., meats and bread are common sources of dietary selenium. Some nuts are also sources of selenium.

Selenium content of foods can vary. For example, Brazil nuts may contain as much as 544 micrograms of selenium per ounce. They also may contain far less selenium. It is wise to eat Brazil nuts only occasionally because of their unusually high intake of selenium.

Recommended Dietary Intake For Selenium

Table 18.5 lists the RDAs for selenium, in micrograms (mcg) per day, for children and adults.

Table 18.5. Recommended Dietary Allowances (RDA) for Selenium for Children and Adults In Micrograms (mcg)

Age (years)	Males and Females (mcg/day)	Pregnancy (mcg/day)	Lactation (mcg/day)
1–3	20		
4–8	30		
9–13	40		
14–18	55	60	70
19+	55	60	70

Selenium Deficiency

Human selenium deficiency is rare in the United States but is seen in other countries, most notably China, where soil concentration of selenium is low. There is evidence that selenium deficiency may contribute to development of a form of heart disease, hypothyroidism, and a weakened immune system. There is also evidence that selenium deficiency does not usually cause illness by itself. Rather, it can make the body more susceptible to illnesses caused by other nutritional, biochemical or infectious stresses.

Three specific diseases have been associated with selenium deficiency:

- Keshan disease, which results in an enlarged heart and poor heart function, occurs in selenium deficient children

- Kashin-Beck disease, which results in osteoarthropathy

- Myxedematous endemic cretinism, which results in mental retardation

Selenium Dietary Supplements

Selenium occurs in staple foods such as corn, wheat, and soybean as selenomethionine, the organic selenium analogue of the amino acid methionine. Selenomethionine can be incorporated into body proteins in place of methionine, and serves as a vehicle for selenium storage in organs and tissues. Selenium supplements may also contain sodium selenite and sodium selenate, two inorganic forms of selenium. Selenomethionine is generally considered to be the best absorbed and utilized form of selenium.

Selenium is also available in "high selenium yeasts," which may contain as much as 1,000 to 2,000 micrograms of selenium per gram. Most of the selenium in these yeasts is in the form of selenomethionine. This form of selenium was used in the large-scale cancer prevention trial in 1983, which demonstrated that taking a daily supplement containing 200 micrograms of selenium per day could lower the risk of developing prostate, lung, and colorectal cancer. However, some yeasts may contain inorganic forms of selenium, which are not utilized as well as selenomethionine.

Zinc

The Body Needs Zinc

Zinc is an essential mineral that is naturally present in some foods, added to others, and available as a dietary supplement. Zinc is also found in many cold lozenges and some over-the-counter drugs sold as cold remedies.

Zinc is involved in numerous aspects of cellular metabolism. It is required for the catalytic activity of approximately 100 enzymes and it plays a role in immune function, protein synthesis, wound healing, DNA synthesis, and cell division. Zinc also supports normal growth and development during pregnancy, childhood, and adolescence and is required for proper sense of taste and smell. A daily intake of zinc is required to maintain a steady state because the body has no specialized zinc storage system.

Table 18.6. Recommended Intakes For Zinc

Age	Male	Female	Pregnancy	Lactation
0–6 months	2 mg*	2 mg*		
7–12 months	3 mg	3 mg		
1–3 years	3 mg	3 mg		
4–8 years	5 mg	5 mg		
9–13 years	8 mg	8 mg		
14–18 years	11 mg	9 mg	12 mg	13 mg
19+ years	11 mg	8 mg	11 mg	12 mg

* Adequate Intake (AI)

Sources Of Zinc

Food: A wide variety of foods contain zinc. Oysters contain more zinc per serving than any other food, but red meat and poultry provide the majority of zinc in the American diet. Other good food sources include beans, nuts, certain types of seafood (such as crab and lobster), whole grains, fortified breakfast cereals, and dairy products.

Phytates—which are present in whole-grain breads, cereals, legumes, and other foods—bind zinc and inhibit its absorption. Thus, the bioavailability of zinc from grains and plant foods is lower than that from animal foods, although many grain- and plant-based foods are still good sources of zinc.

Dietary Supplements: Supplements contain several forms of zinc, including zinc gluconate, zinc sulfate, and zinc acetate. The percentage of elemental zinc varies by form. For example, approximately 23% of zinc sulfate consists of elemental zinc; thus, 220 mg of zinc sulfate contains 50 mg of elemental zinc. The elemental zinc content appears in the supplement facts panel on the supplement container. Research has not determined whether differences exist among forms of zinc in absorption, bioavailability, or tolerability.

In addition to standard tablets and capsules, some zinc-containing cold lozenges are labeled as dietary supplements.

Other Sources: Zinc is present in several products sold over the counter as natural medicines for colds, typically in the form of lozenges and nasal sprays and gels. Numerous case reports of anosmia (loss of smell), in some cases long-lasting or permanent, from the use of zinc-containing nasal gels or sprays raise questions about the safety of intranasal zinc. In June 2009, the U.S. Food and Drug Administration (FDA) warned consumers to stop using three zinc-containing intranasal products because they might cause anosmia. The manufacturer has voluntarily withdrawn these products from the marketplace. These safety concerns do not apply to cold lozenges containing zinc.

Zinc Deficiency

Zinc deficiency is characterized by growth retardation, loss of appetite, and impaired immune function. In more severe cases, zinc deficiency causes hair loss, diarrhea, delayed sexual maturation, impotence, hypogonadism in males, and eye and skin lesions. Weight loss, delayed healing of wounds, taste abnormalities, and mental lethargy can also occur. Many of these symptoms are non-specific and often associated with other health conditions; therefore, a medical examination is necessary to ascertain whether a zinc deficiency is present.

Zinc And The Common Cold

Researchers have hypothesized that zinc could reduce the severity and duration of cold symptoms by directly inhibiting rhinovirus binding and replication in the nasal mucosa and suppressing inflammation. Although studies examining the effect of zinc treatment on cold symptoms have had somewhat conflicting results, overall zinc appears to be beneficial under certain circumstances.

A structured review of the effects of zinc lozenges, nasal sprays, and nasal gels on the common cold reported that seven studies (five using zinc lozenges; two using a nasal gel) showed that the zinc treatment had a beneficial effect, and seven studies (five using zinc lozenges, one using a nasal spray, and one using lozenges and a nasal spray) showed no effect. More recently, another review concluded that zinc can reduce the duration and severity of cold symptoms. More research is needed to determine the optimal dosage, zinc formulation, and duration of treatment before a general recommendation for zinc in the treatment of the common cold can be made.

The safety of intranasal zinc has been called into question, however, because of numerous reports of anosmia (loss of smell), in some cases long-lasting or permanent, from the use of zinc-containing nasal gels or sprays.

Source: Office of Dietary Substances, June 2011.

In North America, overt zinc deficiency is uncommon. When zinc deficiency does occur, it is usually due to inadequate zinc intake or absorption, increased losses of zinc from the body, or increased requirements for zinc. People at risk of zinc deficiency or inadequacy need to include good sources of zinc in their daily diets. Supplemental zinc might also be appropriate in certain situations.

The following groups may be at risk of zinc inadequacy:

- People with gastrointestinal and other diseases

- Vegetarians

- Pregnant and lactating women

- Older infants who are exclusively breastfed

- People with sickle cell disease

- Alcoholics

Chapter 19

What You Should Know About Dietary Supplements

What is a dietary supplement?

Congress defined the term "dietary supplement" in the Dietary Supplement Health and Education Act (DSHEA) of 1994. A dietary supplement is a product taken by mouth that contains a "dietary ingredient" intended to supplement the diet. The "dietary ingredients" in these products may include: vitamins, minerals, herbs or other botanicals, amino acids, and substances such as enzymes, organ tissues, glandulars, and metabolites. Dietary supplements can also be extracts or concentrates, and may be found in many forms such as tablets, capsules, softgels, gelcaps, liquids, or powders. They can also be in other forms, such as a bar, but if they are, information on their label must not represent the product as a conventional food or a sole item of a meal or diet. Whatever their form may be, DSHEA places dietary supplements in a special category under the general umbrella of "foods," not drugs, and requires that every supplement be labeled a dietary supplement.

Where can I get information about a specific dietary supplement?

Manufacturers and distributors do not need U.S. Food and Drug Administration (FDA) approval to sell their dietary supplements. This means that FDA does not keep a list of manufacturers, distributors or the dietary supplement products they sell. If you want more detailed information than the label tells you about a specific product, you may contact the manufacturer of that brand directly. The name and address of the manufacturer or distributor can be found on the label of the dietary supplement.

About This Chapter: Excerpted from "Overview of Dietary Supplements," October 14, 2009; "Dietary Supplements: What You Need to Know," February 2007; and "Fortify Your Knowledge About Vitamins," October 15, 2010; all produced by the U.S. Food and Drug Administration (www.fda.gov).

Who has the responsibility for ensuring that a dietary supplement is safe?

By law, the manufacturer is responsible for ensuring that its dietary supplement products are safe before they are marketed. Unlike drug products that must be proven safe and effective for their intended use before marketing, there are no provisions in the law for FDA to "approve" dietary supplements for safety or effectiveness before they reach the consumer. Under DSHEA, once the product is marketed, FDA has the responsibility for showing that a dietary supplement is "unsafe," before it can take action to restrict the product's use or removal from the marketplace. However, manufacturers and distributors of dietary supplements must record, investigate, and forward to FDA any reports they receive of serious adverse events associated with the use of their products that are reported to them directly. FDA is able to evaluate these reports and any other adverse event information reported directly to us by healthcare providers or consumers to identify early signals that a product may present safety risks to consumers.

How can consumers inform themselves about safety and other issues related to dietary supplements?

It is important to be well informed about products before purchasing them. Because it is often difficult to know what information is reliable and what is questionable, consumers may first want to contact the manufacturer about the product they intend to purchase (see previous question "Where can I get information about a specific dietary supplement?").

In addition, to help consumers in their search to be better informed, FDA provides fact sheets such as "Tips for the Savvy Supplement User: Making Informed Decisions and Evaluating Information," which includes information on how to evaluate research findings and health information on-line (available through a link at www.fda.gov/Food/DietarySupplements /ConsumerInformation/default.htm), and "Claims That Can Be Made for Conventional Foods and Dietary Supplements," which provides information on what types of claims can be made for dietary supplements (available through a link at www.fda.gov/Food/Labeling/ NutritionLabelClaims/default.htm).

What is FDA's oversight responsibility for dietary supplements?

Because dietary supplements are under the "umbrella" of foods, FDA's Center for Food Safety and Applied Nutrition (CFSAN) is responsible for the agency's oversight of these products. FDA's efforts to monitor the marketplace for potential illegal products (that is, products that may be unsafe or make false or misleading claims) include obtaining information from inspections of dietary supplement manufacturers and distributors, the internet, consumer and trade complaints, occasional laboratory analyses of selected products, and adverse events associated with the use of supplements that are reported to the agency.

Does FDA routinely analyze the content of dietary supplements?

In that FDA has limited resources to analyze the composition of food products, including dietary supplements, it focuses these resources first on public health emergencies and products that may have caused injury or illness. Enforcement priorities then go to products thought to be unsafe or fraudulent or in violation of the law. The remaining funds are used for routine monitoring of products pulled from store shelves or collected during inspections of manufacturing firms. The agency does not analyze dietary supplements before they are sold to consumers. The manufacturer is responsible for ensuring that the "Supplement Facts" label and ingredient list are accurate, that the dietary ingredients are safe, and that the content matches the amount declared on the label. FDA does not have resources to analyze dietary supplements sent to the agency by consumers who want to know their content. Instead, consumers may contact the manufacturer or a commercial laboratory for an analysis of the content.

Is it legal to market a dietary supplement product as a treatment or cure for a specific disease or condition?

No, a product sold as a dietary supplement and promoted on its label or in labeling (labeling refers to the label as well as accompanying material that is used by a manufacturer to promote and market a specific product) as a treatment, prevention, or cure for a specific disease or condition would be considered an unapproved, and thus illegal, drug. To maintain the product's status as a dietary supplement, the label and labeling must be consistent with the provisions in the Dietary Supplement Health and Education Act of 1994.

Who validates claims and what kinds of claims can be made on dietary supplement labels?

FDA receives many consumer inquiries about the validity of claims for dietary supplements, including product labels, advertisements, media, and printed materials. The responsibility for ensuring the validity of these claims rests with the manufacturer, FDA, and, in the case of advertising, with the Federal Trade Commission.

By law, manufacturers may make three types of claims for their dietary supplement products: health claims, structure/function claims, and nutrient content claims. Some of these claims describe: the link between a food substance and disease or a health-related condition;

the intended benefits of using the product; or the amount of a nutrient or dietary substance in a product. Different requirements generally apply to each type of claim.

Why do some supplements have a disclaimer that says: "This statement has not been evaluated by the FDA. This product is not intended to diagnose, treat, cure, or prevent any disease"?

This statement or "disclaimer" is required by law when a manufacturer makes a structure/ function claim on a dietary supplement label. In general, these claims describe the role of a nutrient or dietary ingredient intended to affect the structure or function of the body. The manufacturer is responsible for ensuring the accuracy and truthfulness of these claims; they are not approved by FDA. For this reason, the law says that if a dietary supplement label includes such a claim, it must state in a "disclaimer" that FDA has not evaluated this claim. The disclaimer must also state that this product is not intended to "diagnose, treat, cure or prevent any disease," because only a drug can legally make such a claim.

What are the benefits of dietary supplements?

Some supplements can help assure that you get an adequate dietary intake of essential nutrients; others may help you reduce the risk of disease. However, supplements should not replace the variety of foods that are important to a healthful diet—so, be sure you eat a variety of foods as well.

Unlike drugs, supplements are not intended to treat, diagnose, prevent, or cure diseases. That means supplements should not make claims, such as "reduces arthritic pain" or "treats heart disease." Claims like these can only legitimately be made for drugs, not dietary supplements.

Tips For Buying Dietary Supplements

Consider the following tips before buying a dietary supplement:

- Think twice about chasing the latest headline. Sound health advice is generally based on research over time, not a single study touted by the media. Be wary of results claiming a "quick fix" that departs from scientific research and established dietary guidance.
- More may not be better. Some products can be harmful when consumed in high amounts, for a long time, or in combination with certain other substances.
- Learn to spot false claims. If something sounds too good to be true, it probably is.

Source: U.S. Food and Drug Administration (www.fda.gov), October 15, 2010.

Are there any risks in taking supplements?

Yes. Many supplements contain active ingredients that have strong biological effects in the body. This could make them unsafe in some situations, and hurt or complicate your health. For example, the following actions could lead to harmful—even life-threatening—consequences.

- Combining supplements
- Using supplements with medications (whether prescription or over-the-counter)
- Substituting supplements for prescription medicines
- Taking too much of some supplements, such as vitamin A, vitamin D, and iron

Some supplements can also have unwanted effects before, during, and after surgery. So, be sure to inform your health-care provider, including your pharmacist, about any supplements you are taking—especially before surgery.

How can I find out more about the dietary supplement I'm taking?

If you want to know more about the product you are taking, check with the manufacturer or distributor about information to support the claims of the product, information on the safety and effectiveness of the ingredients in the product, and facts about any reports of adverse effects or events from consumers using the product.

How can I be a smart supplement shopper?

Although the benefits of some dietary supplements have been documented, the claims of others may be unproven. If something sounds too good to be true, it usually is. Be a savvy supplement user. Watch out for false statements like these:

- A quick and effective "cure-all"
- Can treat or cure diseases
- "Totally safe" or has "no side effects"

Other red flags include claims about limited availability, offers of "no-risk, money-back guarantees," and requirements for advance payment.

Be aware that the term natural doesn't always mean safe. Don't assume that even if a product may not help you, at least it won't hurt you. When searching for supplements on the internet, use the sites of respected organizations, rather than doing blind searches.

Ask your health-care provider for help in distinguishing between reliable and questionable information. Always remember, safety first.

Why buy vitamins?

There are many good reasons to consider taking vitamin supplements, such as over-the-counter multivitamins. According to the American Academy of Family Physicians (AAFP), a doctor may recommend that you take them for certain health problems, if you eat a vegetarian or vegan diet, or if you are pregnant or breastfeeding.

How do I practice safety with dietary supplements?

When it comes to purchasing dietary supplements, Vasilios Frankos, Ph.D., Director of FDA's Division of Dietary Supplement Programs, offers this advice: "Be savvy!"

Today's dietary supplements are not only vitamins and minerals. "They also include other less familiar substances such as herbals, botanicals, amino acids, and enzymes," Frankos says. "Check with your health care providers before combining or substituting them with other foods or medicines." Frankos adds, "Do not self-diagnose any health condition. Work with your health care providers to determine how best to achieve optimal health."

Also ask yourself, "Is the product worth the money?'" Frankos advises. "Resist the pressure to buy a product or treatment on the spot. Some supplement products may be expensive or may not provide the benefit you expect. For example, excessive amounts of water-soluble vitamins, like vitamins C and B, are not used by the body and are eliminated in the urine."

What's It Mean?

Your body uses vitamins for a variety of biological processes, including growth, digestion, and nerve function. There are 13 vitamins that the body absolutely needs: vitamins A, C, D, E, K, and the B vitamins (thiamine, riboflavin, niacin, pantothenic acid, biotin, vitamin B6, vitamin B12, and folate). The American Academy of Family Physicians (AAFP) cites two categories of vitamins.

Water-soluble vitamins are easily absorbed by the body, which doesn't store large amounts. The kidneys remove those vitamins that are not needed.

Fat-soluble vitamins are absorbed into the body with the use of bile acids, which are fluids used to absorb fat. The body stores these for use as needed.

Source: U.S. Food and Drug Administration (www.fda.gov), October 15, 2010.

How vitamins are regulated?

Vitamin products are regulated by FDA as "dietary supplements." The law defines dietary supplements, in part, as products taken by mouth that contain a "dietary ingredient" intended to supplement the diet.

Listed in the "dietary ingredient" category are not only vitamins, but minerals, botanicals products, amino acids, and substances such as enzymes, microbial probiotics, and metabolites. Dietary supplements can also be extracts or concentrates, and may be found in many forms. The Dietary Supplement Health and Education Act of 1994 requires that all such products be labeled as dietary supplements.

In June 2007, FDA established dietary supplement "current Good Manufacturing Practice" (cGMP) regulations requiring that manufacturers evaluate their products through testing identity, purity, strength, and composition.

What are the risks of overdoing it?

As is the case with all dietary supplements, the decision to use supplemental vitamins should not be taken lightly, says Dr. Vasilios Frankos, Director of FDA's Division of Dietary Supplement Programs.

"Vitamins are not dangerous unless you get too much of them," he says. "More is not necessarily better with supplements, especially if you take fat-soluble vitamins." For some vitamins and minerals, the National Academy of Sciences has established upper limits of intake (ULs) that it recommends not be exceeded during any given day.

Also, the AAFP lists the following side effects that are sometimes associated with taking too much of a vitamin.

Fat-Soluble Vitamins

- *Vitamin A (retinol, retinal, retinoic acid):* Nausea, vomiting, headache, dizziness, blurred vision, clumsiness, birth defects, liver problems, possible risk of osteoporosis. You may be at greater risk of these effects if you drink high amounts of alcohol or you have liver problems, high cholesterol levels or don't get enough protein.

- *Vitamin D (calciferol):* Nausea, vomiting, poor appetite, constipation, weakness, weight loss, confusion, heart rhythm problems, deposits of calcium and phosphate in soft tissues.

If you take blood thinners, talk to your doctor before taking vitamin E or vitamin K pills.

Water-Soluble Vitamins

- *Vitamin B3 (niacin):* Flushing, redness of the skin, upset stomach.

- *Vitamin B6 (pyridoxine, pyridoxal, and pyridoxamine):* Nerve damage to the limbs, which may cause numbness, trouble walking, and pain.

- *Vitamin C (ascorbic acid):* Upset stomach, kidney stones, increased iron absorption.

- *Folic Acid (folate):* High levels may, especially in older adults, hide signs of B12 deficiency, a condition that can cause nerve damage

Taking too much of a vitamin can also cause problems with some medical tests or interfere with how some drugs work.

Part Three
Other Elements Inside Food

Chapter 20

Sodium: Salt By Any Name

Sodium has several functions in the food supply. Various forms of sodium, including sodium chloride or salt, are used as preservatives to inhibit the growth of food-borne pathogens (especially in luncheon meats, fermented foods, salad dressings, and cheese products). Sodium is also an essential nutrient used to modify flavor, plus it binds ingredients, enhances color, and serves as a stabilizer. Sodium is an essential nutrient, but very little is needed in the diet.

Where's The Salt?

Sodium can come from natural sources or be added to foods. Most foods in their natural state contain some sodium. However, the majority (up to 75 percent) of sodium that Americans consume comes from sodium added to processed foods by manufacturers. While some of this sodium is added to foods for safety reasons, the amount of salt added to processed foods is clearly above and beyond what is required for safety and function of the food supply.

Major food sources of sodium include:

- Tomato sauce

- Soups

- Condiments

- Canned foods

- Prepared mixes

About This Chapter: "Sodium (Salt or Sodium Chloride)," reprinted with permission www.heart.org. © 2011 American Heart Association, Inc.

Call It What You Will

When you buy prepared and packaged foods, read the labels. You can tell the sodium content by looking at the Nutrition Facts panel of a food. Listed are the amount for sodium, in milligrams (mg), and the "% Daily Value." Also read the ingredient list to watch for the words "soda" (referring to sodium bicarbonate, or baking soda), "sodium" and the symbol "Na" to see if the product contains sodium.

Furthermore, some products include terms related to sodium. Here are some common terms and their meanings:

- **Sodium-free:** Less than 5 milligrams of sodium per serving

- **Very low-sodium:** 35 milligrams or less per serving

- **Low-sodium:** 140 milligrams or less per serving

- **Reduced sodium:** Usual sodium level is reduced by 25 percent

- **Unsalted, no salt added, or without added salt:** Made without the salt that's normally used, but still contains the sodium that's a natural part of the food itself

The U.S. Food and Drug Administration and U.S. Department of Agriculture state that an individual food that has the claim "healthy" must not exceed 480 mg sodium per reference amount. "Meal type" products must not exceed 600 mg sodium per labeled serving size.

Sodium Equivalents

- 1/4 teaspoon salt = 600 mg sodium

- 1/2 teaspoon salt = 1,200 mg sodium

- 3/4 teaspoon salt = 1,800 mg sodium

- 1 teaspoon salt = 2,300 mg sodium

- 1 teaspoon baking soda = 1,000 mg sodium

Sodium In Medications

Some drugs contain high amounts of sodium. Carefully read the labels on all over-the-counter drugs. Look at the ingredient list and warning statement to see if the product has sodium. A statement of sodium content must be on labels of antacids that have 5 mg or more per dosage unit (tablet, teaspoon, etc.). Some companies are now producing low-sodium over-the-counter products. If in doubt, ask your doctor or pharmacist if the drug is OK for you.

Reducing Sodium In Your Diet

High-sodium diets are linked to an increase in blood pressure and a higher risk for heart disease and stroke. Reducing the amount of sodium you consume can help lower high blood pressure or prevent it from developing in the first place. Keeping your blood pressure at healthy levels is important, because high blood pressure can lead to heart attacks or stroke.

The American Heart Association recommends that you choose and prepare foods with little or no salt to reduce the risk of cardiovascular disease. Aim to eat less than 1,500 mg of sodium per day.

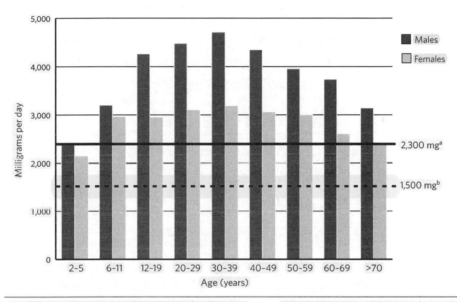

a. 2,300 mg/day is the Tolerable Upper Intake Level (UL) for sodium intake in adults set by the Institute of Medicine (IOM). For children younger than age 14 years, the UL is less than 2,300 mg/day.
b. 1,500 mg/day is the Adequate Intake (AI) for individuals ages 9 years and older.

Source: U.S. Department of Agriculture, Agricultural Research Service and U.S. Department of Health and Human Services, Centers for Disease Control and Prevention. What We Eat In America, NHANES 2005-2006. http://www.ars.usda.gov/Services/docs.htm?docid=13793. Accessed August 11, 2010.

Figure 20.1. Estimated Mean Daily Sodium Intake, By Age–Gender Group, National Health and Nutrition Examination Survey (NHANES) 2005–2006 (*Dietary Guidelines for Americans 2010*, U.S. Department of Agriculture, December 2010.

Reducing Sodium In Our Food Supply

Americans on average consume 3,436 mg sodium daily. Many experts now believe that lowering daily consumption to no more than 1,500 mg of sodium daily would be an effective way to prevent or lower high blood pressure. However, the amount of sodium and salt used in the U.S. food supply makes this goal difficult to achieve for most Americans.

The American Heart Association is working with federal agencies to identify strategies to reduce the amount of sodium in the food supply. The association is encouraging food manufacturers and restaurants to reduce the amount of sodium in foods by 50 percent over a 10-year period. Over the next three years, the association will focus on helping Americans lower the amount of sodium they consume via three strategies:

- Reducing the amount of sodium in the food supply,

- Making more healthy foods available (for example, more fruits and vegetables); and

- Providing consumers with education and decision-making tools to make better choices.

We know that sodium is an acquired taste. As consumers take steps to reduce sodium in their diets, they will appreciate foods for their true flavor, and their taste sensitivities will adapt. It takes about 8–12 weeks for a shift in taste preference in most people.

Tips For Reducing Sodium In The Diet

- Choose fresh, frozen or canned food items without added salts.

- Select unsalted nuts or seeds, dried beans, peas, and lentils.

- Limit salty snacks like chips and pretzels.

- Avoid adding salt and canned vegetables to homemade dishes.

- Select unsalted, lower sodium, fat-free broths, bouillons, or soups.

- Select fat-free or low-fat milk, low-sodium, low-fat cheeses, and low-fat yogurt.

- Learn to use spices and herbs to enhance the taste of your food. Most spices naturally contain very small amounts of sodium.

- Add fresh lemon juice instead of salt to fish and vegetables.

- Specify how you want your food prepared when dining out. Ask for your dish to be prepared without salt.

- Don't use the salt shaker. Use the pepper shaker or mill.

Chapter 21

Carbohydrates

Not sure what to think about carbohydrates these days? You've come to the right chapter. Here are the facts to separate the hype from the truth about carbohydrates.

Basic Facts About Carbohydrates

Your body uses carbohydrates, or carbs, to make glucose, which is the fuel that gives you energy and helps keep everything going.

Your body can use glucose immediately or store it in your liver and muscles for when it is needed. You can find carbohydrates in the following foods:

- Fruits

- Vegetables

- Breads, cereals, and other grains

- Milk and milk products

- Foods containing added sugars (for example, cakes, cookies, and sugar-sweetened beverages)

Healthier foods higher in carbohydrates include ones that provide dietary fiber and whole grains as well as those without added sugars.

What about foods higher in carbohydrates such as sodas and candies that also contain added sugars? Those are the ones that add extra calories but not many nutrients to your diet.

About This Chapter: Excerpted from "Carbohydrates," Centers for Disease Control and Prevention (www.cdc .gov), December 2008.

There are two main types of carbohydrates: complex carbohydrates and simple carbohydrates.

"Good" And "Bad" Carbs

Some diet books use "bad" carbs to talk about foods with refined carbohydrates (this means they're made from white flour and added sugars). Examples include white bread, cakes, and cookies.

"Good" carbs is used to describe foods that have more fiber and complex carbohydrates. Complex carbohydrates are carbohydrates that take longer to break down into glucose.

These terms aren't used in the *Dietary Guidelines for Americans*. Instead, the guidelines recommend choosing fiber-rich carbohydrate choices from the vegetable, fruit, and grain groups and avoid added sugars.

It is also recommended that at least half of your daily grain choices are whole grains. With this plan, you can also choose to have small amounts of added sugars and count them as discretionary calories.

Complex Carbohydrates

Starch and dietary fiber are the two types of complex carbohydrates. Starch must be broken down through digestion before your body can use it as a glucose source. Quite a few foods contain starch and dietary fiber. Starch is also found in breads, cereals, grains, and certain vegetables (like potatoes, dry beans, peas, and corn). Dietary fiber is also found in vegetables, fruits, and whole grain foods.

Dietary Fiber

You may have seen dietary fiber on the label listed as soluble fiber or insoluble fiber.

Soluble fiber is found in the following:

- Oatmeal
- Oat bran
- Nuts and seeds
- Most fruits (for example, strawberries, blueberries, pears, and apples)
- Dry beans and peas

Insoluble fiber found in the following:

- Whole wheat bread
- Barley
- Brown rice
- Couscous
- Bulgur or whole grain cereals
- Wheat bran
- Seeds
- Most vegetables
- Fruits

Which type is best? Both. Each has important health benefits so eat a variety of these foods to get enough of both. You're also more likely to get other nutrients that you might miss if you just chose one or two high-fiber foods.

Table 21.1. Easy Dietary Fiber Estimator

Daily calorie needs	Daily dietary fiber needs
1000	14 grams
1200	17 grams
1400	20 grams
1600	22 grams
1800	25 grams
2000	28 grams
2200	31 grams
2400	34 grams
2600	36 grams
2800	39 grams
3000	42 grams

Dietary Fiber Requirements

It's recommended that you get 14 grams of dietary fiber for every 1,000 calories that you consume each day. If you need 2,000 calories each day, you should try to include 28 grams of dietary fiber.

At first, you may find it challenging to eat all of your daily fiber grams. Just take it slowly and try to choose higher-fiber foods more often. Over time, you'll gradually be eating more fiber. Try the following tips to jump-start your intake of dietary fiber:

- Choose whole fruits more often than fruit juice. Fresh, frozen, or canned—it doesn't matter—they all count.
- Try to eat two vegetables with your evening meal.
- Keep a bowl of veggies already washed and prepared your refrigerator—try carrots, cucumbers, or celery for a quick snack.
- Make a meal around dried beans or peas (also called legumes) instead of meat.

Choose whole grain foods more often. A good guide is to make at least half of your grain choices be whole grains.

Start your day with a whole grain breakfast cereal low in added sugar. Top your cereal with fruit for even more fiber. While bananas may come to your mind first, you can add even more variety by also trying sliced peaches or berries. You can often find these fruits all year in the frozen foods section of your grocery store.

Whole Grains

Whole grains are a good source of fiber and nutrients. Whole grains refer to grains that have all of the parts of the grain seed (sometimes called the kernel). These parts of the kernel are called the bran, the germ, and the endosperm.

If the whole grain has been cracked, crushed, or flaked (as in cracked whole grain bread or flake cereal), then the whole grain must still have about the same proportions of bran, germ, and endosperm to be called a whole grain.

When whole grains are processed, some of the dietary fiber and other important nutrients are removed. A processed grain is called a "refined" grain.

Some refined grain products have key nutrients, such as folic acid and iron, which were removed during the initial processing and added back. These are called enriched grains. White rice and white bread are enriched grain products.

Some enriched grain foods have extra nutrients added. These are called fortified grains.

The *Dietary Guidelines for Americans* recommend that you try to make at least half of your daily grain choices as whole grains.

Less Familiar Grains

The following list describes some of the less-familiar grains:

Bulgur: A staple of Middle Eastern dishes. Bulgur wheat consists of kernels that have been steamed, dried, and crushed. It has a tender and chewy texture.

Millet: A staple grain in parts of Africa and Asia. Millet comes in several varieties and has a bland flavor that is a background to other seasonings.

Quinoa: A grain that has been traditionally used in South American cuisine. Its texture has been compared to that of couscous.

Triticale: A grain that is a hybrid of wheat and rye. It comes in several varieties including whole berry, flakes, and flour.

You can find out if the food you are eating is made of whole grains by looking at the ingredients list of the food label. The whole grain should be the first ingredient listed. The following are some examples of how whole grains could be listed:

- Brown rice
- Bulgur (cracked wheat)
- Wild rice
- Triticale
- Whole-grain corn
- Whole rye
- Buckwheat
- Millet
- Quinoa
- Whole-grain barley
- Whole oats/oatmeal
- Whole wheat

Popcorn is also a whole grain that can have added fat and salt. Try air-popping your popcorn to avoid these extras. If you're buying microwave popcorn, look for a lower-fat variety. You may also want to try the snack size bag to help with portion control.

Simple Carbohydrates

Simple carbohydrates include sugars found naturally in foods such as fruits, vegetables milk, and milk products. Simple carbohydrates also include sugars added during food processing and refining. What's the difference? In general, foods with added sugars have fewer nutrients than foods with naturally occurring sugars.

Avoiding Added Sugars

One way to avoid these sugars is to read the ingredient lists on food labels. Look for the following ingredients as added sugars:

- Brown sugar
- Corn syrup
- Fructose
- Glucose
- Honey
- Lactose
- Malt Syrup
- Raw sugar
- Sugar
- Corn sweetener
- Dextrose
- Fruit juice concentrates
- High-fructose corn syrup
- Invert sugar
- Maltose
- Molasses
- Sucrose
- Syrup

If you see any of these in the ingredient list, you know the food has added sugars. The closer to the top of the list, the more of that sugar is in the food.

Tips For Avoiding Added Sugars

Try the following tips to avoid added sugars:

- Drink water instead of sugar-sweetened sodas.
- Try a half a cup of 100% fruit juice rather than a fruit drink
- Have a piece of fruit for dessert and skip desserts with added sugar.
- Choose breakfast cereals that contain no or less added sugars.

You probably already know sugars and starches can play a role in causing cavities. But it's worth mentioning again, particularly as far as teens are concerned. Be sure to also brush and floss to help prevent cavities.

Chapter 22

Sugars

Naturally Occurring Sugars And Added Sugars

There are two types of sugars in American diets: naturally occurring sugars and added sugars.

- Naturally occurring sugars are found naturally in foods such as fruit (fructose) and milk (lactose).

- Added sugars include any sugars or caloric sweeteners that are added to foods or beverages during processing or preparation (such as putting sugar in your coffee or adding sugar to your cereal). Added sugars (or added sweeteners) can include natural sugars such as white sugar, brown sugar, and honey as well as other caloric sweeteners that are chemically manufactured (such as high fructose corn syrup).

You can use sugars to help enhance your diet. Adding a limited amount of sugar to improve the taste of foods (especially for children) that provide important nutrients, such as whole-grain cereal, low-fat milk, or yogurt, is better than eating nutrient-poor, highly sweetened foods.

Sources Of Added Sugars

The major sources of added sugars in American diets are regular soft drinks, sugars, candy, cakes, cookies, pies, and fruit drinks (fruitades and fruit punch); dairy desserts and milk products (ice cream, sweetened yogurt, and sweetened milk); and other grains (cinnamon toast and honey-nut waffles).

About This Chapter: "Sugars 101," reprinted with permission www.heart.org. © 2011 American Heart Association, Inc.

The U.S. Department of Agriculture has identified some common foods with added sugars. Table 22.1 lists a few examples and the number of calories from added sugars they contain. Note the calories here are only from added sugars in the food, not the total amount of calories in the food.

Table 22.1. Calories From Added Sugars In Common Foods

Food	Calories from added sugars per serving
Carbonated soda, 12 oz. can	132.5
Canned peaches in heavy syrup, 1 cup	115.4
Jelly beans, 10 large	78.4
Non-fat fruit yogurt, 6 oz. container	77.5
Milk chocolate, 1 bar (1.55 oz)	77.4
Cake doughnut (1)	74.2
Sweetened condensed milk, 1 fl oz	73.8
Fruit punch drink, 12 oz can	62.1
Angel food cake, 1 piece	60.4
Chocolate puff cereal, 1 cup	56.4
Vanilla ice cream, 1/2 cup	48.0
Pancake syrup, 1 Tbsp	26.5
Chocolate chip cookies (1)	13.6
Cinnamon raisin bagel (4" diameter)	12.8

Finding Added Sugars In Food

Unfortunately, you can't tell easily by looking at the nutrition facts panel of a food if it contains added sugars. The line for "sugars" includes both added and natural sugars. Naturally occurring sugars are found in milk (lactose) and fruit (fructose). Any product that contains milk (such as yogurt, milk, or cream) or fruit (fresh, dried) contains some natural sugars.

Reading the ingredient list on a processed food's label can tell you if the product contains added sugars, just not the exact amount if the product also contains natural sugars.

Names for added sugars on labels include:

- Brown sugar
- Corn syrup
- High-fructose corn syrup
- Corn sweetener
- Fruit juice concentrates
- Honey

- Invert sugar
- Molasses
- Sugar
- Syrup

- Malt sugar
- Raw sugar
- Sugar molecules ending in "ose" (dextrose, fructose, glucose, lactose, maltose, sucrose)

Furthermore, some products include terms related to sugars. Here are some common terms and their meanings:

- **Sugar-free:** Less than 0.5 grams of sugar per serving

- **Reduced sugar or less sugar:** At least 25% less sugars per serving compared to a standard serving size of the traditional variety

- **No added sugars or without added sugars:** No sugars or sugar-containing ingredient such as juice or dry fruit is added during processing

- **Low sugar:** Not defined or allowed as a claim on food labels

Although you can't isolate the calories per serving from added sugars with the information on a nutrition label, it may be helpful to calculate the calories per serving from total sugars (added sugars and naturally occurring sugars). To do this, multiply the grams of sugar by four (there are four calories per one gram of sugar). For example, a product containing 15 grams of sugar has 60 calories from sugar per serving.

Added Sugars In The Diet

Added sugars contribute an average of 16 percent of the total calories in American diets. As a percent of calories from total added sugars, the major sources of added sugars in the diets of Americans are soda, energy drinks, and sports drinks (36% of added sugar intake), grain-based desserts such as cakes, pies, and cookies (13%), sugar-sweetened fruit drinks (10%), dairy-based desserts such as ice cream, frozen yogurt, and pudding (6%), and candy (6%).

Reducing the consumption of these sources of added sugars will lower the calorie content of the diet, without compromising its nutrient adequacy. Sweetened foods and beverages can be replaced with those that have no or are low in added sugars. For example, sweetened beverages can be replaced with water and unsweetened beverages.

Source: Excerpted from *Dietary Guidelines for Americans 2010*, U.S. Department of Agriculture, December 2010.

Keep in mind that if the product has no fruit or milk products in the ingredients, all of the sugars in the food are from added sugars. If the product contains fruit or milk products, the total sugar per serving listed on the label will include added and naturally occurring sugars.

Need To Reduce Added Sugars

Although sugars are not harmful to the body, our bodies don't need sugars to function properly. Added sugars contribute additional calories and zero nutrients to food.

Over the past 30 years, Americans have steadily consumed more and more added sugars in their diets, which has contributed to the obesity epidemic. Reducing the amount of added sugars we eat cuts calories and can help you improve your heart health and control your weight.

The American Heart Association recommends limiting the amount of added sugars you consume to no more than half of your daily discretionary calorie allowance. [Ed. Note: The updated MyPlate food guidance system announced by the U.S. Department of Agriculture in June 2011 uses the term "empty calories" to describe discretionary calories.] For most American women, this is no more than 100 calories per day and no more than 150 calories per day for men (or about six teaspoons per day for women and nine teaspoons per day for men).

Discretionary Calories And Added Sugars

You have a daily energy need—the amount of calories (or energy units) your body needs to function and provide energy for your activities. Think of your daily energy need as a budget. You'd organize a real budget with "essentials" (things like rent and utilities) and "extras" (such as vacation and entertainment). In a daily calorie budget, the essentials are the minimum number of calories you need to meet your nutrient needs.

Select low-fat and no-sugar-added foods to make good "nutrient buys" with your budget. Depending on the foods you choose and the amount of physical activity you do each day, you may have calories left over for "extras" that can be used on treats like solid fats, added sugars, and alcohol. [Ed. Note: Only adults should consider spending calories on alcohol; teens should not drink.] These are discretionary calories, or calories to be spent at your discretion.

A person's discretionary calorie budget varies depending on how physically active they are and how many calories they need to consume to meet their daily nutrient requirements. The American Heart Association recommends that no more than half of a person's daily discretionary calorie allowance be spent on added sugars.

Common sources of discretionary calories (in addition to added sugars) are fats, oils, and alcohol. Fats are the most concentrated source of calories. Discretionary calories can be used to:

- Eat additional foods from a food group above your daily recommendation;

- Select a higher-calorie form of a food that's higher in fat or contains added sugars (whole milk vs. skim or sweetened vs. unsweetened cereal);

- Add fats or sweeteners to the leanest versions of foods (for example, sauce, dressing, and butter/margarine);

- Eat or drink items that are mostly fat, sugar, or alcohol, such as candy, cake, beer, wine, or regular soda. [Ed. Note: Alcoholic products, such as beer and wine, are appropriate for adults only.]

Tips For Getting Less Added Sugar

Most Americans consume more than double the daily recommended amount of added sugars. A report from the 2001–04 NHANES (National Health and Nutrition Examination Survey) database showed that Americans get about 22.2 teaspoons of sugar a day or about 355 calories. This is well over the recommended amount of no more than 100 calories per day for women and no more than 150 calories per day for men.

Use these simple tips to reduce sugar in your diet:

- Remove sugar (white and brown), syrup, honey, and molasses from the table—out of sight, out of mind.

- Cut back on the amount of sugar added to things you eat or drink regularly like cereal, pancakes, coffee, or tea. Try cutting the usual amount of sugar you add by half and wean down from there, or consider using an artificial sweetener.

- Buy sugar-free or low-calorie beverages.

- Buy fresh fruits or fruits canned in water or natural juice. Avoid fruit canned in syrup, especially heavy syrup.

- Instead of adding sugar to cereal or oatmeal, add fresh fruit (try bananas, cherries, or strawberries) or dried fruit (raisins, cranberries, or apricots).

- When baking cookies, brownies, or cakes, cut the sugar called for in your recipe by one-third to one-half. Often you won't notice the difference.

- Instead of adding sugar in recipes, use extracts such as almond, vanilla, orange, or lemon.

- Enhance foods with spices instead of sugar; try ginger, allspice, cinnamon, or nutmeg.

- Substitute unsweetened applesauce for sugar in recipes (use equal amounts).

- Try zero-calorie sweeteners such as aspartame, sucralose, or saccharin in moderation.

Chapter 23

Which Fats Are Which?

What is dietary fat?

What counts as fat? Are some fats better than other fats? While fats are essential for normal body function, some fats are better for you than others. Trans fats, saturated fats and cholesterol are less healthy than polyunsaturated and monounsaturated fats.

How much total dietary fat do I need?

The *Dietary Guidelines for Americans* recommend that Americans keep their total fat intake within certain limits. This limit is defined as a percentage of your total calorie needs.

You can meet fat intake recommendations by following a healthy meal plan that meets your calorie needs and is designed to provide 20% to 35% of calories from total fat.

The USDA Food Guide (visit ChooseMyPlate.gov) and DASH (Dietary Approaches to Stop Hypertension) eating plan are examples of healthy meal plans that can meet your calorie needs and provide the right amounts of fat. The DASH Eating Plan provides a healthy eating plan with menu examples and recipes to get you started. For proper growth, children and teens need healthy diets that provide the recommended fat intakes.

What is trans fat?

You may have heard about trans fats recently in the news. These fats made headlines when food manufacturers were required to list them on the Nutrition Facts Label by 2006.

About This Chapter: Excerpted from "Dietary Fat," Centers for Disease Control and Prevention, December 2008.

Table 23.1. Fat Intake Guidelines

Age Group	Total Fat Limits
Children ages 2 to 3	30% to 35% of total calories
Children and adolescents ages 4 to 18	25% to 35% of total calories
Adults, ages 19 and older	20% to 35% of total calories

So what's the story with trans fats? These fats are created during food processing when liquid oils are converted into semi-solid fats—a process called hydrogenation. This creates partially hydrogenated oils that tend to keep food fresh longer while on grocery shelves. The problem is that these partially hydrogenated oils contain trans fats which can also increase low-density lipoprotein LDL-cholesterol and decrease high-density lipoprotein (HDL) cholesterol—risk factors for heart disease.

What's the recommendation for eating trans fat?

The *Dietary Guidelines for Americans* recommend keeping the amount of trans fat you consume as low as possible.

Though some fried foods and commercially baked goods may contain trans fats, the good news is that some manufacturers have changed how they process foods to reduce the amounts of trans fats in their products. Be on the look out for foods that contain trans fats, such as commercially baked cookies, crackers, and pies. Some commercial restaurants may also use partially hydrogenated oils when frying their entrees and side items or preparing baking goods and spreads.

How do I control my trans fat intake?

Here are some ideas on how to reduce the trans fat in your diet:

- Look for the trans fat listing on the Nutrition Facts label. Compare brands and choose the one lowest in trans fat, preferably with no trans fat.

How much fat is healthy?

Some fats are healthier than others, but that doesn't mean you can eat as much of those fats as you want. It's best to keep your total fat intake between 20% and 35% of your total calories each day.

A healthy eating plan such as MyPlate or the DASH eating plan contain between 20% and 35% of calories as fat. Check out these plans to get the right amounts of fat you need each day.

- Replace margarine containing trans fat with unsaturated vegetable oil.

- If you use margarine, choose a soft margarine spread instead of stick margarine.

- Check your labels to be sure the soft margarine does contain less trans fat. If possible, find one that says zero grams of trans fat.

What is saturated fat?

You may have heard that saturated fats are the "solid" fats in your diet. For the most part, this is true. For example, if you open a container of meat stew, you will probably find some fat floating on top. This fat is saturated fat.

What's the recommendation for eating saturated fat?

Diets high in saturated fat have been linked to chronic disease, specifically, coronary heart disease. The *Dietary Guidelines for Americans* recommend consuming less than 10% of daily calories as saturated fat.

But other saturated fats can be more difficult to see in your diet. In general, saturated fat can be found in the following foods:

- High-fat cheeses

- High fat cuts of meat

- Whole-fat milk and cream

- Butter

- Ice cream and ice cream products

- Palm and coconut oils

It's important to note that lower-fat versions of these foods usually will contain saturated fats, but typically in smaller quantities than the regular versions.

As you look at this list above, notice two things. First, animal fats are a primary source of saturated fat. Secondly, certain plant oils are another source of saturated fats: palm oils, coconut oils, and cocoa butter. You may think you don't use palm or coconut oils, but they are often added to commercially-prepared foods, such as cookies, cakes, doughnuts, and pies. Solid vegetable shortening often contains palm oils and some whipped dessert toppings contain coconut oil.

How do I control my saturated fat intake?

In general, saturated fat can be found in the following foods:

- High-fat cheeses

- High-fat cuts of meat

- Whole-fat milk and cream

- Butter

- Ice cream and ice cream products

Try these tips:

- Choose leaner cuts of meat that do not have a marbled appearance (where the fat appears embedded in the meat). Leaner cuts include round cuts and sirloin cuts. Trim all visible fat off meats before eating.

- Remove the skin from chicken, turkey, and other poultry before cooking.

- When re-heating soups or stews, skim the solid fats from the top before heating.

> ## Butter Or Margarine?
>
> What should I choose—butter or margarine? Should I choose a stick, tub, or liquid?
>
> With such a variety of products available, it can be a difficult decision. Here are some general rules of thumb to help you compare products:
>
> - Look at the Nutrition Facts label to compare both the trans fat and the saturated fat content. Choose the one that has the fewest grams of trans fat and the fewest grams of saturated fat and dietary cholesterol. If possible, find one that says zero grams of trans fat.
>
> - When looking at the Daily Value for saturated fat and cholesterol remember that 5% is low and 20% is high.
>
> - If you are also trying to reduce calories, you may want to look for a version that says "light." These products contain fewer calories and can help you stay within your calorie goals.
>
> - If you find two products that seem comparable, try them both and choose the one that tastes better.

- Drink low-fat (1%) or fat-free (skim) milk rather than whole or 2% milk.

- Buy low-fat or non-fat versions of your favorite cheeses and other milk or dairy products.

- When you want a sweet treat, reach for a low-fat or fat-free version of your favorite ice cream or frozen dessert. These versions usually contain less saturated fat.

- Use low-fat spreads instead of butter. Most margarine spreads contain less saturated fat than butter. Look for a spread that is low in saturated fat and doesn't contain trans fats.

- Choose baked goods, breads, and desserts that are low in saturated fat. You can find this information on the Nutrition Facts label.

- Pay attention at snack time. Some convenience snacks such as sandwich crackers contain saturated fat. Choose instead to have non-fat or low-fat yogurt and a piece of fruit.

What are polyunsaturated fats and monounsaturated fats?

Most of the fat that you eat should come from unsaturated sources: polyunsaturated fats and monounsaturated fats. In general, nuts, vegetable oils, and fish are sources of unsaturated fats. Table 23.2 provides examples of specific types of unsaturated fats.

Polyunsaturated fats can also be broken down into two types:

- **Omega-6 Polyunsaturated Fats:** These fats provide an essential fatty acid that our bodies need, but can't make.

- **Omega-3 Polyunsaturated Fats:** These fats also provide an essential fatty acid that our bodies need. In addition, omega-3 fatty acids, particularly from fish sources, may have potential health benefits.

How do I control my polyunsaturated fat and monounsaturated fat intake?

Below are tips for including appropriate amounts of unsaturated fats in your diet:

- Replace solid fats used in cooking with liquid oils.

- Remember any type of fat is high in calories. To avoid additional calories, substitute polyunsaturated and monounsaturated fats for saturated fats and trans fats rather than adding these fats to your diet.

- Have an ounce of dry-roasted nuts as a snack. Nuts and seeds count as part of your meat and beans allowance.

Table 23.2. Types Of Unsaturated Fats

Monounsaturated Fat Sources	Omega-6 Polyunsaturated Fat Sources	Omega-3 Polyunsaturated Fat Sources
Nuts	Soybean oil	Soybean oil
Vegetable oils	Corn oil	Canola oil
Canola oil	Safflower oil	Walnuts
Olive oil		Flaxseed
High oleic safflower oil		Fish: trout, herring, and salmon
Sunflower oil		
Avocado		

Chapter 24

Food Additives And Colors

For centuries, ingredients have served useful functions in a variety of foods. Our ancestors used salt to preserve meats and fish, added herbs and spices to improve the flavor of foods, preserved fruit with sugar, and pickled cucumbers in a vinegar solution. Today, consumers demand and enjoy a food supply that is flavorful, nutritious, safe, convenient, colorful, and affordable. Food additives and advances in technology help make that possible.

There are thousands of ingredients used to make foods. The U.S. Food and Drug Administration (FDA) maintains a list of over 3,000 ingredients in its data base "Everything Added to Food in the United States," many of which we use at home every day (for example, sugar, baking soda, salt, vanilla, yeast, spices, and colors).

Still, some consumers have concerns about additives because they may see the long, unfamiliar names and think of them as complex chemical compounds. In fact, every food we eat—whether a just-picked strawberry or a homemade cookie—is made up of chemical compounds that determine flavor, color, texture, and nutrient value. All food additives are carefully regulated by federal authorities and various international organizations to ensure that foods are safe to eat and are accurately labeled.

The purpose of this chapter is to provide helpful background information about food and color additives: what they are, why they are used in foods, and how they are regulated for safe use.

About This Chapter: "Food Ingredients and Colors," 2010. Reprinted with permission from the International Food Information Council (www.foodinsight.org). Prepared under a partnering agreement with the U.S. Food and Drug Administration (FDA).

Why are food and color ingredients added to food?

Additives perform a variety of useful functions in foods that consumers often take for granted. Some additives could be eliminated if we were willing to grow our own food, harvest, and grind it, spend many hours cooking and canning, or accept increased risks of food spoilage. But most consumers today rely on the many technological, aesthetic, and convenient benefits that additives provide.

Following are some reasons why ingredients are added to foods:

To Maintain Or Improve Safety And Freshness: Preservatives slow product spoilage caused by mold, air, bacteria, fungi, or yeast. In addition to maintaining the quality of the food, they help control contamination that can cause foodborne illness, including life-threatening botulism. One group of preservatives—antioxidants—prevents fats and oils and the foods containing them from becoming rancid or developing an off-flavor. They also prevent cut fresh fruits such as apples from turning brown when exposed to air.

To Improve Or Maintain Nutritional Value: Vitamins and minerals (and fiber) are added to many foods to make up for those lacking in a person's diet or lost in processing, or to enhance the nutritional quality of a food. Such fortification and enrichment has helped reduce malnutrition in the U.S. and worldwide. All products containing added nutrients must be appropriately labeled.

Improve Taste, Texture And Appearance: Spices, natural and artificial flavors, and sweeteners are added to enhance the taste of food. Food colors maintain or improve appearance. Emulsifiers, stabilizers, and thickeners give foods the texture and consistency consumers expect. Leavening agents allow baked goods to rise during baking. Some additives help control the acidity and alkalinity of foods, while other ingredients help maintain the taste and appeal of foods with reduced fat content.

What is a food additive?

In its broadest sense, a food additive is any substance added to food. Legally, the term refers to "any substance the intended use of which results or may reasonably be expected to result—directly or indirectly—in its becoming a component or otherwise affecting the characteristics of any food." This definition includes any substance used in the production, processing, treatment, packaging, transportation, or storage of food. The purpose of the legal definition, however, is to impose a premarket approval requirement. Therefore, this definition excludes ingredients whose use is generally recognized as safe (where government approval is not needed), those ingredients approved for use by FDA or the U.S. Department of Agriculture prior to the food additives provisions of law, and color additives and pesticides where other legal premarket approval requirements apply.

Herbs, Spices, And Seasonings

A spice is any root, bud, seed or bark derived from a plant grown in a tropical zone that is used to season foods. A herb comes from a seed plant that has no woody tissue and is grown in a temperate zone. Both herbs and spices vary in color and flavor from crop to crop.

The word "spice" is commonly used to refer to any vegetable substance that flavors food. For example, basil is a herb, but it is often grouped under the spice category.

Functions Of Herbs And Spices

Herbs and spices have the following functions:

- **Flavor:** The flavoring portion of spices is found in their volatile essential oils and their non-volatile oleoresins.
- **Appearance:** Spices make foods appealing by adding a color contrast to products.
- **Antioxidant:** Some spices retard the oxidation of fats in certain food. An example is rosemary in sausages.
- **Preservative:** Certain spices—for example, mustard, cinnamon and cloves—contain antimicrobial compounds that retard or inhibit the growth of moulds, yeasts or bacteria.
- **Medicinal properties:** It is believed that some spices impart beneficial health aspects when they are eaten.

Source: Excerpted from "Your Guide to Food Processing in Ontario," Ontario Ministry of Agriculture, Food and Rural Affairs (www.omafra.gov.ca). © Queen's Printer for Ontario, 2008. Reproduced with permission.

Direct food additives are those that are added to a food for a specific purpose in that food. For example, xanthan gum—used in salad dressings, chocolate milk, bakery fillings, puddings, and other foods to add texture—is a direct additive. Most direct additives are identified on the ingredient label of foods.

Indirect food additives are those that become part of the food in trace amounts due to its packaging, storage, or other handling. For instance, minute amounts of packaging substances may find their way into foods during storage. Food packaging manufacturers must prove to the U.S. Food and Drug Administration (FDA) that all materials coming in contact with food are safe before they are permitted for use in such a manner.

What is a color additive?

A color additive is any dye, pigment, or substance which when added or applied to a food, drug, or cosmetic, or to the human body, is capable (alone or through reactions with other substances) of imparting color. FDA is responsible for regulating all color additives to ensure that foods containing color additives are safe to eat, contain only approved ingredients, and are accurately labeled.

Color additives are used in foods for many reasons: 1) to offset color loss due to exposure to light, air, temperature extremes, moisture, and storage conditions; 2) to correct natural variations in color; 3) to enhance colors that occur naturally; and 4) to provide color to colorless and "fun" foods. Without color additives, colas wouldn't be brown, margarine wouldn't be yellow, and mint ice cream wouldn't be green. Color additives are now recognized as an important part of practically all processed foods we eat.

FDA's permitted colors are classified as subject to certification or exempt from certification, both of which are subject to rigorous safety standards prior to their approval and listing for use in foods.

- Certified colors are synthetically produced (or human made) and used widely because they impart an intense, uniform color, are less expensive, and blend more easily to create a variety of hues. There are nine certified color additives approved for use in the United States (for example, FD&C Yellow No. 6.). Certified food colors generally do not add undesirable flavors to foods.

- Colors that are exempt from certification include pigments derived from natural sources such as vegetables, minerals, or animals. Nature derived color additives are typically more expensive than certified colors and may add unintended flavors to foods. Examples of exempt colors include annatto extract (yellow), dehydrated beets (bluish-red to brown), caramel (yellow to tan), beta-carotene (yellow to orange), and grape skin extract (red, green).

How are additives approved for use in foods?

Today, food and color additives are more strictly studied, regulated, and monitored than at any other time in history. FDA has the primary legal responsibility for determining their safe use. To market a new food or color additive (or before using an additive already approved for one use in another manner not yet approved), a manufacturer or other sponsor must first petition FDA for its approval. These petitions must provide evidence that the substance is safe for the ways in which it will be used. As a result of recent legislation, since 1999, indirect additives have been approved via a premarket notification process requiring the same data as was previously required by petition.

Why are food additives regulated?

During the early part of the first century in America, people lived off the land. They grew their own foods or bought them from someone they knew and trusted. There was no need for food safety laws. As the country grew and became more industrialized, the number of people who produced their own foods decreased drastically. Therefore, the nation depended on the newly emerging food industry to produce and distribute its food. Unfortunately, during the 1850s, there was much dishonesty concerning adding substances to foods.

The first efforts to pass laws to govern foods were state laws (1850 and beyond). These laws were difficult to enforce. The first major Federal law governing food was the 1906 Federal Food and Drug Act. It set the framework for the regulation of foods and stated that it was illegal to sell misbranded or adulterated foods and drugs in interstate commerce. It listed chemicals that were illegal to add to foods, such as borax or formaldehyde. The law was weak in that there was no method of enforcement and no punishment.

In 1938, the Federal Food and Drug Act was revised to account for changes in medical science and food technology, and was renamed the Federal Food, Drug, and Cosmetic Act. Among the many provisions of the law was a requirement for truthful labeling of additives.

Source: Excerpted from "Food Labeling: Additives in Meat and Poultry Products," a fact sheet produced by the Food Safety Inspection Service, U.S. Department of Agriculture (www.fsis.usda.gov), November 2008.

Under the Food Additives Amendment, two groups of ingredients were exempted from the regulation process.

- GROUP I, prior-sanctioned substances, are substances that FDA or USDA had determined safe for use in food prior to the 1958 amendment. Examples are sodium nitrite and potassium nitrite used to preserve luncheon meats.

- GROUP II, GRAS (generally recognized as safe) ingredients, are those that are generally recognized by experts as safe, based on their extensive history of use in food before 1958 or based on published scientific evidence. Among the several hundred GRAS substances are salt, sugar, spices, vitamins, and monosodium glutamate (MSG). Manufacturers may also request that FDA review the industry's determination of GRAS status.

When evaluating the safety of a substance and whether it should be approved, FDA considers: 1) the composition and properties of the substance, 2) the amount that would typically be consumed, 3) immediate and long-term health effects, and 4) various safety factors. The evaluation determines an appropriate level of use that includes a built-in safety margin—a factor that allows for uncertainty about the levels of consumption that are expected to be harmless. In other words, the levels of use that gain approval are much lower than what would be expected to have any adverse effect.

Because of inherent limitations of science, FDA can never be absolutely certain of the absence of any risk from the use of any substance. Therefore, FDA must determine—based on the best science available—if there is a reasonable certainty of no harm to consumers when an additive is used as proposed.

If an additive is approved, FDA issues regulations that may include the types of foods in which it can be used, the maximum amounts to be used, and how it should be identified on food labels. In 1999, procedures changed so that FDA now consults with USDA during the review process for ingredients that are proposed for use in meat and poultry products. Federal officials then monitor the extent of Americans' consumption of the new additive and results of any new research on its safety to ensure its use continues to be within safe limits.

If new evidence suggests that a product already in use may be unsafe, or if consumption levels have changed enough to require another look, federal authorities may prohibit its use or conduct further studies to determine if the use can still be considered safe.

Regulations known as Good Manufacturing Practices (GMP) limit the amount of food ingredients used in foods to the amount necessary to achieve the desired effect.

Questions And Answers About Food And Color Additives

How are ingredients listed on a product label?

Food manufacturers are required to list all ingredients in the food on the label. On a product label, the ingredients are listed in order of predominance, with the ingredients used in the greatest amount first, followed in descending order by those in smaller amounts. The label must list the names of any FDA-certified color additives (for example, FD&C Blue No. 1 or the abbreviated name, Blue 1). But some ingredients can be listed collectively as "flavors," "spices," "artificial flavoring," or in the case of color additives exempt from certification, "artificial colors", without naming each one. Declaration of an allergenic ingredient in a collective or single color, flavor, or spice could be accomplished by simply naming the allergenic ingredient in the ingredient list.

What are dyes and lakes in color additives?

Certified color additives are categorized as either dyes or lakes. Dyes dissolve in water and are manufactured as powders, granules, liquids, or other special-purpose forms. They can be used in beverages, dry mixes, baked goods, confections, dairy products, pet foods, and a variety of other products.

Lakes are the water insoluble form of the dye. Lakes are more stable than dyes and are ideal for coloring products containing fats and oils or items lacking sufficient moisture to dissolve dyes. Typical uses include coated tablets, cake and donut mixes, hard candies, and chewing gums.

Do additives cause childhood hyperactivity?

Although this hypothesis was popularized in the 1970s, results from studies on this issue either have been inconclusive, inconsistent, or difficult to interpret due to inadequacies in study design. A Consensus Development Panel of the National Institutes of Health concluded in 1982 that for some children with attention deficit hyperactivity disorder (ADHD) and confirmed food allergy, dietary modification has produced some improvement in behavior. Although the panel said that elimination diets should not be used universally to treat childhood hyperactivity, since there is no scientific evidence to predict which children may benefit, the panel recognized that initiation of a trial of dietary treatment or continuation of a diet in patients whose families and physicians perceive benefits may be warranted. However, a 1997 review published in the *Journal of the American Academy of Child & Adolescent Psychiatry* noted there is minimal evidence of efficacy and extreme difficulty inducing children and adolescents to comply with restricted diets.

Thus, dietary treatment should not be recommended, except possibly with a small number of preschool children who may be sensitive to tartrazine, known commonly as FD&C Yellow No. 5. In 2007, synthetic certified color additives again came under scrutiny following publication of a study commissioned by the UK Food Standards Agency to investigate whether certain color additives cause hyperactivity in children. Both the FDA and the European Food Safety Authority independently reviewed the results from this study and each has concluded that the study does not substantiate a link between the color additives that were tested and behavioral effects. [Ed. Note: In March 2011, an FDA advisory panel reconsidered this issue. The panel decided against adding warning labels to foods with color additives, but it did recommend additional research to evaluate the safety of color additives.]

What is the difference between natural and artificial ingredients? Is a naturally produced ingredient safer than an artificially manufactured ingredient?

Natural ingredients are derived from natural sources (for example, soybeans and corn provide lecithin to maintain product consistency; beets provide beet powder used as food coloring). Other ingredients are not found in nature and, therefore, must be synthetically produced as artificial ingredients. Also, some ingredients found in nature can be manufactured artificially and produced more economically, with greater purity and more consistent quality, than their natural counterparts. For example, vitamin C or ascorbic acid may be derived from an orange or produced in a laboratory. Food ingredients are subject to the same strict safety standards regardless of whether they are naturally or artificially derived.

Are certain people sensitive to FD&C Yellow No. 5 in foods?

FD&C Yellow No. 5 is used to color beverages, dessert powders, candy, ice cream, custards, and other foods. FDA's Committee on Hypersensitivity to Food Constituents concluded in 1986 that FD&C Yellow No. 5 might cause hives in fewer than one out of 10,000 people. It also concluded that there was no evidence the color additive in food provokes asthma attacks. The law now requires Yellow No. 5 to be identified on the ingredient line. This allows the few who may be sensitive to the color to avoid it.

Do low-calorie sweeteners cause adverse reactions?

No. Food safety experts generally agree there is no convincing evidence of a cause and effect relationship between these sweeteners and negative health effects in humans. The FDA has monitored consumer complaints of possible adverse reactions for more than 15 years.

For example, in carefully controlled clinical studies, aspartame has not been shown to cause adverse or allergic reactions. However, persons with a rare hereditary disease known as phenylketonuria (PKU) must control their intake of phenylalanine from all sources, including aspartame. Although aspartame contains only a small amount of phenylalanine, labels of aspartame-containing foods and beverages must include a statement advising phenylketonurics of the presence of phenylalanine.

Individuals who have concerns about possible adverse effects from food additives or other substances should contact their physicians.

How do they add vitamins and minerals to fortified cereals?

Adding nutrients to a cereal can cause taste and color changes in the product. This is especially true with added minerals. Since no one wants cereal that tastes like a vitamin supplement, a variety of techniques are employed in the fortification process. In general, those nutrients that are heat stable (such as vitamins A and E and various minerals) are incorporated into the cereal itself (they're baked right in). Nutrients that are not stable to heat (such as B-vitamins) are applied directly to the cereal after all heating steps are completed. Each cereal is unique—some can handle more nutrients than others can. This is one reason why fortification levels are different across all cereals.

What is the role of modern technology in producing food additives?

Many new techniques are being researched that will allow the production of additives in ways not previously possible. One approach is the use of biotechnology, which can use simple organisms to produce food additives. These additives are the same as food components found in nature. In 1990, FDA approved the first bioengineered enzyme, rennin, which traditionally had been extracted from calves' stomachs for use in making cheese.

Types Of Food Ingredients

The following summary lists the types of common food ingredients, why they are used, and some examples of the names that can be found on product labels. Some additives are used for more than one purpose.

Preservatives

What They Do: Prevent food spoilage from bacteria, molds, fungi, or yeast (antimicrobials); slow or prevent changes in color, flavor, or texture and delay rancidity (antioxidants); maintain freshness.

Examples Of Uses: Fruit sauces and jellies, beverages, baked goods, cured meats, oils and margarines, cereals, dressings, snack foods, fruits and vegetables.

Names Found On Product Labels: Ascorbic acid, citric acid, sodium benzoate, calcium propionate, sodium erythorbate, sodium nitrite, calcium sorbate, potassium sorbate, BHA, BHT, EDTA, tocopherols (Vitamin E).

Sweeteners

What They Do: Add sweetness with or without the extra calories.

Examples Of Uses: Beverages, baked goods, confections, table-top sugar, substitutes, many processed foods.

What's It Mean?

Commonly Used Meat And Poultry Additives And Terms

Antioxidant: Substances added to foods to prevent the oxygen present in the air from causing undesirable changes in flavor or color. BHA, BHT, and tocopherols are examples of antioxidants.

Binder: A substance that may be added to foods to thicken or improve texture.

Carrageenan: Seaweed is the source of this additive. It may be used in products as binder.

Gelatin: Thickener from collagen which is derived from the skin, tendons, ligaments, or bones of livestock. It may be used in canned hams or jellied meat products.

Monosodium Glutamate (MSG): MSG is a flavor enhancer. It comes from a common amino acid, glutamic acid, and must be declared as monosodium glutamate on meat and poultry labels.

Phosphates: The two beneficial effects of phosphates in meat and poultry products are moisture retention and flavor protection.

Sodium Nitrite: Used alone or in conjunction with sodium nitrate as a color fixative in cured meat and poultry products (bologna, hot dogs, bacon). Helps prevent growth of *Clostridium botulinum*, which can cause botulism in humans.

Whey, Dried: The dried form of a component of milk that remains after cheese making. Can be used as a binder or extender in various meat products, such as sausage and stews.

Source: Excerpted from "Food Labeling: Additives in Meat and Poultry Products," a fact sheet produced by the Food Safety Inspection Service, U.S. Department of Agriculture (www.fsis.usda.gov), November 2008.

Names Found On Product Labels: Sucrose (sugar), glucose, fructose, sorbitol, mannitol, corn syrup, high fructose corn syrup, saccharin, aspartame, sucralose, acesulfame potassium (acesulfame-K), neotame.

Color Additives

What They Do: Offset color loss due to exposure to light, air, temperature extremes, moisture, and storage conditions; correct natural variations in color; enhance colors that occur naturally; provide color to colorless and "fun" foods.

Examples Of Uses: Many processed foods, (candies, snack foods, margarine, cheese, soft drinks, jams/jellies, gelatins, pudding, and pie fillings).

Names Found On Product Labels: FD&C Blue Nos. 1 and 2, FD&C Green No. 3, FD&C Red Nos. 3 and 40, FD&C Yellow Nos. 5 and 6, Orange B, Citrus Red No. 2, annatto extract, beta-carotene, grape skin extract, cochineal extract or carmine, paprika oleoresin, caramel color, fruit and vegetable juices, saffron (Note: Exempt color additives are not required to be declared by name on labels but may be declared simply as colorings or color added).

Flavors And Spices

What They Do: Add specific flavors (natural and synthetic).

Examples Of Uses: Pudding and pie fillings, gelatin dessert mixes, cake mixes, salad dressings, candies, soft drinks, ice cream, BBQ sauce.

Names Found On Product Labels: Natural flavoring, artificial flavor, and spices.

Flavor Enhancers

What They Do: Enhance flavors already present in foods (without providing their own separate flavor)

Examples Of Uses: Many processed foods

Names Found On Product Labels: Monosodium glutamate (MSG), hydrolyzed soy protein, autolyzed yeast extract, disodium guanylate. or inosinate

Fat Replacers (and components of formulations used to replace fats)

What They Do: Provide expected texture and a creamy "mouth-feel" in reduced-fat foods

Examples Of Uses: Baked goods, dressings, frozen desserts, confections, cake and dessert mixes, dairy products

Names Found On Product Labels: Olestra, cellulose gel, carrageenan, polydextrose, modified food starch, microparticulated egg white protein, guar gum, xanthan gum, whey protein concentrate

Nutrients

What They Do: Replace vitamins and minerals lost in processing (enrichment), add nutrients that may be lacking in the diet (fortification)

Examples Of Uses: Flour, breads, cereals, rice, macaroni, margarine, salt, milk, fruit beverages, energy bars, instant breakfast drinks

Names Found On Product Labels: Thiamine hydrochloride, riboflavin (Vitamin B2), niacin, niacinamide, folate or folic acid, beta carotene, potassium iodide, iron or ferrous sulfate, alpha tocopherols, ascorbic acid, Vitamin D, amino acids (L-tryptophan, L-lysine, L-leucine, L-methionine)

Emulsifiers

What They Do: Allow smooth mixing of ingredients, prevent separation; keep emulsified products stable, reduce stickiness, control crystallization, keep ingredients dispersed, and to help products dissolve more easily

Examples Of Uses: Salad dressings, peanut butter, chocolate, margarine, frozen desserts

Names Found On Product Labels: Soy lecithin, mono- and diglycerides, egg yolks, polysorbates, sorbitan monostearate

Stabilizers And Thickeners, Binders, Texturizers

What They Do: Produce uniform texture, improve "mouth-feel"

Examples Of Uses: Frozen desserts, dairy products, cakes, pudding and gelatin mixes, dressings, jams and jellies, sauces

Names Found On Product Labels: Gelatin, pectin, guar gum, carrageenan, xanthan gum, whey

pH Control Agents And Acidulants

What They Do: Control acidity and alkalinity, prevent spoilage

Examples Of Uses: Beverages, frozen desserts, chocolate, low acid canned foods, baking powder

Names Found On Product Labels: Lactic acid, citric acid, ammonium hydroxide, sodium carbonate

Leavening Agents

What They Do: Promote rising of baked goods

Examples Of Uses: Breads and other baked goods

Names Found On Product Labels: Baking soda, monocalcium phosphate, calcium carbonate

Anti-Caking Agents

What They Do: Keep powdered foods free-flowing, prevent moisture absorption

Examples Of Uses: Salt, baking powder, confectioner's sugar

Names Found On Product Labels: Calcium silicate, iron ammonium citrate, silicon dioxide

Humectants

What They Do: Retain moisture

Examples Of Uses: Shredded coconut, marshmallows, soft candies, confections

Names Found On Product Labels: Glycerin, sorbitol

Yeast Nutrients

What They Do: Promote growth of yeast

Examples Of Uses: Breads and other baked goods

Names Found On Product Labels: Calcium sulfate, ammonium phosphate

Dough Strengtheners And Conditioners

What They Do: Produce more stable dough

Examples Of Uses: Breads and other baked goods

Names Found On Product Labels: Ammonium sulfate, azodicarbonamide, L-cysteine

Firming Agents

What They Do: Maintain crispness and firmness

Examples Of Uses: Processed fruits and vegetables

Names Found On Product Labels: Calcium chloride, calcium lactate

Enzyme Preparations

What They Do: Modify proteins, polysaccharides, and fats

Examples Of Uses: Cheese, dairy products, meat

Names Found On Product Labels: Enzymes, lactase, papain, rennet, chymosin

Gases

What They Do: Serve as propellant, aerate, or create carbonation

Examples Of Uses: Oil cooking spray, whipped cream, carbonated beverages

Names Found On Product Labels: Carbon dioxide, nitrous oxide

Chapter 25

Artificial Sweeteners

Abstract

America's obesity epidemic has gathered much media attention recently. A rise in the percent of the population who are obese coincides with an increase in the widespread use of noncaloric artificial sweeteners, such as aspartame (for example, in Diet Coke) and sucralose (for example, in Pepsi One), in food products (see Figure 25.1). Both forward and reverse causalities have been proposed. While people often choose "diet" or "light" products to lose weight, research studies suggest that artificial sweeteners may contribute to weight gain. In this minireview, inspired by a discussion with Dr. Dana Small at Yale's Neuroscience 2010 conference in April, I first examine the development of artificial sweeteners in a historic context. I then summarize the epidemiological and experimental evidence concerning their effects on weight. Finally, I attempt to explain those effects in light of the neurobiology of food reward.

Sweeteners

We owe the discovery of several artificial sweeteners to a few brave scientists who violated the code of laboratory hygiene and tasted their samples, often inadvertently. Saccharin, the oldest artificial sweetener, was discovered by Constantine Fahlberg at Johns Hopkins in 1879 while working on coal tar derivatives. For decades after its debut, saccharin remained a specialty product for diabetics on stores' medicinal shelves. A sugar shortage during World War II and shift of esthetics toward favoring a thin figure encouraged women to turn to artificial

About This Chapter: "Gain weight by 'going diet?' Artificial sweeteners and the neurobiology of sugar cravings," by Qing Yang. *Yale Journal of Biology and Medicine*, Volume 83, Number 2, pp 101-108. June 2010. Reprinted with permission. The complete text of this article including references is available at http://www.ncbi.nlm.nih.gov/pmc/articles/PMC2892765/.

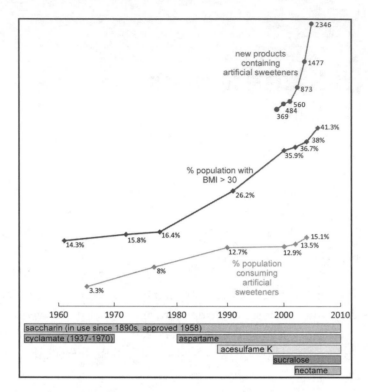

Figure 25.1. Time line of artificial sweetener use and obesity trends in the United States. Middle line: changes in the percentage of the population who are obese (BMI >30) from 1961 to 2006. Source: National Health and Nutrition Examination Survey.[1] Bottom line: changes in the percentage of the population who are regular artificial sweetener users from 1965 to 2004. Source: National Household Survey.[2] Top line: changes in the number of new artificial sweetener containing food products introduced to the American market from 1999 to 2004. Source: Mintel Market Analysis.[3] Bars below the time axis indicates the type and availability of artificial sweeteners in the United States over time. Source: Kroger et al.[4]

1. National Center for Health Statistics. Prevalence of overweight, obesity and extreme obesity among adults: United States, trends 1960–62 through 2005–2006. National Health and Nutrition Examination Survey.

2. Mattes RD, Popkin BM. Nonnutritive sweetener consumption in humans: effects on appetite and food intake and their putative mechanisms. Am J Clin Nutr. 2009;89:1–14.

3. Mintel. Ingredient Trends—US, December 2004, Market Research Report.

4. Kroger M, Meister K, Kava R. Low-calorie Sweeteners and Other Sugar Substitutes: A Review of the Safety Issues. Comprehensive Reviews in Food Science and Food Safety. 2006;5:35-47.

substitutes as well. Around this time, the wording on diet soda bottles subtly changed from "for use only in people who must limit sugar intake" to "for use in people who desire to limit sugar intake." Saccharin is about 300 times sweeter than sucrose but has a bitter aftertaste. Cyclamate, which was discovered in 1937 by Michael Sveda at the University of Illinois, was often blended with saccharin to improve the taste. Both compounds were deemed "generally recognized as safe" in the 1958 Food Additives Amendment to the Federal Food, Drug, and Cosmetics Act. After the Food and Drug Administration (FDA) banned cyclamate in 1969 because of its carcinogenic potentials, concern about saccharin's safety also intensified. Eventually, the FDA announced its intention to ban saccharin in 1977. Avid consumer protests led to a moratorium from Congress on the final ban decision. A warning label was nonetheless required on all saccharin products. Subsequent studies refuted the link between cyclamate and cancer. Bladder cancer associated with saccharin ingestion was also found to be specific to rodent physiology. Cyclamate continues to be marketed in about 50 countries, including Canada. The saccharin warning label was removed in 2000.

Even though saccharin stayed on the U.S. market, regular artificial sweetener users were relatively few until the next generation of compounds arrived (see Figure 25.1). Rigorous safety testing preceded FDA approval for those new artificial sweeteners. In 1965, James Schlatter at Searle discovered aspartame. He was trying to make new ulcer drugs. Aspartame consists of two amino acids, phenylalanine and aspartate, linked to a methanol backbone. Unlike the other artificial sweeteners that are usually excreted unchanged, aspartame can be metabolized. Therefore, it is not strictly non-caloric (4 Kcal/g) and forbidden in people with phenylketonuria. Aspartame is about 200 times sweeter than sucrose. Due to the small amount ingested at a time, its caloric contribution is negligible. The FDA approved aspartame first for use in dry foods in 1981, then as a general sweetener in 1996. Monsanto bought Searle and converted it into NutraSweet in 1984. The patent on aspartame expired in 1992. Amid competition from generic manufacturers, NutraSweet engineered neotame, which was approved in 2002. Neotame is the most potent sweetener on the market, at 7,000 times the sweetness of sucrose.

What's It Mean?

Artificial Sweeteners: Also called sugar substitutes; substances that are used instead of sucrose (table sugar) to sweeten foods and beverages. Because artificial sweeteners are many times sweeter than table sugar, smaller amounts are needed to create the same level of sweetness.

Source: Excerpted from "Artificial Sweeteners and Cancer," National Cancer Institute, August 2009.

Acesulfame potassium resembles saccharin and cyclamate in structure and taste. Karl Clauss at Hoechst discovered it in 1967. The FDA approved its use in dry foods in 1988 and as a general sweetener in 2003.

The most recent structural advance came in 1979, when Shashikant Phadnis, a graduate student working for Tate & Lyle, discovered sucralose. It is synthesized from sucrose by substituting chlorine for three of its hydroxyl groups, generating 600 times the sweetness. It was approved in 1999. Sucralose sales amounted to £148 million in 2008, generating 23 percent of Tate & Lyle's total operating profit.

The last decade saw an explosive increase in the number of food products containing non-caloric artificial sweeteners. More than 6,000 new products were launched in the United States between 1999 and 2004. Currently, an ingredient search on foodfacts.com yields 3,648 products containing one or more of the five FDA approved artificial sweeteners. Sucralose is the most popular (1,500 products), followed by acesulfame potassium (1,103 products), and aspartame (974 products). Artificial sweeteners are most commonly used in carbonated drinks. They also are found in a variety of other products, from baby food (for example, Pedialyte) to frozen food (for example, Lean Pockets). With such a diverse selection, it is more likely that people will encounter artificially sweetened items when making the day-to-day choices on food and beverages. The National Household Nutritional Survey estimated that as of 2004, 15 percent of the population regularly were using artificial sweetener. IRI Consumer Report stated that 65 percent of American households bought at least one sucralose-containing product in 2008. Therefore, the total number of artificial sweetener consumers, either regular or sporadic, is probably much greater.

How are artificial sweeteners regulated in the United States?

Artificial sweeteners are regulated by the U.S. Food and Drug Administration (FDA). The FDA, like the National Cancer Institute (NCI), is an agency of the Department of Health and Human Services. The FDA regulates food, drugs, medical devices, cosmetics, biologics, and radiation-emitting products. The Food Additives Amendment to the Food, Drug, and Cosmetic Act, which was passed by Congress in 1958, requires the FDA to approve food additives, including artificial sweeteners, before they can be made available for sale in the United States. However, this legislation does not apply to products that are "generally recognized as safe." Such products do not require FDA approval before being marketed.

Source: Excerpted from "Artificial Sweeteners and Cancer," National Cancer Institute, August 2009.

Do artificial sweeteners affect weight?

Intuitively, people choose non-caloric artificial sweeteners over sugar to lose or maintain weight. Sugar provides a large amount of rapidly absorbable carbohydrates, leading to excessive energy intake, weight gain, and metabolic syndrome. Sugar and other caloric sweeteners such as high fructose corn syrup have been cast as the main culprits of the obesity epidemic. Whether due to a successful marketing effort on the part of the diet beverage industry or not, the weight conscious public often consider artificial sweeteners "health food." But do artificial sweeteners actually help reduce weight?

Surprisingly, epidemiologic data suggest the contrary. Several large scale prospective cohort studies found positive correlation between artificial sweetener use and weight gain. The San Antonio Heart Study examined 3,682 adults over a seven- to eight-year period in the 1980s. When matched for initial body mass index (BMI), gender, ethnicity, and diet, drinkers of artificially sweetened beverages consistently had higher BMIs at the follow-up, with dose dependence on the amount of consumption. Average BMI gain was +1.01 kg/m2 for control and 1.78 kg/m2 for people in the third quartile for artificially sweetened beverage consumption. The American Cancer Society study conducted in early 1980s included 78,694 women who were highly homogenous with regard to age, ethnicity, socioeconomic status, and lack of preexisting conditions. At one-year follow-up, 2.7 percent to 7.1 percent more regular artificial sweetener users gained weight compared to non-users matched by initial weight. The difference in the amount gained between the two groups was less than two pounds, albeit statistically significant. Saccharin use was also associated with eight-year weight gain in 31,940 women from the Nurses' Health Study conducted in the 1970s.

Similar observations have been reported in children. However, childhood studies often were complicated by the more dynamic growth-associated diet changes. Consumption of both sugar-sweetened and artificially sweetened soda increased and milk consumption decreased with age. A strict differentiation between artificial sweetener users and non-users was not possible. A two-year prospective study involving 166 school children found that increased diet soda consumption was associated with higher BMI Z-scores at follow-up, indicating weight gain. The Growing Up Today Study, involving 11,654 children aged 9 to 14 also reported positive association between diet soda and weight gain for boys. For each daily serving of diet beverage, BMI increased by 0.16 kg/m2. The correlation was not significant for girls. The National Heart, Lung, and Blood Institute Growth and Health Study followed 2,371 girls from age 9 to 19 for 10 years. Both diet and regular soda drinking was associated with increase in total daily energy intake. Soda intake also predicted the greatest increase in BMI, although the correlation between diet soda and BMI was not significant. A cross-sectional study looking at 3,111 children and youth found diet soda drinkers had significantly elevated BMI.

In addition, consensus from interventional studies suggests that artificial sweeteners do not help reduce weight when used alone. BMI did not decrease after 25 weeks of substituting diet beverages for sugar-sweetened beverages in 103 adolescents in a randomized controlled trial, except among the heaviest participants. A double blind study subjected 55 overweight youth to 13 weeks of a 1,000 Kcal diet accompanied by daily capsules of aspartame or lactose placebo. Both groups lost weight, and the difference was not significant. Weight loss was attributed to caloric restriction. Similar results were reported for a 12-week, 1,500 Kcal program using either regular or diet soda. Interestingly, when sugar was covertly switched to aspartame in a metabolic ward, a 25 percent immediate reduction in energy intake was achieved. Conversely, knowingly ingesting aspartame was associated with increased overall energy intake, suggesting overcompensation for the expected caloric reduction. Vigilant monitoring, caloric restriction, and exercise were likely involved in the weight loss seen in multidisciplinary programs that included artificial sweeteners.

Is there an association between artificial sweeteners and cancer?

Questions about artificial sweeteners and cancer arose when early studies showed that cyclamate in combination with saccharin caused bladder cancer in laboratory animals. However, results from subsequent carcinogenicity studies (studies that examine whether a substance can cause cancer) of these sweeteners have not provided clear evidence of an association with cancer in humans. Similarly, studies of other FDA-approved sweeteners have not demonstrated clear evidence of an association with cancer in humans.

Source: Excerpted from "Artificial Sweeteners and Cancer," National Cancer Institute, August 2009.

Experimental Studies On Artificial Sweeteners And Energy

Preload experiments generally have found that sweet taste, whether delivered by sugar or artificial sweeteners, enhanced human appetite. Aspartame-sweetened water, but not aspartame capsule, increased subjective appetite rating in normal weight adult males. Aspartame also increased subjective hunger ratings compared to glucose or water. Glucose preload reduced the perceived pleasantness of sucrose, but aspartame did not. In another study, aspartame, acesulfame potassium, and saccharin were all associated with heightened motivation to eat and more items selected on a food preference list. Aspartame had the most pronounced effect, possibly because it does not have a bitter aftertaste. Unlike glucose or sucrose, which decreased the energy intake at the test meal, artificial sweetener preloads either had no effect or increased subsequent energy intake. Those findings suggest that the calorie contained in natural sweeteners may trigger a response to keep the overall energy consumption constant.

Human research must rely on subjective ratings and voluntary dietary control. Rodent models helped elucidate how artificial sweeteners contribute to energy balance. Rats conditioned with saccharin supplement had significantly elevated total energy intake and gained more weight with increased body adiposity compared to controls conditioned with glucose. Saccharin-conditioned rats also failed to curb their chow intake following a sweet pre-meal. When a flavor was arbitrarily associated with high or low caloric content, rats ate more chow following a pre-meal with the flavor predictive of low caloric content. These studies pose a hypothesis: Inconsistent coupling between sweet taste and caloric content can lead to compensatory overeating and positive energy balance.

Neuronal Responses To Artificial Sweeteners

What drives the desire to eat? Food reward shares brain circuitry with other pleasurable activities such as sex and drug administration. It also shares the same behavioral paradigm with other forms of addiction: binging, withdrawal, craving, and cross-sensitization. A period of abstinence greatly increased sucrose self-administration in rats, similar to binging behavior in humans.

Food reward consists of two branches: sensory and postingestive. In humans, gustatory information perceived by taste receptors on the tongue ascends through the thalamus and eventually terminates in the anterior insula/frontal operculum and the orbitofrontal cortex. Amygdala makes reciprocal connections along all levels of the gustatory pathway. Mesolimbic dopamine system is also crucial for the hedonic recognition of the stimulus and feeling of satisfaction following ingesting food with pleasant tastes.

The postingestive component depends on metabolic products of the food. When food deprived, rats preferred glucose solution over saccharin solution, regardless of flavor that can be masked by adding quinine. The postingestive effects contained both positive and negative neuronal signals separate from mechanical satiety. For moderately concentrated nutrients, rats learned to prefer the food associated with regular feeding than "sham feeding," in which the ingested food flowed out of the body through a gastric fistula. However, rats did not show preference if highly concentrated nutrients were used. Hypothalamus has been shown to mediate the postingestive food reward. Hypothalamus secretes various neuropeptides to regulate energy, osmotic balance, and feeding behavior.

The separation of brain areas in food reward is not exclusive, as dopaminergic activation was associated in sucrose preference in mice lacking sweet taste perception.

Increasing evidence suggests that artificial sweeteners do not activate the food reward pathways in the same fashion as natural sweeteners. Lack of caloric contribution generally eliminates the postingestive component. Functional magnetic imaging in normal weight men showed that glucose ingestion resulted in a prolonged signal depression in the hypothalamus. This response was not observed with sucralose ingestion. Natural and artificial sweeteners also activate the gustatory branch differently. The sweet taste receptor, a heterodimer of two G protein coupled transmembrane receptors, contain several ligand-binding sites. For instance, aspartame and cyclamate, respectively, bind to each of the two monomers. On the functional level, sucrose ingestion, compared to saccharin ingestion, was associated with greater activation of the higher gustatory areas such as the insula, orbitofrontal cortex, and amygdala.

These pilot investigations are consistent with a revised hypothesis: Sweetness decoupled from caloric content offers partial, but not complete, activation of the food reward pathways. Activation of the hedonic component may contribute to increased appetite. Animals seek food to satisfy the inherent craving for sweetness, even in the absence of energy need. Lack of complete satisfaction, likely because of the failure to activate the postingestive component, further fuels the food seeking behavior. Reduction in reward response may contribute to obesity. Impaired activation of the mesolimbic pathways following milkshake ingestion was observed in obese adolescent girls.

Lastly, artificial sweeteners, precisely because they are sweet, encourage sugar craving and sugar dependence. Repeated exposure trains flavor preference. A strong correlation exists between a person's customary intake of a flavor and his preferred intensity for that flavor. Systematic reduction of dietary salt or fat without any flavorful substitution over the course of several weeks led to a preference for lower levels of those nutrients in the research subjects. In light of these findings, a similar approach might be used to reduce sugar intake. Unsweetening the world's diet may be the key to reversing the obesity epidemic.

Part Four
Smart Eating Plans

Chapter 26

MyPlate: A New Food Guidance Icon

MyPlate

The federal government unveiled a new food icon, MyPlate, on June 2, 2011 to serve as a reminder to help consumers make healthier food choices. MyPlate is a new generation icon with the intent to prompt consumers to think about building a healthy plate at meal times and to seek more information to help them do that by going to www.ChooseMyPlate.gov. The new MyPlate icon emphasizes the fruit, vegetable, grains, protein and dairy food groups.

Replacing Pyramids

The Food Guide Pyramid (in use from 1992 to 2005) became one of the most recognized, used, and influential food guides in history. It was widely adopted and used by nutrition educators, food industry, Federal food and nutrition programs, schools, among others, and a large majority of the American public was familiar with the graphic. However, qualitative research in 2002 and 2004 indicated that, while key concepts of the Pyramid were understood, specific knowledge about it was limited. Because consumers preferred images and messages that were perceived as new, personal, and active, and desired some continuity with the original Pyramid shape, USDA simplified the Food Guide Pyramid infographic to create the MyPyramid graphic in 2005.

About This Chapter: "MyPlate" is excerpted from "First Lady, Agriculture Secretary Launch MyPlate Icon as a New Reminder to Help Consumers to Make Healthier Food Choices," a press release from the U.S. Department of Agriculture (USDA), June 2, 2011. "Replaced Pyramids" is excerpted from "Development of 2010 Dietary Guidelines for Americans, Consumer Messages and New Food Icon: Executive Summary of Formative Research," USDA, Center for Nutrition Policy and Promotion, June 2011. "How to Build a Healthy Plate" is excerpted from "Let's Eat for the Health of It," USDA, June 2011.

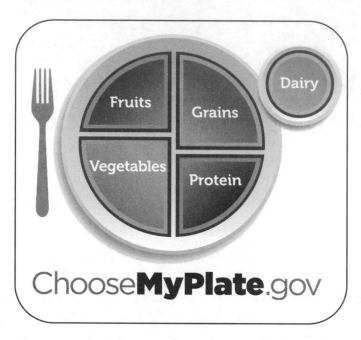

Figure 26.1. MyPlate: The food guidance icon introduced in 2011 (Source: USDA, June 2011).

MyPyramid was designed as a simple icon to represent the MyPyramid Food Guidance System and to direct consumers to information, resources, and tools on MyPyramid.gov, recognizing the difficulty of teaching all pertinent nutrition concepts through a graphic alone.

Over time, confusion arose with some still using the "old Pyramid" and others the "new Pyramid." The Pyramid became simultaneously critiqued for being too complicated and too simplistic. Additionally, concern remained that consumers were so familiar with the Pyramid, that they were not paying attention and implementing its advice.

In May of 2010, the White House Childhood Obesity Task Force released a report that recommended "The Federal government, working with local communities, should disseminate information about the 2010 *Dietary Guidelines for Americans* through simple, easily actionable messages for consumers and a next generation Food Pyramid." While it was recognized that the Pyramid has significant brand equity among nutrition education intermediaries and consumers, some felt that an entirely new image was needed to refocus attention on healthy eating. A plate was identified as a potential alternative image to the food pyramid due to its association with eating and its frequent use in the marketplace to demonstrate to consumers how to build a healthy meal.

A Brief History Of USDA Food Guides

- **1916 to 1930s:** "Food for Young Children" and "How to Select Food" established guidance based on food groups and household measures and focused on "protective foods."

- **1940s:** "A Guide to Good Eating (Basic Seven)" suggested a diet for nutrient adequacy and included the daily number of servings from each of seven food groups: (1) Leafy, green, and yellow vegetables; (2) Citrus fruit, tomatoes, and raw cabbage; (3) Potatoes and other fruits and vegetables; (4) Milk, cheese, and ice cream; (5) Meat, poultry, fish, eggs, dried peas, and beans; (6) Bread, flour, cereals; and (7) Butter and fortified margarine.

- **1956 to 1970s:** "Food for Fitness, A Daily Food Guide (Basic Four)" focused goals for nutrient adequacy and specified amounts from four food groups: (1) Milk group; (2) Meat group; (3); Vegetable and fruit group; and (4) Bread/cereal group.

- **1979:** The "Hassle-Free Daily Food Guide" was based on the Basic Four, but also included a fifth group to highlight the need to moderate intake of fats, sweets, and alcohol.

- **1984:** "Food Wheel: A Pattern for Daily Food Choices" included goals for nutrient adequacy and recommended servings in five food groups: (1) Breads; (2) Fruits; (3); Vegetables; (4) Meat; and (5) Milk. It also called for moderation of alcohol, fats, and sweets.

- **1992:** The "Food Guide Pyramid" illustration focused on variety, moderation, and proportion. It provided visualization of added fats and sugars throughout five food groups and in the tip. It included ranges for daily amounts of food across three calorie levels.

- **2005:** The updated "MyPyramid Food Guidance System" featured a simplified illustration with an added a band for oils and a figure to represent physical activity. Detailed information, including daily amounts of food at 12 calorie levels, was provided through the website MyPyramid.gov [which has been replaced by ChooseMyPlate.gov].

- **2011:** "MyPlate" introduced a different shape to help grab consumers' attention and serve as a reminder for healthy eating.

Source: Excerpted and adapted from "A Brief History of USDA Food Guides," USDA, June 2011.

How To Build A Healthy Meal

Before you eat, think about what goes on your plate or in your cup or bowl. Foods like vegetables, fruits, whole grains, low-fat dairy products, and lean protein foods contain the nutrients you need without too many calories. Try some of these options.

Make half your plate fruits and vegetables: Eat red, orange, and dark-green vegetables, such as tomatoes, sweet potatoes, and broccoli, in main and side dishes. Eat fruit, vegetables, or unsalted nuts as snacks—they are nature's original fast foods.

Switch to skim or 1% milk: They have the same amount of calcium and other essential nutrients as whole milk, but less fat and calories. Try calcium-fortified soy products as an alternative to dairy foods.

Make at least half your grains whole: Choose 100% whole-grain cereals, breads, crackers, rice, and pasta. Check the ingredients list on food packages to find whole-grain foods.

Vary your protein food choices: Twice a week, make seafood the protein on your plate. Eat beans, which are a natural source of fiber and protein, and keep meat and poultry portions small and lean.

Where To Cut Back

Many people eat foods with too much solid fats, added sugars, and salt (sodium). Added sugars and fats load foods with extra calories you don't need. Too much sodium may increase your blood pressure.

Choose foods and drinks with little or no added sugars: Drink water instead of sugary drinks. There are about 10 packets of sugar in a 12-ounce can of soda. Select fruit for dessert. Eat sugary desserts less often. Choose 100% fruit juice instead of fruit-flavored drinks.

Look out for salt (sodium) in foods you buy—it all adds up: Compare sodium in foods like soup, bread, and frozen meals—and choose the foods with lower numbers. Add spices or herbs to season food without adding salt.

Eat fewer foods that are high in solid fats: Make major sources of saturated fats—such as cakes, cookies, ice cream, pizza, cheese, sausages, and hot dogs—occasional choices, not everyday foods. Select lean cuts of meats or poultry and fat-free or low-fat milk, yogurt, and cheese. Switch from solid fats to oils when preparing food.

The Right Amount Of Calories

Everyone has a personal calorie limit. Staying within yours can help you get to or maintain a healthy weight. People who are successful at managing their weight have found ways to keep track of how much they eat in a day, even if they don't count every calorie.

Enjoy your food, but eat less: Get your personal daily calorie limit at www.ChooseMy Plate.gov and keep that number in mind when deciding what to eat. Think before you eat: Is it worth the calories? Avoid oversized portions. Use a smaller plate, bowl, and glass. Stop eating when you are satisfied, not full.

Cook more often at home: At home you are in control of what's in your food.

When eating out, choose lower calorie menu options: Check posted calorie amounts. Choose dishes that include vegetables, fruits, and/or whole grains. Order a smaller portion or share when eating out.

Write it down: Write down what you eat to keep track of how much you eat.

Be Physically Active

Pick activities you like and start by doing what you can, at least 10 minutes at a time. Every bit adds up, and the health benefits increase as you spend more time being active.

Use Food Labels

Most packaged foods have a Nutrition Facts label and an ingredients list. For a healthier you, use this tool to make smart food choices quickly and easily.

- Check for calories. Be sure to look at the serving size and how many servings you are actually consuming. If you double the servings you eat, you double the calories.

- Choose foods with lower calories, saturated fat, trans fat, and sodium.

- Check for added sugars using the ingredients list. When a sugar is close to first on the ingredients list, the food is high in added sugars. Some names for added sugars include sucrose, glucose, high fructose corn syrup, corn syrup, maple syrup, and fructose.

Chapter 27

Eating Well To Live Well

Take Charge

This chapter is designed to help you take small and simple steps to keep a healthy weight. It gives you basic facts about nutrition and physical activity, and offers practical tools that you can use in your everyday life, from reading food labels and selecting how much and what foods to eat, to replacing TV time with physical activities.

Life Can Move At A Hectic Pace

You may feel stressed from school, after-school activities, peer pressure, and family relationships. Your busy schedule may lead you to skip breakfast, buy lunch from vending machines, and grab whatever is in the refrigerator for dinner when you get home.

Make The Time To Think About Your Health

Healthy behaviors, like nutritious eating and regular physical activity, may help you meet the challenges of your life. In fact, healthy eating and regular exercise may help you feel energized, learn better, and stay alert in class. These healthy habits may also lower your risk for diseases such as diabetes, asthma, heart disease, and some forms of cancer.

Healthy Eating

Eating healthfully means getting the right balance of nutrients your body needs to perform every day. You can find out more about your nutritional needs by checking out the *Dietary*

About This Chapter: Excepted from, "Take Charge of Your Health," National Institute of Diabetes and Digestive and Kidney Diseases, August 2009.

Wrong Ways To Lose Weight

From 2003 to 2004, approximately 17.4 percent of U.S. teens between the ages of 12 and 19 were overweight. Overweight children and teens are at high risk for developing serious diseases. Type 2 diabetes and heart disease were considered adult diseases, but they are now being reported in children and teens.

Dieting is not the answer.

The best way to lose weight is to eat healthfully and be physically active. It is a good idea to talk with your health care provider if you want to lose weight.

Many teens turn to unhealthy dieting methods to lose weight, including eating very little, cutting out whole groups of foods (like grain products), skipping meals, and fasting. These methods can leave out important foods you need to grow. Other weight-loss tactics such as smoking, self-induced vomiting, or using diet pills or laxatives can lead to health problems.

In fact, unhealthy dieting can actually cause you to gain more weight because it often leads to a cycle of eating very little, then overeating or binge eating. Also, unhealthy dieting can put you at greater risk for growth and emotional problems.

Source: National Institute of Diabetes and Digestive and Kidney Diseases, August 2009.

Guidelines for Americans. Published by the U.S. Government, this publication explains how much of each type of food you should eat, along with great information on nutrition and physical activity. The guidelines suggest the number of calories you should eat daily based on your gender, age, and activity level.

According to the guidelines, a healthy eating plan includes the following components:

- Fruits and vegetables
- Fat-free or low-fat milk and milk products
- Lean meats, poultry, fish, beans, eggs, and nuts
- Whole grains

In addition, a healthy diet is low in saturated and trans fats, cholesterol, salt, and added sugars.

When it comes to food portions, the *Dietary Guidelines* use the word "servings" to describe a standard amount of food. Serving sizes are measured as "ounce-" or "cup-equivalents." Listed below are some tips based on the guidelines that can help you develop healthy eating habits for a lifetime.

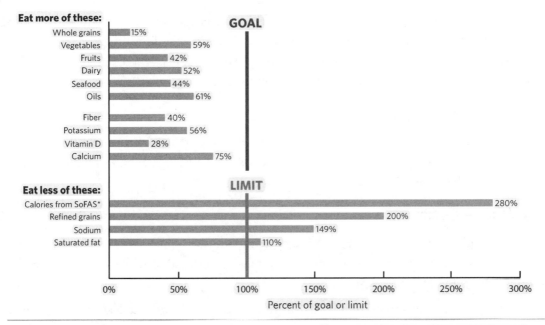

Figure 27.1. How Do Typical American Diets Compare To Recommended Intake Levels Or Limits? (Source: *Dietary Guidelines for Americans 2010*, U.S. Department of Agriculture, December 2010.)

Eat Fruits And Vegetables Every Day

When consumed as part of a well-balanced and nutritious eating plan, fruits and vegetables can help keep you healthy.

You may get your servings from fresh, frozen, dried, and canned fruits and vegetables. Teenagers who are consuming 2,000 calories per day should aim for two cups of fruit and two and a half cups of vegetables every day. You may need fewer or more servings depending on your individual calorie needs, which your health care provider can help you determine.

Count Your Calcium

Calcium helps strengthen bones and teeth. This nutrient is very important, since getting enough calcium now can reduce the risk for broken bones later in life. Yet most teens get less than the recommended 1,200 mg of calcium per day. Aim for at least three one cup-equivalents of low-fat or fat-free calcium-rich foods and beverages each day.

Power Up With Protein

Protein builds and repairs body tissue like muscles and organs. Eating enough protein can help you grow strong and sustain your energy levels. Teens need five and one-half 1 ounce-equivalents of protein-rich foods each day.

Go Whole Grain

Grain foods help give you energy. Whole-grain foods like whole-wheat bread, brown rice, and oatmeal usually have more nutrients than refined grain products. They give you a feeling of fullness and add bulk to your diet.

Try to get six one ounce-equivalents of grains every day, with at least three 1 ounce-equivalents coming from whole-grain sources.

Know Your Fats

Fat is also an important nutrient. It helps your body grow and develop, and it is a source of energy as well—it even keeps your skin and hair healthy. But be aware that some fats are better for you than others. Limit your fat intake to 25 to 35 percent of your total calories each day.

Unsaturated fat can be part of a healthy diet—as long as you do not eat too much since it is still high in calories. Good sources include the following:

- Olive, canola, safflower, sunflower, corn, and soybean oils
- Fish like salmon, trout, tuna, and whitefish
- Nuts like walnuts, almonds, peanuts, and cashews

Limit saturated fat, which can clog your arteries and raise your risk for heart disease. Saturated fat is found primarily in animal products and in a few plant oils like these:

- Butter
- Full-fat cheese
- Whole milk
- Fatty meats
- Coconut, palm, and palm kernel oils

Limit trans fat, which is also bad for your heart. Trans fat is often found in products such as these:

- Baked goods like cookies, muffins, and doughnuts
- Snack foods like crackers and chips
- Vegetable shortening
- Stick margarine
- Fried foods

Look for words like "shortening," "partially hydrogenated vegetable oil," or "hydrogenated vegetable oil" in the list of ingredients. These ingredients tell you that the food contains trans fat. Packaged food products are required to list trans fat on their nutrition facts label.

Replenish Your Body With Iron

Teen boys need iron to support their rapid growth—most boys double their lean body mass between the ages of 10 and 17. Teen girls also need iron to support growth and replace blood lost during menstruation. To get the iron you need, try eating these foods:

- Fish and shellfish
- Lean beef
- Iron-fortified cereals
- Enriched and whole-grain breads
- Cooked dried beans and peas like black beans, kidney beans, black-eyed peas, and chick-peas/garbanzo beans
- Spinach

Control Your Food Portions

The portion sizes that you get away from home at a restaurant, grocery store, or school event may contain more food than you need to eat in one sitting. Research shows that when people are served more food, they eat more food. So, how can you control your food portions? Try these tips:

- When eating out, share your meal, order a half-portion, or order an appetizer as a main meal. Be aware that some appetizers are larger than others and can have as many calories as an entree.

- Take at least half of your meal home.

- When eating at home, take one serving out of a package (read the nutrition facts label to find out how big a serving is) and eat it off a plate instead of eating straight out of a box or bag.

- Avoid eating in front of the TV or while you are busy with other activities. It is easy to lose track of how much you are eating if you eat while doing other things.

- Eat slowly so your brain can get the message that your stomach is full.

- Do not skip meals. Skipping meals may lead you to eat more high-calorie, high-fat foods at your next meal or snack. Eat breakfast every day.

- Read food labels.

When you read a food label, pay special attention to this information:

- **Serving Size:** Check the amount of food in a serving. Do you eat more or less? The "servings per container" line tells you the number of servings in the food package.

- **Calories and Other Nutrients:** Remember, the number of calories and other listed nutrients are for one serving only. Food packages often contain more than one serving.

- **Percent Daily Value:** Look at how much of the recommended daily amount of a nutrient (% DV) is in one serving of food—5% DV or less is low and 20% DV or more is high. For example, if your breakfast cereal has 25% DV for iron, it is high in iron.

Plan Meals And Snacks

You and your family have busy schedules, which can make eating healthfully a challenge. Planning ahead can help. Think about the meals and snacks you would like for the week—including bag lunches to take to school—and help your family make a shopping list. You may even want to go grocery shopping and cook together.

Jumpstart Your Day With Breakfast

Did you know that eating breakfast can help you do better in school? By eating breakfast you can increase your attention span and memory, have more energy, and feel less irritable and restless. A breakfast that is part of a healthy diet can also help you maintain an appropriate weight now and in the future.

Pack Your Own Lunch

Whether you eat lunch from school or pack your own, this meal should provide you with one-third of the day's nutritional needs. A lunch of chips, cookies, candy, or soda just gives you lots of calories, but not many nutrients. Instead of buying snacks from vending machines at school, bring food from home. Try packing your lunch with a lean turkey sandwich on whole-grain bread, healthy foods like fruits, vegetables, low-fat yogurt, and nuts.

Snack Smart

A healthy snack can contribute to a healthy eating plan and give you the energy boost you need to get through the day. Try these snack ideas, but keep in mind that most of these foods should be eaten in small amounts:

- Fruit (any kind—fresh, canned, dried, or frozen)
- Peanut butter on rice cakes or whole-wheat crackers
- Baked potato chips or tortilla chips with salsa
- Veggies with low-fat dip
- String cheese, low-fat cottage cheese, or low-fat yogurt

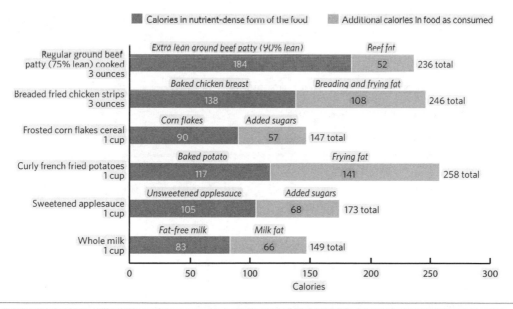

Based on data from the U.S. Department of Agriculture, Agricultural Research Service, Food and Nutrient Database for Dietary Studies 4.1. http://www.ars.usda.gov/Services/docs.htm?docid=20511 and USDA National Nutrient Database for Standard Reference, Release 23. http://www.nal.usda.gov/fnic/foodcomp/search/.

Figure 27.2. Examples Of The Calories In Food Choices That Are Not Nutrient Dense Forms And The Calories In Nutrient Dense Forms Of These Foods. (Source: *Dietary Guidelines for Americans 2010*, U.S. Department of Agriculture, December 2010.)

- Frozen fruit bars, fruit sorbet, or low-fat frozen yogurt
- Vanilla wafers, graham crackers, animal crackers, or fig bars
- Popcorn (air popped or low-fat microwave)

Eat Dinner With Your Family

For many teens, dinner consists of eating on the run, snacking in front of the TV, or nonstop munching from after school to bedtime. Try to eat dinner as a family instead. Believe it or not, when you eat with your family you are more likely to get more fruits, vegetables, and other foods with the vitamins and minerals your body needs. Family meals also help you reconnect after a busy day. Talk to your family about fitting in at least a few meals together throughout the week.

Limit Fast Food And Choose Wisely

Like many teens, you may eat at fast food restaurants often. If so, you are probably taking in a lot of extra calories from added sugar and fat. Just one value-sized fast food meal of a sandwich, fries, and sweetened soda can have more calories, fat, and added sugar than anyone.

The best approach is to limit the amount of fast food you eat. If you do order fast food, try these tips:

- Skip "value-sized" or "super-sized" meals.
- Choose a grilled chicken sandwich or a plain, small burger.
- Use mustard instead of mayonnaise.
- Limit fried foods or remove breading from fried chicken, which can cut half the fat.
- Order garden or grilled chicken salads with light or reduced-calorie dressings.
- Choose water, fat-free, or low-fat milk instead of sweetened soda.
- Rethink your drinks.

Soda and other sugary drinks have replaced milk and water as the drinks of choice for teens and adults alike. Yet these drinks are actually more like desserts because they are high in added sugar and calories. In fact, soda and sugar-laden drinks may contribute to weight problems in kids and teens. Try sticking to water, low-fat milk, or fat-free milk.

Physical Activity

Like eating well, physical activity may help you feel good. Being physically active may benefit you in several ways:

- Help you control your weight, build lean muscle, and reduce your body fat
- Strengthen your bones
- Increase flexibility and balance
- Reduce your risk for chronic diseases like type 2 diabetes, heart disease, and high blood pressure

Physical activity also has possible emotional and social benefits, including the following:

- Improving your self-esteem and mood
- Decreasing feelings of anxiety and depression
- Helping you do better in school
- Improving your teamwork skills through sports

Be Active Every Day

Physical activity should be part of your daily life, whether you play sports, take P.E. or other exercise classes, or even get from place to place by walking or bicycling. Teens should be physically active for 60 minutes or more on most, preferably all, days of the week.

Turn Off The TV And Get Moving

Can too much TV contribute to weight problems? Several research studies say yes. In fact, one study noted that boys and girls who watched the most TV had more body fat than those who watched TV less than two hours a day.

Try to cut back on your TV, computer, and video game time and get moving instead.

Break The TV Habit

Here are some tips to help you break the TV habit:

- Tape your favorite shows and watch them later. This cuts down on TV time because you plan to watch specific shows instead of zoning out and flipping through the channels indefinitely.
- Replace after-school TV watching and video game use with physical activities. Get involved with activities at your school or in your community.

Source: National Institute of Diabetes and Digestive and Kidney Diseases, August 2009.

Making It Work

Look for chances to move more and eat better at home, at school, and in the community.

It is not easy to maintain a healthy weight in today's environment. Fast food restaurants on every corner, vending machines at schools, and not enough safe places for physical activity can make it difficult to eat healthfully and be active. Busy schedules may also keep families from fixing and eating dinners together.

Understanding your home, school, and community is an important step in changing your eating and activity habits. Your answers to the questions on this checklist can help you identify barriers and ways to change your behavior to support your success.

Home

1. Is the kitchen stocked with fruits, vegetables, low-fat or fat-free milk and milk products, whole-grain items, and other foods you need to eat healthy?

2. Can you get water and low-fat or fat-free milk instead of soda, sweetened tea, and sugary fruit drinks?

3. Do you pack healthy lunches to take to school?

4. Does your family eat dinner together a few times per week?

5. Do you have sports or exercise equipment at home, including balls, bikes, and jump ropes?

6. Do you limit the hours you spend watching TV or playing video or computer games?

School

1. Does the cafeteria offer healthy foods such as salads and fruit?

2. Are there vending machines in school where you can buy snacks and drinks like baked chips, fig bars, and bottled water?

3. Do you take gym class on a regular basis?

4. Are there after-school sports or other physical activities available aside from gym class?

Community

1. Are there bike paths, hiking trails, swimming pools, parks, or open fields that are safe to use?

2. Is there a community center, church, or other place that offers classes such as dance, self-defense, or other physical activities?

3. Are there grocery stores that offer fruits, vegetables, and other healthy foods?

4. Do the streets have sidewalks so you can walk safely?

Change Occurs Slowly

Old habits are hard to break and new ones, especially those related to eating and physical activity, can take months to develop and stick with. Here are some tips to help you in the process:

- **Make changes slowly.** Do not expect to change your eating or activity habits overnight. Changing too much too fast can hurt your chances of success. Look at your current eating and physical activity habits and at ways you can make them healthier. Use a food and activity journal for four or five days, and write down everything you eat, your activities, and your emotions. Review your journal to get a picture of your habits. Do you skip breakfast? Are you eating fruits and vegetables every day? Are you physically active most days of the week? Do you eat when you are stressed? Can you substitute physical activity for eating at these times?

- **Set a few realistic goals for yourself.** First, try cutting back the number of sweetened sodas you drink by replacing a couple of them with unsweetened beverages. Once you have reduced your sweetened soda intake, try eliminating these drinks from your diet. Then set a few more goals, like drinking low-fat or fat-free milk, eating more fruits, or getting more physical activity each day.

- **Identify your barriers.** Are there unhealthy snack foods at home that are too tempting? Is the food at your cafeteria too high in fat and added sugars? Do you find it hard to resist drinking several sweetened sodas a day because your friends do it? Use the tips above to identify changes you can make.

- **Get a buddy at school or someone at home to support your new habits.** Ask a friend, sibling, parent, or guardian to help you make changes and stick with your new habits.

- **Know that you can do it.** Use the information in this chapter and the resources listed at the end to help you. Stay positive and focused by remembering why you wanted to be healthier—to look, feel, move, and learn better. Accept relapses—if you fail at one of your nutrition or physical activity goals one day, do not give up. Just try again the next day. Also, share this information with your family. They can support you in adopting healthier behaviors.

Chapter 28

Begin At The Grocery Store

Get Smart As You Shop

Fruits and vegetables can fit into any budget. The following tips can help you save money as you strive to eat more fruits and vegetables.

Before You Shop

- Look for store ads and use them when planning your weekly grocery list. Plan to buy the fruits and vegetables that are on sale and use them in meals and snacks that week.

- Plan your weekly meals and snacks before you go shopping. Look through your freezer and pantry to see what fruits and vegetables you have at home that you can use.

- Make a point to try a new fruit or vegetable each week. Purchase fresh fruits and vegetables in season when they tend to be less expensive.

After You Shop

- Buy whole fruits and vegetables instead of pre-cut or pre-packaged forms, which tend to be more expensive. Consider frozen and canned if fresh are too expensive. Frozen and canned fruits and vegetables keep longer than fresh.

- As you are putting your groceries away, chop some fruits and vegetables and place in bags or storage containers. Keep them in the refrigerator so they will be ready to grab for lunches and snacks.

About This Chapter: Excerpted from "Get Smart As You Shop," an undated document produced by the Centers for Disease Control and Prevention (www.cdc.gov). Information under the heading "Tips for Affordable Vegetables and Fruits" is from "Smart Shopping for Veggies and Fruits," Center for Nutrition Policy and Promotion, U.S. Department of Agriculture, June 2011.

While You Shop

- Consider generic or store brands instead of name brands. Store brands tend to cost less and have similar taste and nutrition.

- Look out for added sugar in canned fruits; look for fruit packed in water or juice. Choose veggies with low sodium.

- If your budget allows, buy larger bags of frozen fruits and vegetables. They may be a better bargain and you can use what you need and keep the rest for later use.

- Buy canned or dried beans and use them in recipes instead of meat, which is more expensive.

- Traditional recipes made with meat such as chili, soups, and Mexican dishes like burritos are delicious with beans.

- Use fresh fruits and vegetables within a few days after shopping and use frozen and canned fruits and vegetables later in the week.

Many varieties of fresh fruit and vegetables are available all year in almost every part of the state, because of excellent transportation and storage facilities. For the greatest nutritional value and flavor, however, choose fruits and vegetables at the peak of their freshness.

Tips For Affordable Vegetables And Fruits

It is possible to fit vegetables and fruits into any budget. Making nutritious choices does not have to hurt your wallet. Getting enough of these foods promotes health and can reduce your risk of certain diseases. There are many low-cost ways to meet your fruit and vegetable needs.

Celebrate the season: Use fresh vegetables and fruits that are in season. They are easy to get, have more flavor, and are usually less expensive. Your local farmer's market is a great source of seasonal produce.

Why pay full price? Check the local newspaper, online, and at the store for sales, coupons, and specials that will cut food costs. Often, you can get more for less by visiting larger grocery stores (discount grocers if available).

Stick to your list: Plan out your meals ahead of time and make a grocery list. You will save money by buying only what you need. Don't shop when you're hungry. Shopping after eating will make it easier to pass on the tempting snack foods. You'll have more of your food budget for vegetables and fruits.

Try canned or frozen: Compare the price and the number of servings from fresh, canned, and frozen forms of the same veggie or fruit. Canned and frozen items may be less expensive than fresh. For canned items, choose fruit canned in 100% fruit juice and vegetables with "low sodium" or "no salt added" on the label.

Buy small amounts frequently: Some fresh vegetables and fruits don't last long. Buy small amounts more often to ensure you can eat the foods without throwing any away.

Buy in bulk when items are on sale: For fresh vegetables or fruits you use often, a large size bag is the better buy. Canned or frozen fruits or vegetables can be bought in large quantities when they are on sale, since they last much longer.

Disparities In Access To Healthy Choices

Ultimately, Americans make their own food and physical activity choices at the individual (and family) level. In order for Americans to make healthy choices, however, they need to have opportunities to purchase and consume healthy foods and engage in physical activity.

Disparities in health among racial and ethnic minorities, individuals with disabilities, and different socioeconomic groups are of substantial concern. Research has demonstrated that some Americans lack access to affordable nutritious foods and/or opportunities for safe physical activity in their neighborhoods. This lack of access makes it a challenge for many Americans to consume a diet consistent with the *Dietary Guidelines for Americans 2010* and maintain physical activity levels consistent with the *2008 Physical Activity Guidelines for Americans*. Thus, access may be related to overall disparities in health. In order for individuals and families to be able to make healthy lifestyle choices, they first need to be aware of and have access to those healthy choices. Access includes not only availability of these choices, but also affordability and safety. Acceptability of the choices is also important.

Source: Excerpted from *Dietary Guidelines for Americans 2010*, U.S. Department of Agriculture, December 2010.

Store brands equal savings: Opt for store brands when possible. You will get the same or similar product for a cheaper price. If your grocery store has a membership card, sign up for even more savings.

Keep it simple: Buy vegetables and fruits in their simplest form. Pre-cut, pre-washed, ready-to-eat, and processed foods are convenient, but often cost much more than when purchased in their basic forms.

Plant your own: Start a garden—in the yard or a pot on the deck—for fresh, inexpensive, flavorful additions to meals. Herbs, cucumbers, peppers, or tomatoes are good options for beginners. Browse through a local library or online for more information on starting a garden.

Plan and cook smart: Prepare and freeze vegetable soups, stews, or other dishes in advance. This saves time and money. Add leftover vegetables to casseroles or blend them to make soup. Overripe fruit is great for smoothies or baking.

Seasonal Chart For Fresh Fruits And Vegetables

Many of the listed fruits and vegetables are available year round, but their cost will be higher and quality may be less. (Sources: Information can be found at www.fruitsandveggiesmatter .gov and University of Tennessee Extension, 2002. A Guide To Buying Fruits & Vegetables at www.utextension.utk.edu/publications/spfiles/SP527.pdf.)

Apples

- **Peak Season:** September through May
- **Tips:** Choose firm apples with no soft spots.

Avocado

- **Peak Season:** Year round
- **Tips:** Ripe fruit will be slightly firm, but yield to gentle pressure.

Banana

- **Peak Season:** Year round
- **Tips:** Select bananas that are firm, with no bruises.

Bell Pepper

- **Peak Season:** Year round
- **Tips:** Choose peppers with firm skin, with no wrinkles.

Broccoli

- **Peak Season:** October through May
- **Tips:** Select bunches that are dark green.

Cantaloupe

- **Peak Season:** May through September
- **Tips:** Select melons that are slightly golden with a light fragrant smell.

Carrots

- **Peak Season:** Year round
- **Tips:** Pick carrots that are deep orange in color. Avoid carrots that are cracked or wilted.

Corn

- **Peak Season:** May through September
- **Tips:** Husks should be green, tight, and fresh looking. The car should have tightly packed rows of plump kernels.

Cucumber

- **Peak Season:** May through August
- **Tips:** Choose firm cucumbers with rich green color and no soft spots.

Eggplant

- **Peak Season:** July through October
- **Tips:** Pick symmetrical eggplant; avoid oversized eggplants with may be tough and bitter.

Grapes

- **Peak Season:** June through December
- **Tips:** Look for firm, plump, well-colored clusters.

Lettuce

- **Peak Season:** Year round
- **Tips:** Choose fresh, crisp leaves with no wilting.

Mushrooms

- **Peak Season:** November through May
- **Tips:** Mushrooms should be firm, moisture-free (not dry), and blemish-free.

Onion

- **Peak Season:** Year round
- **Tips:** Onions should feel dry and solid with no soft spots or sprouts.

Orange

- **Peak Season:** November through June
- **Tips:** Pick oranges that are firm, heavy for their size and have bright colorful skins.

Peach

- **Peak Season:** June through September
- **Tips:** Choose peaches that are soft to the touch with a fragrant smell.

Pear

- **Peak Season:** August through May
- **Tips:** Ripe pears will yield slightly to gently pressure a the stem end.

Strawberries

- **Peak Season:** April through July
- **Tips:** Strawberries should be dry, firm and well shaped and be a bright shade of red.

Summer Squash

- **Peak Season:** June through August
- **Tips:** Look for squash that are firm with bright, glossy exteriors.

Tips For Making Healthy Meat Choices

When shopping, start with a lean choice:

- The leanest beef cuts include round steaks and roasts (eye of round, top round, bottom round, round tip), top loin, top sirloin, and chuck shoulder and arm roasts.

- The leanest pork choices include pork loin, tenderloin, center loin, and ham.

- Choose extra lean ground beef. The label should say at least "90% lean." You may be able to find ground beef that is 93% or 95% lean.

- Buy skinless chicken parts, or take off the skin before cooking.

- Boneless skinless chicken breasts and turkey cutlets are the leanest poultry choices.

- Choose lean turkey, roast beef, ham, or low-fat luncheon meats for sandwiches instead of luncheon/deli meats with more fat, such as regular bologna or salami.

Source: Excerpted from "Food Groups: Protein Foods," U.S. Department of Agriculture (ChooseMyPlate.gov), June 8, 2011.

Sweet Potato

- **Peak Season:** September through December
- **Tips:** Choose firm, dark, smooth sweet potatoes.

Tomato

- **Peak Season:** May through August

- **Tips:** Select plump tomatoes with smooth skins, free [of blemishes].

Chapter 29

Eating Well While Eating Out

If I Eat Well At Home, What's Wrong With Splurging When I Eat Out?

A slice of pizza once in a while won't do you any harm. What's important is a person's average food intake over a few days, not just in a single meal. So if you eat a less-than-healthy meal once in a while, try to balance it with healthier foods the rest of that day and week.

But if pizza (or any fast food) is all you eat, that can lead to problems. The most obvious health threat of eating too much fast food is weight gain—or even obesity.

But weight gain isn't the only problem. Too much fast food can drag a person's body down in other ways. Because the food we eat affects all aspects of how the body functions, eating the right (or wrong) foods can influence any number of things, including:

- mental functioning
- emotional well-being
- energy
- strength
- weight
- future health

Eating On The Go

It's actually easier than you think to make good choices at a fast-food restaurant, the mall, or even the school cafeteria. Most cafeterias and fast-food places offer healthy choices that are also tasty, like grilled chicken or salads. Be mindful of portion sizes and high fat add-ons, like dressings, sauces or cheese. Here are some pointers to remember that can help you make wise choices when eating out:

Go for balance: Choose meals that contain a balance of lean proteins (like fish, chicken, or beans if you're a vegetarian), fruits and vegetables (fries and potato chips don't qualify as veggies), and whole-grains (like whole wheat bread and brown rice). That's why a turkey sandwich on whole wheat with lettuce and tomato is a better choice than a cheeseburger on a white bun.

Watch portion sizes: The portion sizes of American foods have increased over the past few decades so that we are now eating way more than we need. The average size of a hamburger in the 1950s was just one and a half ounces, compared with today's hamburgers, which weigh in at eight ounces or more.

Drink water or low-fat milk: Regular sodas, juices, and energy drinks usually contain "empty" calories that you don't need—not to mention other stuff, like caffeine.

Tips For Eating At A Restaurant

Most restaurant portions are way larger than the average serving of food at home. Ask for half portions, share an entrée with a friend, or take half of your dish home.

Here are some other restaurant survival tips:

- Ask for sauces and salad dressings on the side and use them sparingly.

- Use salsa and mustard instead of mayonnaise or oil.

- Ask for olive or canola oil instead of butter, margarine, or shortening.

- Use nonfat or low-fat milk instead of whole milk or cream.

- Order baked, broiled, or grilled (not fried) lean meats including turkey, chicken, seafood, or sirloin steak.

- Salads and vegetables make healthier side dishes than french fries.

- Use a small amount of sour cream instead of butter if you order a baked potato.

- Choose fresh fruit instead of sugary, high-fat desserts.

> ## Remember
> It can be easy to eat well, even on the run. If you develop the skills to make healthy choices now, your body will thank you later. And the good news is you don't have to eat perfectly all the time. It's okay to splurge every once in a while, as long as your food choices are generally good.

Tips For Eating At The Mall Or Fast-Food Place

It's tempting to pig out while shopping, but with a little planning, it's easy to eat healthy foods at the mall. Here are some choices:

- A single slice of veggie pizza
- Grilled, not fried, sandwiches (for example, a grilled chicken breast sandwich)
- Deli sandwiches on whole-grain bread
- A small hamburger
- A bean burrito
- A baked potato
- A side salad
- Frozen yogurt

Choose the smaller sizes, especially when it comes to drinks and snacks if you have a craving for something unhealthy, try sharing the food you crave with a friend.

Tips For Eating In The School Cafeteria

The suggestions for eating in a restaurant and at the mall apply to cafeteria food as well. Add vegetables and fruit whenever possible, and opt for leaner, lighter items. Choose sandwiches on whole-grain bread or a plain hamburger over fried foods or pizza. Go easy on the high-fat, low-nutrition items, such as mayonnaise and heavy salad dressings.

You might want to consider packing your own lunch occasionally. Here are some lunch items that pack a healthy punch:

- Sandwiches with lean meats or fish, like turkey, chicken, tuna salad (made with low-fat mayo), lean ham, or lean roast beef (for variety, try other sources of protein, like peanut butter, hummus, or meatless chili)

- Low-fat or nonfat milk, yogurt, or cheese

- Any fruit that's in season

- Raw baby carrots, green and red pepper strips, tomatoes, or cucumbers

- Whole-grain breads, pita, bagels, or crackers

Chapter 30

Ordering Fast Food

Fast foods are quick, reasonably priced, and readily available alternatives to home cooking. While convenient and inexpensive for a busy lifestyle, fast foods are typically high in calories, fat, saturated fat, sugar, and salt.

Fast food chains and restaurants have responded to the public's increasing awareness about nutrition and have attempted to help people concerned about health. For example, they now make ingredient and nutrition information available on their menus. Despite these changes, however, in order to maintain a healthy diet, it is necessary to choose fast foods carefully.

Function

Most people today have less time to select, prepare, and eat food than their grandparents did. Fast foods are very appealing because they are widely available and inexpensive.

Food Sources

Fast food items have been modified to reflect consumers' concern about the fat content of their food. Many fast food restaurants have switched from beef tallow or lard to hydrogenated vegetable oils for frying.

Some restaurants offer low calorie choices like salad bars and assorted take-out salads with low calorie dressing, low-fat milkshakes, whole grain buns, lean meats, and grilled chicken items.

About This Chapter: "Fast Foods," © 2011 A.D.A.M., Inc. Reprinted with permission.

Fast Food And Obesity

Studies examining the relationship between the food environment and body mass index (BMI) have found that communities with a larger number of fast food or quick-service restaurants tend to have higher BMIs. Since the 1970s, the number of fast food restaurants has more than doubled. Further, the proportion of daily calorie intake from foods eaten away from home has increased, and evidence shows that children, adolescents, and adults who eat out, particularly at fast food restaurants, are at increased risk of weight gain, overweight, and obesity.

The strongest association between fast food consumption and obesity is when one or more fast food meals are consumed per week. As a result of the changing food environment, individuals need to deliberately make food choices, both at home and away from home, that are nutrient dense, low in calories, and appropriate in portion size.

Source: Excerpted from *Dietary Guidelines for Americans 2010*, U.S. Department of Agriculture, December 2010.

Side Effects

Maintaining nutritional balance is not easy with fast food, because there is no control over how they are cooked. For example, some are cooked with a lot of oil and butter, and there may be no option if you want your selection with reduced fat.

The large portions often served at restaurants also encourage overeating. Fast food also tend to lack fresh fruits and vegetables.

In general, people with high blood pressure, diabetes, and heart disease must be much more careful about choosing fast food, due to the high content of fat, sodium, and sugar.

Recommendations

Knowing the number of calories and the amount of fat and salt in the fast food can help you decide which items are better choices. Many fast food restaurants have published the nutrient content of their foods. These are often available on request. You can plan a convenient yet healthful meal with the following information.

Make better choices when eating at fast food restaurants. In general eat at places that offer a variety of salads, soups, and vegetables.

Choose smaller-sized servings. Consider splitting some fast food items to reduce the amount of calories and fat. Ask for a "doggy bag," or simply leave the excess on your plate.

To help supplement and balance a fast food meal, make nutritious options such as fresh fruits, vegetables, and yogurt available as snacks.

When chosen carefully and not used in excess, fast foods can offer reasonably good quality nutrition. By being aware of what and how much you eat, and paying attention to how it affects your health. As always, variety and moderation are the key principles in providing a healthy diet for children as well as adults.

Consider these general tips:

Pizza: Ask for less cheese, and choose low-fat toppings such as onions, mushrooms, green peppers, tomatoes, and other vegetables.

Sandwiches: Healthier choices include regular or junior-size lean roast beef, turkey, or chicken breast, or lean ham. Extras, such as, bacon, cheese, or mayo will increase the fat and calories of the item. Select whole-grain breads over high-fat croissants or biscuits.

Hamburgers: A single, plain meat patty without the cheese and sauces is the best choice. Ask for extra lettuce, tomatoes, and onions. Limit your intake of french fries.

Meat, chicken, and fish: Look for items that are roasted, grilled, baked, or broiled. Avoid meats that are breaded or fried. Ask for heavy sauces, such as gravy, on the side. Better still, avoid heavy sauces and dressings altogether.

Salads: High-fat food items such as dressing, bacon bits, and shredded cheese add fat and calories. Choose lettuce and assorted vegetables to make up the majority of your salad. Select low-fat or fat-free salad dressings, vinegar, or lemon juice when available. Ask for the salad dressing on the side.

Desserts: Choose low-fat frozen yogurt, fruit ices, sorbets, and sherbets. Occasional indulgent desserts add fun to a carefully selected, well-balanced diet.

Chapter 31

Eating In The School Cafeteria

You're sitting in class and your stomach is starting to rumble. Finally, the bell rings and it's time for lunch. After all that time in class, you deserve a chance to head to the cafeteria and sit down, relax, and enjoy the company of your friends over a lunchtime meal. But wait a minute—what exactly are you eating?

More than at other meals, kids have a lot of control over what they eat for lunch at school. A kid can choose to eat the green beans or throw them out. A kid also can choose to eat an apple instead of an ice cream sandwich.

When choosing what to eat for lunch, making a healthy choice is really important. Here's why: Eating a variety of healthy foods gives you energy to do stuff, helps you grow the way you should, and can even keep you from getting sick.

Think of your school lunch as the fuel you put in your tank. If you choose the wrong kind of fuel, you might run out of energy before the day is over. So what is the right kind of fuel? What does a healthy lunch look like? Unlike that killer question on your math test, there are many right answers to these questions.

To Buy Or Not To Buy

Most kids have the choice of packing lunch or buying one at school. The good news is that a kid can get a healthy lunch by doing either one. But it's not a slam-dunk. Chances are, some meals and foods served in the school cafeteria are healthier than others.

About This Chapter: "School Lunches," April 2007, reprinted with permission from www.kidshealth.org. Copyright © 2007 The Nemours Foundation. This information was provided by KidsHealth, one of the largest resources online for medically reviewed health information written for parents, kids, and teens. For more articles like this one, visit www.KidsHealth.org, or www.TeensHealth.org.

The typical school lunch is still higher in fat than it should be, according to a recent study. That doesn't mean you shouldn't buy your lunch, it just means you might want to give the cafeteria menu a closer look. Read the cafeteria menu the night before. Knowing what's for lunch beforehand will let you know if you want to eat it! Bring home a copy of the menu or figure out how to find it on the school website.

If you want to pack your lunch, you'll need some help from your parents. Talk to them about what you like to eat in your lunch so they can stock up on those foods. A parent may offer to pack your lunch for you. This is nice of them, but you may want to watch how they do it and ask if you can start making your lunches yourself. It's a way to show that you're growing up.

Remember

A packed lunch isn't automatically healthier than one you buy at school. If you pack chocolate cake and potato chips, that's not a nutritious meal! But a packed lunch, if you do it right, does have a clear advantage. When you pack your lunch, you can be sure it includes your favorite healthy foods—stuff you know you like. It's not a one-size-fits-all lunch. It's a lunch just for you. If your favorite sandwich is peanut butter and banana, just make it and pack it—then you can eat it for lunch. Or maybe you love olives. Go ahead and pack them.

Ten Steps To A Great Lunch

Whether you pack or buy your lunch, follow these guidelines:

1. **Choose fruits and vegetables.** Fruits and vegetables are like hitting the jackpot when it comes to nutrition. They make your plate more colorful and they're packed with vitamins and fiber. It's a good idea to eat at least five servings of fruits and vegetables every day, so try to fit in one or two at lunch. A serving isn't a lot. A serving of carrots is half cup or about six baby carrots. A fruit serving could be one medium orange.

2. **Know the facts about fat.** Kids need some fat in their diets to stay healthy—it also helps keep you feeling full—but you don't want to eat too much of it. Fat is found in butter, oils, cheese, nuts, and meats. Some higher-fat lunch foods include french fries, hot dogs, cheeseburgers, macaroni and cheese, and chicken nuggets. Don't worry if you like these foods. No food is bad, but you may want to eat them less often and in smaller portions. Foods that are lower in fat are usually baked or grilled. Some of the best low-fat foods are fruits, vegetables, and skim and low-fat milk.

3. **Let whole grains reign.** "Grains" include breads, cereals, rice, and pasta. But as we learn more about good nutrition, it's clear that whole grains are better than refined grains. What's the difference? Brown rice is a whole grain, but white rice is not. Likewise, wheat bread contains whole grains, whereas 100% white bread does not.

4. **Slurp sensibly.** It's not just about what you eat—drinks count, too! Milk has been a favorite lunchtime drink for a long time. If you don't like milk, choose water. Avoid juice drinks and sodas.

5. **Balance your lunch.** When people talk about balanced meals, they mean meals that include a mix of food groups: some grains, some fruits, some vegetables, some meat or protein foods, and some dairy foods such as milk and cheese. Try to do this with your lunch. If you don't have a variety of foods on your plate, it's probably not balanced. A double order of french fries, for example, would not make for a balanced lunch.

6. **Steer clear of packaged snacks.** Many schools make salty snacks, candy, and soda available in the cafeteria or in vending machines. It's okay to have these foods once in a while, but they shouldn't be on your lunch menu.

7. **Mix it up.** Do you eat the same lunch every day? If that lunch is a hot dog, it's time to change your routine. Keep your taste buds from getting bored and try something new. Eating lots of different kinds of food gives your body a variety of nutrients.

8. **Quit the clean plate club.** Because lunch can be a busy time, you might not stop to think whether you're getting full. Try to listen to what your body is telling you. If you feel full, it's okay to stop eating.

9. **Use your manners.** Cafeterias sometimes look like feeding time at the zoo. Don't be an animal. Follow those simple rules your parents are always reminding you about: Chew with your mouth closed. Don't talk and eat at the same time. Use your utensils. Put your napkin on your lap. Be polite. And don't make fun of what someone else is eating.

10. **Don't drink milk and laugh at the same time.** Whatever you do at lunch, don't tell your friends a funny joke when they're drinking milk. Before you know it, they'll be laughing and that milk will be coming out their noses.

Chapter 32

Healthy Snacking

A common misconception is that snacking isn't a healthy habit for growing teens. The truth is that most teens need snacks—the trick is making healthy food choices in the right amounts. Eating too many calories can cause teens to become overweight, which puts them at higher risk for developing type 2 diabetes, a disease that's now being diagnosed in teens.

Teens can lower their risk for type 2 diabetes if they stay at a healthy weight by being physically active and choosing the right amounts of healthy foods—including snacks. When making snacks, use a small plate or bowl and snack at the table instead of in front of the TV or computer. These habits help teens control portion size and take their time while eating so they don't eat too much. Teens should also be active. One strategy is to participate in fun family outings, another is to join active youth recreation programs.

Smart Snack Suggestions

1. Make a fruit pizza by spreading two tablespoons of nonfat cream cheese on a toasted English muffin. Top with ¼ cup of sliced strawberries, handful of grapes, or ¼ cup of any fruit canned in its own juice. Or top with broccoli, carrots, and tomatoes for a veggie twist.

2. Eat a small bag or handful of baked chips, pretzels, or single-serving bag of air-popped popcorn.

3. Create a homemade fruit smoothie by combining ½ cup frozen vanilla yogurt, ½ cup 100% orange juice, and one peeled orange in a blender.

About This Chapter: Excerpted from, "Ten Smart Snacks For Teens," an undated document produced by the National Diabetes Education Program (http://ndep.nih.gov).

Snack Tips

Try to pick snacks to fill in your dietary gaps:

- Hit your day's grain target by snacking on a bagel, pretzels, popcorn, muffin, breakfast cereal, or oatmeal cookies, among others.

- If your day's meals come up short in vegetables and fruits, reach for crunchy raw vegetables, frozen fruit juice bars, dried fruit, or a piece of whole fruit.

- Short on dairy? Grab string cheese, a carton of reduced fat yogurt, frozen yogurt, or guzzle a glass of milk.

- If you have a gap in your proteins, try a hard-boiled egg, a slice of meat, or a handful of peanuts.

Excerpted from "Snack Attack," From yourSELF Middle School Nutrition Education Kit, U.S. Department of Agriculture (USDA), 1998. Despite the older date of this document, the snack suggestions are still helpful.

4. Have two rice cakes, six whole-grain crackers, or one slice of whole-grain bread served with low-fat cheese, fruit spread, hummus, or peanut butter.

5. Opt for an individual serving size of sugar-free, nonfat pudding instead of regular ice cream.

Remember These Suggestions

- Take time to enjoy your snacks, as well as your meals.

- It takes a while for your brain to know your stomach is full. Slow down, eat, and enjoy.

- If you snack on foods that have some fat or sugars, no problem—just keep your helpings sensible.

- Make snack drinks count toward food-group servings. Drinking reduced fat milk, fruit juice, or a shake as a snack can help meet your day's requirements.

- Do you reach for a snack when you're bored, nervous, happy, angry, or tense? If you do, you may be eating when you're not hungry. Find other ways to handle your feelings. Go for a walk, listen to music, or call a friend.

- Use food labels to make smart snack choices. The Nutrition Facts tell you the calories, fat, and other nutrients in one serving. (Double the numbers for two servings.)

Excerpted from "Snack Attack," From yourSELF Middle School Nutrition Education Kit, U.S. Department of Agriculture (USDA), 1998. Despite the older date of this document, the snack suggestions are still helpful.

Snacks Can Help You Eat More Fruits And Vegetables

Use these easy tips and recipes to help you eat a colorful variety of fruits and vegetables everyday.

- Try hummus and whole wheat pitas.
- Snack on vegetables like bell pepper strips and broccoli with a low-fat or fat-free ranch dip.
- Try baked tortilla chips with black bean and corn salsa.
- Stash bags of dried fruit at your desk for a convenient snack.
- Keep a bowl of fruit on your desk or counter.
- Drink a fruit smoothie made with whole fruit, ice cubes, and low-fat or fat-free yogurt.
- Top a cup of fat-free or low-fat yogurt with sliced fresh fruit.
- For quick and easy snacks, stock up on fresh, dried, frozen, and canned fruits and vegetables.
- Pick up ready-packed salad greens from the produce shelf for a quick salad any time.
- Store cleaned, cut-up vegetables in the fridge at eye level and keep a low-fat or fat-free dip on hand.
- Canned, dried, and frozen fruits and vegetables are also good options. Look for fruit without added sugar or syrups and vegetables without added salt, butter, or cream sauces.

Sweet Potato Fries

1. Preheat oven to 425° F.
2. Cut uncooked sweet potatoes into thin slices.
3. Dip slices in a mixture of egg substitute and nutmeg.
4. Spray a baking pan lightly with a non-stick cooking spray. Arrange the slices in a single layer on the baking pan.
5. Bake for 20 minutes or until slices are tender.

Bean Quesadillas

1. Spread low-fat cheese and low-fat or fat-free refried beans between two tortillas.
2. Brown on both sides in a pan until cheese melts.

Source: Excerpted from "Snacks," an undated document produced by the Centers for Disease Control and Prevention (www.cdc.gov).

6. Choose a small tortilla with one or two slices of low-fat cheese or turkey, or a small bowl of vegetable soup and a few crackers.

7. Snack on one cup of whole-grain cereal with nonfat or low-fat milk and add ¼ cup of blueberries, strawberries, or peaches.

8. Spread one tablespoon of peanut butter on a tortilla and then sprinkle one tablespoon of whole grain cereal on top. Peel and place one banana on the tortilla and then roll the tortilla for a crunchy treat.

9. Try an apple, banana, or plum with one or two reduced-fat or low-fat string cheese sticks.

10. Combine 1/8 cup of almonds and 1/8 cup of dried cranberries, cherries, or raisins with ½ cup of whole-grain cereal for a fun trail mix.

Chapter 33

What You Should Know About Caffeine And Energy Drinks

It's 11 p.m. and Aaron has already had a full day of school, work, and after-school activities. He's tired and knows he could use some sleep. But he still hasn't finished his homework. So he reaches for his headphones—and some caffeine.

What Is Caffeine?

Caffeine is a drug that is naturally produced in the leaves and seeds of many plants. It's also produced artificially and added to certain foods. Caffeine is defined as a drug because it stimulates the central nervous system, causing increased alertness. Caffeine gives most people a temporary energy boost and elevates mood.

Caffeine is in tea, coffee, chocolate, many soft drinks, and pain relievers and other over-the-counter medications. In its natural form, caffeine tastes very bitter. But most caffeinated drinks have gone through enough processing to camouflage the bitter taste.

Teens usually get most of their caffeine from soft drinks and energy drinks. (In addition to caffeine, these also can have added sugar and artificial flavors.) Caffeine is not stored in the body, but you may feel its effects for up to six hours.

Got The Jitters?

Many people feel that caffeine increases their mental alertness. Higher doses of caffeine can cause anxiety, dizziness, headaches, and the jitters. Caffeine can also interfere with normal sleep.

About This Chapter: "Caffeine," January 2008, reprinted with permission from www.kidshealth.org. Copyright © 2008 The Nemours Foundation. This information was provided by KidsHealth, one of the largest resources online for medically reviewed health information written for parents, kids, and teens. For more articles like this one, visit www.KidsHealth.org, or www.TeensHealth.org.

Caffeine sensitivity (the amount of caffeine that will produce an effect in someone) varies from person to person. On average, the smaller the person, the less caffeine needed to produce side effects. Caffeine sensitivity is most affected by the amount of caffeine a person has daily. People who regularly take in a lot of caffeine soon develop less sensitivity to it. This means they may need more caffeine to achieve the same effects.

Caffeine is a diuretic, meaning it causes a person to urinate (pee) more. It's not clear whether this causes dehydration or not. To be safe, it's probably a good idea to stay away from too much caffeine in hot weather, during long workouts, or in other situations where you might sweat a lot.

Caffeine may also cause the body to lose calcium, and that can lead to bone loss over time. Drinking caffeine-containing soft drinks and coffee instead of milk can have an even greater impact on bone density and the risk of developing osteoporosis.

Caffeine can aggravate certain heart problems. It may also interact with some medications or supplements. If you are stressed or anxious, caffeine can make these feelings worse. Although caffeine is sometimes used to treat migraine headaches, it can make headaches worse for some people.

Moderation Is The Key

Caffeine is usually thought to be safe in moderate amounts. Experts consider 200–300 mg of caffeine a day to be a moderate amount for adults. But consuming as little as 100 milligrams (mg) of caffeine a day can lead a person to become "dependent" on caffeine. This means that someone may develop withdrawal symptoms (like tiredness, irritability, and headaches) if he or she quits caffeine suddenly.

Teens should try to limit caffeine consumption to no more than 100 mg of caffeine daily, and kids should get even less. Table 33.1 shows common caffeinated products and the amounts of caffeine they contain:

Too Wired

People can now buy drinks with a whopping 500 mg of caffeine. This amount is risky for some people—even more so when these drinks are combined with other foods that contain caffeine (like a chocolate bar or soda) or medications.

Source: Copyright © 2008 The Nemours Foundation.

Table 33.1. Amounts Of Caffeine In Common Caffeinated Products In Milligrams (mg)

Drink/Food/Supplement	Amt. of Drink/Food	Amt. of Caffeine
SoBe No Fear	8 ounces	83 mg
Monster energy drink	16 ounces	160 mg
Rockstar energy drink	8 ounces	80 mg
Red Bull energy drink	8.3 ounces	80 mg
Jolt cola	12 ounces	72 mg
Mountain Dew	12 ounces	55 mg
Coca-Cola	12 ounces	54 mg
Diet Coke	12 ounces	45 mg
Pepsi	12 ounces	38 mg
7-Up	12 ounces	0 mg
Brewed coffee (drip method)	5 ounces	115 mg*
Iced tea	12 ounces	70 mg*
Cocoa beverage	5 ounces	4 mg*
Chocolate milk beverage	8 ounces	5 mg*
Dark chocolate	1 ounce	20 mg*
Milk chocolate	1 ounce	6 mg*
Jolt gum	1 stick	33 mg
Cold relief medication	1 tablet	30 mg*
Vivarin	1 tablet	200 mg
Excedrin extra strength	2 tablets	130 mg

*denotes average amount of caffeine

Source of data: U.S. Food and Drug Administration, National Soft Drink Association, Center for Science in the Public Interest.

Cutting Back

If you're taking in too much caffeine, you may want to cut back. The best way is to cut back slowly. Otherwise you could get headaches and feel tired, irritable, or just plain lousy.

Try cutting your intake by replacing caffeinated sodas and coffee with non-caffeinated drinks. Options include water, decaffeinated coffee, caffeine-free sodas, and caffeine-free teas. Start by keeping track of how many caffeinated drinks you have each day, then substitute one of these daily drinks with a caffeine-free alternative. Continue this for a week. Then, if you are still drinking too much caffeine, substitute another of your daily drinks, again, keeping it up for a week. Do this for as many weeks as it takes to bring your daily caffeine intake below the 100-milligram mark. Taking a gradual approach like this can help you wean yourself from caffeine without unwanted side effects like headaches.

As you cut back on the amount of caffeine you consume, you may find yourself feeling tired. Your best bet is to hit the sack, not the sodas: It's just your body's way of telling you it needs more rest. Your energy levels will return to normal in a few days.

Energy Drinks May Hurt Kids

Energy drinks such as Red Bull, AMP, and Rockstar have no health value and may even harm some children and teens, a new review finds.

The increasingly popular, highly caffeinated drinks are especially risky for children with heart abnormalities, attention deficit hyperactivity disorder (ADHD), or other health or emotional problems, said Dr. Steven E. Lipshultz, co-author of the study, published online February 14, 2011 in the journal *Pediatrics*.

"It's a set of products that are totally unregulated and have no therapeutic benefit," said Lipshultz, chairman of pediatrics at the University of Miami.

Surveys suggest that 30 percent to 50 percent of U.S. teenagers and young people consume energy drinks, despite warnings about their safety. Many users mix the energy drinks with alcohol, further heightening the potential for ill effects, say the researchers.

But even without the addition of alcohol, the beverages carry some measure of risk, according to the study authors, who reviewed numerous articles for their report.

For one thing, safe levels of energy drinks, which contain stimulants such as caffeine, taurine, and guarana, have not been established for children and teens, the authors said.

An 8-ounce energy drink may contain dozens or hundreds of milligrams of caffeine, compared to 100 milligrams of caffeine in a generic cup of coffee. An 8-ounce serving of Red Bull contains 77 milligrams of caffeine, compared to 28 milligrams in an equal amount of Mountain Dew, the report noted.

Energy-drink manufacturers often add other ingredients, such as sugar and herbal supplements, whose effects haven't been well-studied. And, some ingredients can interfere with medications, the authors added.

Chapter 34

Fast Facts About Sports Nutrition

Water, Water Everywhere

You can survive for a month without food, but only a few days without water. Water is the most important nutrient for active people.

When you sweat, you lose water, which must be replaced. Drink fluids before, during, and after workouts. Water is a fine choice for most workouts. However; during continuous workouts of greater than 90 minutes, your body may benefit from a sports drink.

Sports drinks have two very important ingredients: electrolytes and carbohydrates. Sports drinks replace electrolytes lost through sweat during workouts lasting several hours. Carbohydrates in sports drinks provide extra energy. The most effective sports drinks contain 15 to 18 grams of carbohydrate in every eight ounces of fluid.

Rev Up Your Engine With Carbohydrates

Carbohydrates are your body's main source of energy. Carbohydrates are sugars and starches, and they are found in foods such as breads, cereals, fruits, vegetables, pasta, milk, honey, syrups and table sugar.

Sugars and starches are broken down by your body into glucose, which is used by your muscles for energy. For health and peak performance, more than half your daily calories should come from carbohydrates.

About This Chapter: This chapter begins with excerpts from, "Fast Facts About Sports Nutrition," President's Council on Physical Fitness and Sports (http://www.fitness.gov), 2010. It continues with excerpts from "Questions Most Frequently Asked about Sports Nutrition," an undated document also produced by the President's Council on Physical Fitness and Sports.

Sugars and starches have four calories per gram, while fat has nine calories per gram. In other words, carbohydrates have less than half the calories of fat.

If you regularly eat a carbohydrate-rich diet you probably have enough carbohydrate stored to fuel activity. Even so, be sure to eat a precompetition meal for fluid and additional energy. What you eat as well as when you eat your precompetition meal will be entirely individual.

Flexing Your Options To Build Bigger Muscles

It is a myth that eating lots of protein and/or taking protein supplements and exercising vigorously will definitely turn you into a big, muscular person. Building muscle depends on your genes, how hard you train, and whether you get enough calories.

The average American diet has more than enough protein for muscle building. Extra protein is eliminated from the body or stored as fat.

Score With Vitamins And Minerals

Eating a varied diet will give you all the vitamins and minerals you need for health and peak performance. Exceptions include active people who follow strict vegetarian diets, avoid an entire group of foods, or eat less than 1,800 calories a day. If you fall into any of these categories, a multivitamin and mineral pill may provide the vitamins and minerals missing in your diet.

Taking large doses of vitamins and minerals will not help your performance and may be bad for your health. Vitamins and minerals do not supply the body with energy and, therefore, are not a substitute for carbohydrates.

Popeye And All That Spinach

Iron supplies working muscles with oxygen. If your iron level is low, you may tire easily and not have enough stamina for activity. The best sources of iron are animal products, but plant foods such as fortified breads, cereals, beans and green leafy vegetables also contain iron.

Iron supplements may have side effects, so take them only if your doctor tells you to.

A Weighty Matter

Your calorie needs depend on your age, body size, sport and training program. The best way to make sure you are not getting too many or too few calories is to check your weight from time to time. If you're keeping within your ideal weight range, you're probably getting the right amount of calories.

No Bones About It: You Need Calcium Everyday

Many people do not get enough of the calcium needed for strong bones and proper muscle function. Lack of calcium can contribute to stress fractures and the bone disease, osteoporosis.

The best sources of calcium are dairy products, but many other foods such as salmon with bones, sardines, collard greens, and okra also contain calcium. Additionally, some brands of bread, tofu, and orange juice are fortified with calcium.

Source: President's Council on Physical Fitness and Sports (http://www.fitness.gov), 2010.

Questions Most Frequently Asked About Sports Nutrition

Do the nutritional needs of athletes differ from non-athletes?

Competitive athletes, sedentary individuals, and people who exercise for health and fitness all need the same nutrients. However, because of the intensity of their sport or training program, some athletes have higher calorie and fluid requirements. Eating a variety of foods to meet increased calorie needs helps to ensure that the athlete's diet contains appropriate amounts of carbohydrate, protein, vitamins and minerals.

Are there certain dietary guidelines athletes should follow?

Health and nutrition professionals recommend that 55–60% of the calories in our diet come from carbohydrate, no more than 30% from fat and the remaining 10–15% from protein. While the exact percentages may vary slightly for some athletes based on their sport or training program, these guidelines will promote health and serve as the basis for a diet that will maximize performance.

How many calories do I need a day?

This depends on your age, body size, sport and training program. For example, a 250-pound weight lifter needs more calories than a 98-pound gymnast. Exercise or training may increase calorie needs by as much as 1,000 to 1,500 calories a day. The best way to determine if you're getting too few or too many calories is to monitor your weight. Keeping within your ideal competitive weight range means that you are getting the right amount of calories.

Which is better for replacing fluids—water or sports drinks?

Depending on how muscular you are, 55–70% of your body weight is water. Being "hydrated" means maintaining your body's fluid level. When you sweat, you lose water which must be replaced if you want to perform your best. You need to drink fluids before, during and after all workouts and events.

Whether you drink water or a sports drink is a matter of choice. However, if your workout or event lasts for more than 90 minutes, you may benefit from the carbohydrates provided by sports drinks. A sports drink that contains 15–18 grams of carbohydrate in every 8 ounces of fluid should be used. Drinks with a higher carbohydrate content will delay the absorption of water and may cause dehydration, cramps, nausea or diarrhea. There are a variety of sports drinks on the market. Be sure to experiment with sports drinks during practice instead of trying them for the first time the day of an event.

What are electrolytes?

Electrolytes are nutrients that affect fluid balance in the body and are necessary for our nerves and muscles to function. Sodium and potassium are the two electrolytes most often added to sports drinks. Generally, electrolyte replacement is not needed during short bursts of exercise since sweat is approximately 99% water and less than 1% electrolytes. Water, in combination with a well-balanced diet, will restore normal fluid and electrolyte levels in the body. However, replacing electrolytes may be beneficial during continuous activity of longer than two hours, especially in a hot environment.

What do muscles use for energy during exercise?

Most activities use a combination of fat and carbohydrate as energy sources. How hard and how long you work out, your level of fitness and your diet will affect the type of fuel your body uses.

For short-term, high-intensity activities like sprinting, athletes rely mostly on carbohydrate for energy. During low-intensity exercises like walking, the body uses more fat for energy.

Is it true that athletes should eat a lot of carbohydrates?

When you are training or competing, your muscles need energy to perform. One source of energy for working muscles is glycogen which is made from carbohydrates and stored in your muscles.

Every time you work out, you use some of your glycogen. If you don't consume enough carbohydrates, your glycogen stores become depleted, which can result in fatigue. Both sugars and starches are effective in replenishing glycogen stores.

When and what should I eat before I compete?

Performance depends largely on the foods consumed during the days and weeks leading up to an event. If you regularly eat a varied, carbohydrate-rich diet you are in good standing and probably have ample glycogen stores to fuel activity. The purpose of the pre-competition meal is to prevent hunger and to provide the water and additional energy the athlete will need during competition.

Most athletes eat two to four hours before their event. However, some athletes perform their best if they eat a small amount 30 minutes before competing, while others eat nothing for six hours beforehand. For many athletes, carbohydrate-rich foods serve as the basis of the meal. However, there is no magic pre-event diet. Simply choose foods and beverages that you enjoy and that don't bother your stomach. Experiment during the weeks before an event to see which foods work best for you.

Will eating sugary foods before an event hurt my performance?

In the past, athletes were warned that eating sugary foods before exercise could hurt performance by causing a drop in blood glucose levels. Recent studies, however, have shown that consuming sugar up to 30 minutes before an event does not diminish performance. In fact, evidence suggests that a sugar-containing pre-competition beverage or snack may improve performance during endurance workouts and events.

What is carbohydrate loading?

Carbohydrate loading is a technique used to increase the amount of glycogen in muscles. For five to seven days before an event, the athlete eats 10–12 grams of carbohydrate per kilogram body weight and gradually reduces the intensity of the workouts. (To find out how much you weigh in kilograms, simply divide your weight in pounds by 2.2.) The day before the event, the athlete rests and eats the same high-carbohydrate diet.

Although carbohydrate loading may be beneficial for athletes participating in endurance sports which require 90 minutes or more of non-stop effort, most athletes needn't worry about carbohydrate loading. Simply eating a diet that derives more than half of its calories from carbohydrates will do.

As an athlete, do I need to take extra vitamins and minerals?

Athletes need to eat about 1,800 calories a day to get the vitamins and minerals they need for good health and optimal performance. Since most athletes eat more than this amount, vitamin and mineral supplements are needed only in special situations.

Athletes who follow vegetarian diets or who avoid an entire group of foods (for example, never drink milk) may need a supplement to make up for the vitamins and minerals not being supplied by food. A multivitamin-mineral pill that supplies 100% of the Recommended Dietary Allowance (RDA) will provide the nutrients needed.

An athlete who frequently cuts back on calories, especially below the 1,800 calorie level, is not only at risk for inadequate vitamin and mineral intake, but also may not be getting enough carbohydrate. Since vitamins and minerals do not provide energy, they cannot replace the energy provided by carbohydrates.

Chapter 35

Healthy Eating For Vegetarians And Vegans

Becoming A Vegetarian

Why Do People Become Vegetarians?

For much of the world, vegetarianism is largely a matter of economics: Meat costs a lot more than, say, beans or rice, so meat becomes a special-occasion dish (if it's eaten at all). Even where meat is more plentiful, it's still used in moderation, often providing a side note to a meal rather than taking center stage.

In countries like the United States where meat is not as expensive, though, people choose to be vegetarians for reasons other than cost. Parental preferences, religious or other beliefs, and health issues are among the most common reasons for choosing to be a vegetarian. Many people choose a vegetarian diet out of concern over animal rights or the environment. And lots of people have more than one reason for choosing vegetarianism.

Vegetarian And Semi-Vegetarian Diets

Different people follow different forms of vegetarianism. A true vegetarian eats no meat at all, including chicken and fish. A lacto-ovo vegetarian eats dairy products and eggs, but excludes meat, fish, and poultry. It follows, then, that a lacto vegetarian eats dairy products but not eggs, whereas an ovo vegetarian eats eggs but not dairy products.

A stricter form of vegetarianism is veganism (pronounced: vee-gun-izm). Not only are eggs and dairy products excluded from a vegan diet, so are animal products like honey and gelatin.

Some macrobiotic diets fall into the vegan category. Macrobiotic diets restrict not only animal products but also refined and processed foods, foods with preservatives, and foods that contain caffeine or other stimulants.

Following a macrobiotic or vegan diet could lead to nutritional deficiencies in some people. Teens need to be sure their diets include enough nutrients to fuel growth, particularly protein and calcium. If you're interested in following a vegan or macrobiotic diet it's a good idea to talk to a registered dietitian. He or she can help you design meal plans that include adequate vitamins and minerals.

Some people consider themselves semi-vegetarians and eat fish and maybe a small amount of poultry as part of a diet that's primarily made up of vegetables, fruits, grains, legumes, seeds, and nuts. A pesci-vegetarian eats fish, but not poultry.

Hidden Animal Products

Some foods that appear to be vegetarian aren't. Most cheeses are made using an animal-derived product called rennet. Other ingredients that show up in seemingly vegetarian foods include gelatin, which is made from meat byproducts, and enzymes, which may be animal derived.

Source: Nemours Foundation, September 2009.

Are These Diets OK For Teens?

In the past, choosing not to eat meat or animal-based foods was considered unusual in the United States. Times and attitudes have changed dramatically, however. Vegetarians are still a minority in the United States, but a large and growing one. The American Dietetic Association (ADA) has officially endorsed vegetarianism, stating "appropriately planned vegetarian diets, including total vegetarian or vegan diets, are healthful, nutritionally adequate, and may provide health benefits in the prevention and treatment of certain diseases."

So what does this mean for you? If you're already a vegetarian, or are thinking of becoming one, you're in good company. There are more choices in the supermarket than ever before, and an increasing number of restaurants and schools are providing vegetarian options—way beyond a basic peanut butter and jelly sandwich.

Nutrients To Focus On For Vegetarians

- Protein has many important functions in the body and is essential for growth and maintenance. Protein needs can easily be met by eating a variety of plant-based foods. Combining different protein sources in the same meal is not necessary. Sources of protein for vegetarians include beans, nuts, nut butters, peas, and soy products (tofu, tempeh, veggie burgers). Milk products and eggs are also good protein sources for lacto-ovo vegetarians.

- Iron functions primarily as a carrier of oxygen in the blood. Iron sources for vegetarians include iron-fortified breakfast cereals, spinach, kidney beans, black-eyed peas, lentils, turnip greens, molasses, whole wheat breads, peas, and some dried fruits (dried apricots, prunes, raisins).

- Calcium is used for building bones and teeth and in maintaining bone strength. Sources of calcium for vegetarians include calcium-fortified soymilk, calcium-fortified breakfast cereals and orange juice, tofu made with calcium sulfate, and some dark-green leafy vegetables (collard greens, turnip greens, bok choy, mustard greens). The amount of calcium that can be absorbed from these foods varies. Consuming enough plant foods to meet calcium needs may be unrealistic for many. Milk products are excellent calcium sources for lacto vegetarians. Calcium supplements are another potential source.

- Zinc is necessary for many biochemical reactions and also helps the immune system function properly. Sources of zinc for vegetarians include many types of beans (white beans, kidney beans, and chickpeas), zinc-fortified breakfast cereals, wheat germ, and pumpkin seeds. Milk products are a zinc source for lacto vegetarians.

- Vitamin B12 is found in animal products and some fortified foods. Sources of vitamin B12 for vegetarians include milk products, eggs, and foods that have been fortified with vitamin B12. These include breakfast cereals, soymilk, veggie burgers, and nutritional yeast.

Source: Excerpted from "Tips and Resources: Vegetarian Diets," U.S. Department of Agriculture (www.choosemyplate.gov), June 21, 2011.

If you're choosing a vegetarian diet, the most important thing you can do is to educate yourself. That's why the ADA says that a vegetarian diet needs to be "appropriately planned." Simply dropping certain foods from your diet isn't the way to go if you're interested in maintaining good health, a high energy level, and strong muscles and bones.

Vegetarians have to be careful to include the following key nutrients that may be lacking in a vegetarian diet:

- Iron
- Calcium
- Protein
- Vitamin D
- Vitamin B12
- Zinc

If meat, fish, dairy products, and/or eggs are not going to be part of your diet, you'll need to know how to get enough of these nutrients, or you may need to take a daily multiple vitamin and mineral supplement.

Iron

Sea vegetables like nori, wakame, and dulse are very high in iron. Less exotic but still good options are iron-fortified breakfast cereals, legumes (chickpeas, lentils, and baked beans), soybeans and tofu, dried fruit (raisins and figs), pumpkin seeds, broccoli, and blackstrap molasses. Eating these foods along with a food high in vitamin C (citrus fruits and juices, tomatoes, and broccoli) will help you to absorb the iron better.

Girls need to be particularly concerned about getting adequate iron because some iron is lost during menstruation. Some girls who are vegetarians may not get adequate iron from vegetable sources and they may require a daily supplement. Check with your doctor about your own iron needs.

Calcium

Milk and yogurt are tops if you're eating dairy products—although vegetarians will want to look for yogurt that does not contain the meat by-product gelatin. Tofu, fortified soy milk, calcium-fortified orange juice, green leafy vegetables, and dried figs are also excellent ways for vegetarians (and vegans) to get calcium. Remember that as a teen you're building up your bones for the rest of your life.

Because women have a greater risk for getting osteoporosis (weak bones) as adults, it's particularly important for girls to make sure they get enough calcium. Again, taking a supplement may be necessary to ensure this.

Vitamin D

People need vitamin D to get calcium into our bones. Your body manufactures vitamin D when your skin is exposed to sunlight. Cow's milk is top on the list for food sources of this vitamin. Vegans can try fortified soy milk and fortified breakfast cereals. Some people may need a supplement that includes vitamin D, especially during the winter months. Everyone should have some exposure to the sun to help the body produce vitamin D.

Protein

Some people believe that vegetarians must combine incomplete plant proteins in one meal—like red beans and rice—to make the type of complete proteins found in meat. We now know that it's not that complicated. Current recommendations are that vegetarians eat a wide variety of foods during the course of a day. Eggs and dairy products are good sources of protein, but also try nuts, peanut butter, tofu, beans, seeds, soy milk, grains, cereals, and vegetables to get all the protein your body needs.

Vitamin B12

B12 is an essential vitamin found only in animal products, including eggs and dairy. Fortified soy milk and fortified breakfast cereals also have this important vitamin. It's hard to get enough vitamin B12 in your diet if you are vegan, so a supplement may be needed.

Zinc

If you're not eating dairy foods, make sure fortified cereals, dried beans, nuts, and soy products like tofu and tempeh are part of your diet so you can meet your daily requirement for this important mineral.

Fat, Calories, And Fiber

In addition to vitamins and minerals, vegetarians need to keep an eye on their total intake of calories and fat. Vegetarian diets tend to be high in fiber and low in fat and calories. That may be good for people who need to lose weight or lower their cholesterol but it can be a problem for kids and teens who are still growing and people who are already at a healthy weight.

Some vegetarians (especially vegans) may not get enough omega-3 fatty acids. Omega-3 fats are good for heart health and are found in fish and eggs. Some products, such as soy milk and breakfast bars, are fortified with docosahexaenoic acid (DHA), an omega-3 fatty acid.

Diets that are high in fiber tend to be more filling, and as a result strict vegetarians may feel full before they've eaten enough calories to keep their bodies healthy and strong. It's a good idea to let your doctor know that you're a vegetarian so that he or she can keep on eye on your growth and make sure you're still getting adequate amounts of calories and fat.

Getting Some Guidance

If you're thinking about becoming a vegetarian, consider making an appointment to talk with a registered dietitian who can go over lists of foods that would give you the nutrients you need. A dietitian can discuss ways to prevent conditions such as iron-deficiency anemia that you might be at an increased risk for if you stop eating meat.

Also, remember to take a daily standard multivitamin, just in case you miss getting enough vitamins or minerals that day.

Tips For Dining Out

Eating at restaurants can be difficult for vegetarians sometimes, but if you do eat fish, you can usually find something suitable on the menu. If not, opt for salad and an appetizer or two—or ask if the meat can be removed. Even fast-food places sometimes have vegetarian choices, such as bean tacos and burritos, veggie burgers, and soy cheese pizza.

Vegetarians can opt for pasta, along with plenty of vegetables, grains, and fruits. You may also find that the veggie burgers, hot dogs, and chicken substitutes available in your local grocery store taste very much like the real thing. Try the ground meat substitute as a stand-in for beef in foods like tacos and spaghetti sauce.

Regardless of whether you choose a vegetarian way of life, it's always a healthy idea to eat a wide variety of foods and try out new foods when you can.

Source: Nemours Foundation, September 2009.

Vegan Food Guide

A vegan (pronounced: vee-gun) doesn't consume any animal-derived foods or use animal products or byproducts, and eats only plant-based foods. In addition to not eating meat, poultry, seafood, eggs, or dairy, vegans avoid using products made from animal sources, such as fur, leather, and wool.

While those are obvious animal products, many animal byproducts are things we might not even realize come from animals. These include:

- gelatin (made using meat byproducts)

- lanolin (made from wool)

- rennet (an enzyme found in the stomach of calves, young goats, and lambs that's used in cheese-making)

- honey and beeswax (made by bees)

- silk (made by silkworms)

- shellac (the resinous secretion of the tiny lac insect)

- cochineal (a red dye derived from the cochineal insect)

Why Vegan?

Veganism (also known as strict vegetarianism or pure vegetarianism), as defined by the Vegan Society, is "a philosophy and way of living which seeks to exclude—as far as is possible and practical—all forms of exploitation of, and cruelty to, animals for food, clothing, or any other purpose."

Vegans also avoid toothpaste with calcium extracted from animal bones, if they are aware of it. Similarly, soap made from animal fat rather than vegetable fats is avoided. Vegans generally oppose the violence and cruelty involved in the meat, dairy, cosmetics, clothing, and other industries.

What About Nutrition?

Vegetarian diets offer a number of advantages, says the ADA, including lower levels of total fat, saturated fat, and cholesterol, and higher levels of fiber, magnesium, potassium, folate, and antioxidants. As a result, the health benefits of a vegetarian diet may include the prevention of certain diseases, including heart disease, diabetes, and some cancers.

But any restrictive diet can make it more difficult to get all the nutrients your body needs. A vegan diet eliminates food sources of vitamin B12, which is found almost exclusively in animal products, including milk, eggs, and cheese. A vegan diet also eliminates milk products, which are good sources of calcium.

To ensure that "well-planned" diet, vegans must find alternative sources for B12 and calcium, as well as vitamin D, protein, iron, zinc, and occasionally riboflavin. Here's how:

Vitamin B12: Vegans can get vitamin B12, needed to produce red blood cells and maintain normal nerve function, from enriched breakfast cereals, fortified soy products, nutritional yeast, or supplements.

Calcium: We all need calcium for strong teeth and bones. You can get calcium from dark green vegetables (spinach, bok choy, broccoli, collards, kale, turnip greens), sesame seeds, almonds, red and white beans, soy foods, dried figs, blackstrap molasses, and calcium-fortified foods like fruit juices and breakfast cereals.

Vitamin D: Vitamin D helps our bodies absorb calcium and is synthesized by exposing skin to sunlight. But vitamin D deficiency can occur, especially if you don't spend a lot of time outside. Vitamin D is not found in most commonly eaten plant foods; best dietary sources are fortified dairy products. Vegans can also get vitamin D from fortified foods, including vitamin D-fortified soy milk or rice milk.

Protein: Not getting enough protein is a concern when switching to a vegetarian diet. Protein needs can be met while following a vegan diet if you consume adequate calories and eat a variety of plant foods, including good plant sources of protein such as soy, other legumes, nuts, and seeds.

Iron: Iron from plant sources is less easily absorbed than iron in meat. This lower bioavailability means that iron intake for vegetarians should be higher than the recommended daily allowance (RDA) for nonvegetarians. Vegetarian food sources of iron include soy foods like soybeans, tempeh, and tofu; legumes like lentils and chickpeas; and fortified cereals. Iron absorption is enhanced by vitamin C.

Zinc: Zinc plays a role in many key body functions, including immune system response, so it's important to get enough of it, which vegans can do by eating nuts, legumes, miso and other soy products, pumpkin and sunflower seeds, tahini, wheat germ, and whole-grain breads and cereals.

Riboflavin: This B vitamin, which is important for growth and red blood cell production, can be found in almonds, mushrooms, broccoli, figs, sweet potatoes, soybeans, wheat germ, and fortified cereals and enriched bread.

Eating A Vegan Diet

Anyone following a vegan diet has to be a meticulous label-reader. No federal regulation dictates the use of the words "vegetarian" or "vegan" in the United States. To be sure a food truly is "suitable for vegans," check the label—what might be vegetarian isn't necessarily vegan.

Vegans are by no means stuck eating boring foods with little variety. But if you're considering becoming a vegan, or wondering whether it's realistic to eliminate animal-based foods from your diet, it might pay to start slowly, especially if you've been a cheeseburger fan most of your life.

Try some of the wide array of meat alternatives that are found in almost every grocery store. Tasty frozen veggie burgers, chicken and meat substitutes, sausage alternative, fake bacon, and tofu dogs will make the transition to a vegan diet convenient and easy.

If you need help, talk to a registered dietician familiar with vegan diets and look for vegetarian cookbooks that can help you plan and prepare healthy meatless meals.

And remember, many foods you probably already have are suitable for a vegan diet. For instance, most breakfast cereals are vegan as are many crackers, cookies, and baked goods. Choose ones made with whole grains and low in fat, pair them with healthy salads, fresh fruits, and some colorful veggies, and you might not ever miss that ham and cheese sandwich.

Meal Time Tips For Vegetarians

- Build meals around protein sources that are naturally low in fat, such as beans, lentils, and rice. Don't overload meals with high-fat cheeses to replace the meat.

- Calcium-fortified soymilk provides calcium in amounts similar to milk. It is usually low in fat and does not contain cholesterol.

- Many foods that typically contain meat or poultry can be made vegetarian. This can increase vegetable intake and cut saturated fat and cholesterol intake. Consider pasta primavera or pasta with marinara or pesto sauce, veggie pizza, vegetable lasagna, tofu-vegetable stir fry, vegetable lo mein, vegetable kabobs, and bean burritos or tacos.

- A variety of vegetarian products look (and may taste) like their non-vegetarian counterparts, but are usually lower in saturated fat and contain no cholesterol. For breakfast, try soy-based sausage patties or links. Rather than hamburgers, try veggie burgers. A variety of kinds are available, made with soy beans, vegetables, and/or rice. Add vegetarian meat substitutes to soups and stews to boost protein without adding saturated fat or cholesterol. These include tempeh (cultured soybeans with a chewy texture), tofu, or wheat gluten (seitan). For barbecues, try veggie burgers, soy hot dogs, marinated tofu or tempeh, and veggie kabobs. Make bean burgers, lentil burgers, or pita halves with falafel (spicy ground chick pea patties).

- Some restaurants offer soy options (texturized vegetable protein) as a substitute for meat, and soy cheese as a substitute for regular cheese. Most restaurants can accommodate vegetarian modifications to menu items by substituting meatless sauces, omitting meat from stir-fries, and adding vegetables or pasta in place of meat. These substitutions are more likely to be available at restaurants that make food to order. Many Asian and Indian restaurants offer a varied selection of vegetarian dishes.

Source: Excerpted from "Tips and Resources: Vegetarian Diets," U.S. Department of Agriculture (www.choosemyplate .gov), June 21, 2011.

Part Five
Eating And Weight-Related Concerns

Chapter 36

What's The Right Weight For My Height?

"What's the right weight for my height?" is one of the most common questions girls and guys have. It seems like a simple question. But, for teens, it's not always an easy one to answer. Why not? People have different body types, so there's no single number that's the right weight for everyone. Even among people who are the same height and age, some are more muscular or more developed than others. That's because not all teens have the same body type or develop at the same time.

It is possible to find out if you are in a healthy weight range for your height, though—it just takes a little effort. Read on to discover how this works. You'll also be able to put your measurements into the KidsHealth calculator and get an idea of how you're doing [see p. 257].

Growth And Puberty

Not everyone grows and develops on the same schedule, but teens do go through a period of faster growth. During puberty, the body begins making hormones that spark physical changes like faster muscle growth (particularly in guys) and spurts in height and weight gain in both guys and girls.

Once these changes start, they continue for several years. The average person can expect to grow as much as 10 inches (25 centimeters) during puberty before he or she reaches full adult height.

Most guys and girls gain weight more rapidly during this time as the amounts of muscle, fat, and bone in their bodies changes. All that new weight gain can be perfectly fine—as long as body fat, muscle, and bone are in the right proportion.

About This Chapter: "What's the Right Weight for My Height?" June 2008, reprinted with permission from www.kidshealth.org. Copyright © 2008 The Nemours Foundation. This information was provided by KidsHealth, one of the largest resources online for medically reviewed health information written for parents, kids, and teens. For more articles like this one, visit www.KidsHealth.org, or www.TeensHealth.org.

Why You Need More Than A Scale

People overweight for their height can have major differences in body composition (the amounts of muscle, fat, and bone they have). An athlete might have a high BMI because of extra muscle, so may not be overweight. But a less fit person of the same height and weight may be considered overweight because of too much body fat.

Because some kids start developing as early as age 8 and some not until age 14 or so, it can be normal for two people who are the same height and age to have very different weights.

It can feel quite strange adjusting to suddenly feeling heavier or taller. So it's perfectly normal to feel self-conscious about weight during adolescence—a lot of people do.

Figuring Out Fat Using BMI

Experts have developed a way to help figure out if a person is in the healthy weight range for his or her height. It's called the body mass index, or BMI. BMI is a formula that doctors use to estimate how much body fat a person has based on his or her weight and height.

The BMI formula uses height and weight measurements to calculate a BMI number. This number is then plotted on a chart, which tells a person whether he or she is underweight, average weight, overweight, or obese.

Figuring out the body mass index is a little more complicated for teens than it is for adults (that puberty thing again). BMI charts for teens use percentile lines to help individuals compare their BMIs with those of a very large group of people the same age and gender. There are different BMI charts for guys and girls under the age of 20.

A person's BMI number is plotted on the chart for their age and gender. A teen whose BMI is at the 50th percentile is close to the average of the age group. A teen whose weight falls between the 85th and 95th percentile is considered overweight because 85% to 95% of the age group has a lower BMI. A teen above the 95th percentile is considered obese. A teen below the 5th percentile is considered underweight because 95% of the age group has a higher BMI.

Remember

Some teens, especially those who go through puberty on a later time schedule, may feel too skinny. The good news is that their growth, development, and weight gain almost always catch up to other people their age later on.

BMI Calculator

To figure out your BMI, use the KidsHealth BMI Calculator tool available online at http://kidshealth.org/teen/food_fitness/dieting/weight_height.html (click on page 3). Before you start, you'll need an accurate height and weight measurement. Bathroom scales and tape measures aren't always precise. So the best way to get accurate measurements is by being weighted and measured at your doctor's office or school.

What Does BMI Tell Us?

Although you can calculate BMI on your own, it's a good idea to ask your doctor, school nurse, or fitness counselor to help you figure out what it means. That's because a doctor can do more than just use BMI to assess a person's current weight. He or she can take into account where a girl or guy is during puberty and use BMI results from past years to track whether that person may be at risk for becoming overweight. Spotting this risk early on can be helpful because the person can then make changes in diet and exercise to help avert developing a weight problem.

People think of weight as a looks issue, but weight problems be more serious than someone's appearance. People who are overweight as teens increase their risk of developing health problems, such as diabetes and high blood pressure.

Being overweight as a teen also makes a person more likely to be overweight as an adult. And adults who are overweight may develop other serious health conditions, such as heart disease.

Although BMI can be a good indicator of a person's body fat, it doesn't always tell the full story. People can have a high BMI because they have a large frame or a lot of muscle (like a bodybuilder or athlete) instead of excess fat. Likewise, a small person with a small frame may have a normal BMI but could still have too much body fat. These are other good reasons to talk about your BMI with your doctor.

How Can I Be Sure I'm Not Overweight Or Under-weight?

If you think you've gained too much weight or are too skinny, a doctor should help you decide whether it's normal for you or whether you really have a weight problem. Your doctor has measured your height and weight over time and knows whether you're growing normally.

If concerned about your height, weight, or BMI, your doctor may ask questions about your health, physical activity, and eating habits. Your doctor may also ask about your family background to find out if you've inherited traits that might make you taller, shorter, or a late bloomer (someone who develops later than other people the same age). The doctor can then put all this information together to decide whether you might have a weight or growth problem.

If your doctor thinks your weight isn't in a healthy range, you will probably get specific dietary and exercise recommendations based on your individual needs. Following a doctor's or dietitian's plan that's designed especially for you will work way better than following fad diets. For teens, fad diets or starvation plans can actually slow down growth and sexual development, and the weight loss usually doesn't last.

What if you're worried about being too skinny? Most teens who weigh less than other teens their age are just fine. They may be going through puberty on a different schedule than some of their peers, and their bodies may be growing and changing at a different rate. Most underweight teens catch up in weight as they finish puberty during their later teen years and there's rarely a need to try to gain weight.

In a few cases, teens can be underweight because of a health problem that needs treatment. If you feel tired or ill a lot, or if you have symptoms like a cough, stomachache, diarrhea, or other problems that have lasted for more than a week or two, be sure to let your parents or your doctor know. Some teens are underweight because of eating disorders, like anorexia or bulimia, that require attention.

Getting Into Your Genes

Heredity plays a role in body shape and what a person weighs. People from different races, ethnic groups, and nationalities tend to have different body fat distribution (meaning they accumulate fat in different parts of their bodies) or body composition (amounts of bone and muscle versus fat).

But genes are not destiny. (That may be a relief if you're looking at Aunt Mildred and wondering if you'll end up with her physique.) No matter whose genes you inherit, you can have a healthy body and keep your weight at a level that's normal for you by eating right and being active.

Genes aren't the only things that family members may share. It's also true that unhealthy eating habits can be passed down, too. The eating and exercise habits of people in the same household probably have an even greater effect than genes on a person's risk of becoming overweight. If your family eats a lot of high-fat foods or snacks or doesn't get much exercise, you may tend to do the same. The good news is these habits can be changed for the better. Even simple forms of exercise, such as walking, have huge benefits on a person's health.

It can be tough dealing with the physical changes our bodies go through during puberty. But at this time, more than any other, it's not a specific number on the scale that's important. It's keeping your body healthy—inside and out.

Chapter 37

Body Mass Index For Children And Teens

What is BMI?

Body mass index (BMI) is a number calculated from a child's weight and height. BMI is a reliable indicator of body fatness for most children and teens. BMI does not measure body fat directly, but research has shown that BMI correlates to direct measures of body fat, such as underwater weighing and dual energy x-ray absorptiometry (DXA). BMI can be considered an alternative for direct measures of body fat. Additionally, BMI is an inexpensive and easy-to-perform method of screening for weight categories that may lead to health problems.

For children and teens, BMI is age and sex-specific and is often referred to as BMI-for-age.

What is a BMI percentile?

After BMI is calculated for children and teens, the BMI number is plotted on the Centers for Disease Control and Prevention (CDC) BMI-for-age growth charts (for either girls or boys) to obtain a percentile ranking. Percentiles are the most commonly used indicator to assess the size and growth patterns of individual children in the United States. The percentile indicates the relative position of the child's BMI number among children of the same sex and age. The growth charts show the weight status categories used with children and teens (underweight, healthy weight, overweight, and obese).

BMI-for-age weight status categories and the corresponding percentiles are shown in Table 37.1.

About This Chapter: Excerpted from, "About BMI for Children and Teens," Centers for Disease Control and Prevention, January 2009.

Table 37.1. BMI-For-Age Percentiles

Weight Status Category	Percentile Range
Underweight	Less than the 5th percentile
Healthy Weight	5th percentile to less than the 85th percentile
Overweight	85th to less than the 95th percentile
Obese	Equal to or greater than the 95th percentile

How is BMI used with children and teens?

BMI is used as a screening tool to identify possible weight problems for children. CDC and the American Academy of Pediatrics (AAP) recommend the use of BMI to screen for overweight and obesity in children beginning at two years old.

For children, BMI is used to screen for obesity, overweight, healthy weight, or underweight. However, BMI is not a diagnostic tool. For example, a child may have a high BMI for age and sex, but to determine if excess fat is a problem, a health care provider would need to perform further assessments. These assessments might include skinfold thickness measurements, evaluations of diet, physical activity, family history, and other appropriate health screenings.

How is BMI calculated and interpreted for children and teens?

Calculating and interpreting BMI using the BMI Percentile Calculator involves the following steps:

1. Before calculating BMI, obtain accurate height and weight measurements.

2. Calculate the BMI and percentile using the Child and Teen BMI Calculator. The BMI number is calculated using standard formulas.

3. Review the calculated BMI-for-age percentile and results. The BMI-for-age percentile is used to interpret the BMI number because BMI is both age-and sex-specific for children and teens. These criteria are different from those used to interpret BMI for adults—which do not take into account age or sex. Age and sex are considered for children and teens for two reasons:

   - The amount of body fat changes with age. (BMI for children and teens is often referred to as BMI-for-age.)
   - The amount of body fat differs between girls and boys.

The CDC BMI-for-age growth charts for girls and boys take into account these differences and allow translation of a BMI number into a percentile for a child's or teen's sex and age.

4. Find the weight status category for the calculated BMI-for-age percentile as shown in Table 37.1. These categories are based on expert committee recommendations.

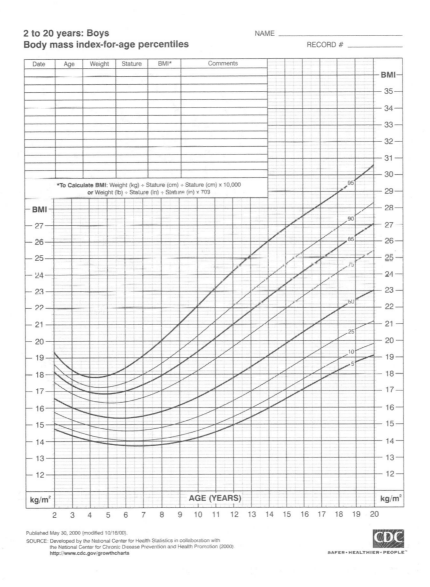

2 to 20 years: Boys
Body mass index-for-age percentiles

NAME _____

RECORD # _____

*To Calculate BMI: Weight (kg) ÷ Stature (cm) ÷ Stature (cm) x 10,000 or Weight (lb) ÷ Stature (in) ÷ Stature (in) x 703

AGE (YEARS)

Published May 30, 2000 (modified 10/16/00).
SOURCE: Developed by the National Center for Health Statistics in collaboration with the National Center for Chronic Disease Prevention and Health Promotion (2000)
http://www.cdc.gov/growthcharts

CDC
SAFER·HEALTHIER·PEOPLE™

Figure 37.1. Boys: BMI for Age (2–20)

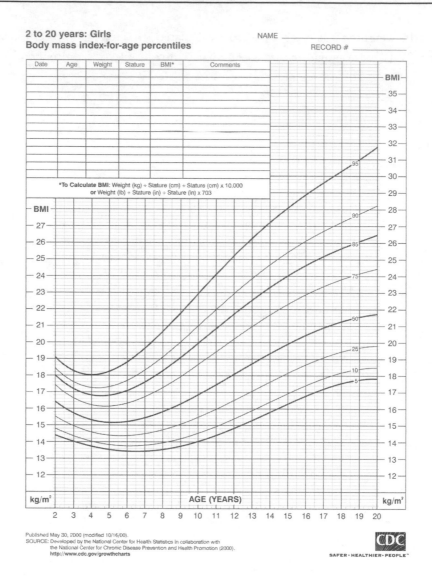

2 to 20 years: Girls
Body mass index-for-age percentiles

NAME _____

RECORD # _____

*To Calculate BMI: Weight (kg) ÷ Stature (cm) ÷ Stature (cm) x 10,000
or Weight (lb) ÷ Stature (in) ÷ Stature (in) x 703

Published May 30, 2000 (modified 10/16/00).
SOURCE: Developed by the National Center for Health Statistics in collaboration with
the National Center for Chronic Disease Prevention and Health Promotion (2000).
http://www.cdc.gov/growthcharts

Figure 37.2. Girls: BMI for Age (2–20)

Why can't healthy weight ranges be provided for children and teens?

Healthy weight ranges cannot be provided for children and teens for the following reasons:

- Healthy weight ranges change with each month of age for each sex.

- Healthy weight ranges change as height increases.

BMI Is Not Interpreted The Same Way For Teens As It Is For Adults

Although the BMI number is calculated the same way for children and adults, the criteria used to interpret the meaning of the BMI number for children and teens are different from those used for adults. For children and teens, BMI age- and sex-specific percentiles are used for two reasons:

- The amount of body fat changes with age.
- The amount of body fat differs between girls and boys.

The CDC BMI-for-age growth charts take into account these differences and allow translation of a BMI number into a percentile for a child's sex and age.

For adults, on the other hand, BMI is interpreted through categories that do not take into account sex or age.

How can I tell if a teen is overweight or obese?

CDC and the American Academy of Pediatrics (AAP) recommend the use of Body Mass Index (BMI) to screen for overweight and obesity in children and teens aged two through 19 years. Although BMI is used to screen for overweight and obesity in children and teens, BMI is not a diagnostic tool.

For example, a child who is relatively heavy may have a high BMI for his or her age. To determine whether the child has excess fat, further assessment would be needed. Further assessment might include skinfold thickness measurements. To determine a counseling strategy, assessments of diet, health, and physical activity are needed.

Can I determine if a teen is obese by using an adult BMI calculator?

No. The adult calculator provides only the BMI number and not the BMI age- and sex-specific percentile that is used to interpret BMI and determine the weight category for children and teens. It is not appropriate to use the BMI categories for adults to interpret BMI numbers for children and teens.

How can two teens have the same BMI values, but one is considered obese and the other is not?

The interpretation of BMI-for-age varies by age and sex so if the children are not exactly the same age and of the same sex, the BMI numbers have different meanings. Calculating BMI-for-age for children of different ages and sexes may yield the same numeric result, but that number will fall at a different percentile for each child for one or both of the following reasons:

- The normal BMI-related changes that take place as children age and as growth occurs.

- The normal BMI-related differences between sexes.

Chapter 38

Body Image And Self-Esteem

I'm fat. I'm too skinny. I'd be happy if I were taller, shorter, had curly hair, straight hair, a smaller nose, bigger muscles, longer legs.

Do any of these statements sound familiar? Are you used to putting yourself down? If so, you're not alone. As a teen, you're going through a ton of changes in your body. And as your body changes, so does your image of yourself. Lots of people have trouble adjusting, and this can affect their self-esteem.

Why Are Self-Esteem And Body Image Important?

Self-esteem is all about how much people value themselves, the pride they feel in themselves, and how worthwhile they feel. Self-esteem is important because feeling good about yourself can affect how you act. A person who has high self-esteem will make friends easily, is more in control of his or her behavior, and will enjoy life more.

Body image is how someone feels about his or her own physical appearance.

For many people, especially those in their early teens, body image can be closely linked to self-esteem. That's because as kids develop into teens, they care more about how others see them.

About This Chapter: "Body Image and Self-Esteem," May 2009, reprinted with permission from www.kidshealth .org. Copyright © 2009 The Nemours Foundation. This information was provided by KidsHealth, one of the largest resources online for medically reviewed health information written for parents, kids, and teens. For more articles like this one, visit www.KidsHealth.org, or www.TeensHealth.org.

What Influences A Person's Self-Esteem?

Puberty

Some teens struggle with their self-esteem when they begin puberty because the body goes through many changes. These changes, combined with a natural desire to feel accepted, mean it can be tempting for people to compare themselves with others. They may compare themselves with the people around them or with actors and celebs they see on TV, in movies, or in magazines.

But it's impossible to measure ourselves against others because the changes that come with puberty are different for everyone. Some people start developing early; others are late bloomers. Some get a temporary layer of fat to prepare for a growth spurt, others fill out permanently, and others feel like they stay skinny no matter how much they eat. It all depends on how our genes have programmed our bodies to act.

The changes that come with puberty can affect how both girls and guys feel about themselves. Some girls may feel uncomfortable or embarrassed about their maturing bodies. Others may wish that they were developing faster. Girls may feel pressure to be thin but guys may feel like they don't look big or muscular enough.

Outside Influences

It's not just development that affects self-esteem, though. Many other factors (like media images of skinny girls and bulked-up guys) can affect a person's body image too.

Family life can sometimes influence self-esteem. Some parents spend more time criticizing their kids and the way they look than praising them, which can reduce kids' ability to develop good self-esteem.

People also may experience negative comments and hurtful teasing about the way they look from classmates and peers. Sometimes racial and ethnic prejudice is the source of such comments. Although these often come from ignorance, sometimes they can affect someone's body image and self-esteem.

Healthy Self-Esteem

If you have a positive body image, you probably like and accept yourself the way you are. This healthy attitude allows you to explore other aspects of growing up, such as developing good friendships, growing more independent from your parents, and challenging yourself physically and mentally. Developing these parts of yourself can help boost your self-esteem.

Resilience

People who believe in themselves are better able to recognize mistakes, learn from them, and bounce back from disappointment. This skill is called resilience.

A positive, optimistic attitude can help people develop strong self-esteem—for example, saying, "Hey, I'm human" instead of "Wow, I'm such a loser" when you've made a mistake, or not blaming others when things don't go as expected.

Knowing what makes you happy and how to meet your goals can help you feel capable, strong, and in control of your life. A positive attitude and a healthy lifestyle (such as exercising and eating right) are a great combination for building good self-esteem.

Tips For Improving Your Body Image

Some people think they need to change how they look or act to feel good about themselves. But actually all you need to do is change the way you see your body and how you think about yourself.

The first thing to do is recognize that your body is your own, no matter what shape, size, or color it comes in. If you're very worried about your weight or size, check with your doctor to verify that things are okay. But it's no one's business but your own what your body is like—ultimately, you have to be happy with yourself.

Next, identify which aspects of your appearance you can realistically change and which you can't. Everyone (even the most perfect-seeming celeb) has things about themselves that they can't change and need to accept—like their height, for example, or their shoe size.

If there are things about yourself that you want to change and can (such as how fit you are), do this by making goals for yourself. For example, if you want to get fit, make a plan to exercise every day and eat nutritious foods. Then keep track of your progress until you reach your goal. Meeting a challenge you set for yourself is a great way to boost self-esteem.

When you hear negative comments coming from within yourself, tell yourself to stop. Try building your self-esteem by giving yourself three compliments every day. While you're at it, every evening list three things in your day that really gave you pleasure. It can be anything from the way the sun felt on your face, the sound of your favorite band, or the way someone laughed at your jokes. By focusing on the good things you do and the positive aspects of your life, you can change how you feel about yourself.

Where Can I Go If I Need Help?

Sometimes low self-esteem and body image problems are too much to handle alone. A few teens may become depressed, lose interest in activities or friends—and even hurt themselves or resort to alcohol or drug abuse.

If you're feeling this way, it can help to talk to a parent, coach, religious leader, guidance counselor, therapist, or an adult friend. A trusted adult—someone who supports you and doesn't bring you down—can help you put your body image in perspective and give you positive feedback about your body, your skills, and your abilities.

If you can't turn to anyone you know, call a teen crisis hotline (check the yellow pages under social services or search online). The most important thing is to get help if you feel like your body image and self-esteem are affecting your life.

Chapter 39

Weight-Loss And Nutrition Myths

Diet Myths

- "Lose 30 pounds in 30 days!"
- "Eat as much as you want and still lose weight!"
- "Try the thigh buster and lose inches fast!"

And so on, and so on. With so many products and weight-loss theories out there, it is easy to get confused.

The information in this chapter may help clear up confusion about weight loss, nutrition, and physical activity. It may also help you make healthy changes in your eating and physical activity habits. If you have questions not answered here, or if you want to lose weight, talk to your health care provider. A registered dietitian or other qualified health professional can give you advice on how to follow a healthy eating plan, lose weight safely, and keep the weight off.

Myth: Fad diets work for permanent weight loss.

Fact: Fad diets are not the best way to lose weight and keep it off. Fad diets often promise quick weight loss or tell you to cut certain foods out of your diet. You may lose weight at first on one of these diets. But diets that strictly limit calories or food choices are hard to follow. Most people quickly get tired of them and regain any lost weight.

Fad diets may be unhealthy because they may not provide all of the nutrients your body needs. Also, losing weight at a very rapid rate (more than three pounds a week after the first

About This Chapter: Excerpted from "Weight-Loss And Nutrition Myths," National Institute of Diabetes and Digestive and Kidney Diseases, March 2009.

couple of weeks) may increase your risk for developing gallstones (clusters of solid material in the gallbladder that can be painful). Diets that provide less than 800 calories per day also could result in heart rhythm abnormalities, which can be fatal.

Tip: Research suggests that losing one half to two pounds a week by making healthy food choices, eating moderate portions, and building physical activity into your daily life is the best way to lose weight and keep it off. By adopting healthy eating and physical activity habits, you may also lower your risk for developing type 2 diabetes, heart disease, and high blood pressure.

Myth: High-protein/low-carbohydrate diets are a healthy way to lose weight.

Fact: The long-term health effects of a high-protein/low-carbohydrate diet are unknown. But getting most of your daily calories from high-protein foods like meat, eggs, and cheese is not a balanced eating plan. You may be eating too much fat and cholesterol, which may raise heart disease risk. You may be eating too few fruits, vegetables, and whole grains, which may lead to constipation due to lack of dietary fiber. Following a high-protein/low-carbohydrate diet may also make you feel nauseous, tired, and weak.

Eating fewer than 130 grams of carbohydrate a day can lead to the buildup of ketones in your blood. Ketones are partially broken-down fats. A buildup of these in your blood (called ketosis) can cause your body to produce high levels of uric acid, which is a risk factor for gout (a painful swelling of the joints) and kidney stones. Ketosis may be especially risky for pregnant women and people with diabetes or kidney disease. Be sure to discuss any changes in your diet with a health care professional, especially if you have health conditions such as cardiovascular disease, kidney disease, or type 2 diabetes.

Tip: High-protein/low-carbohydrate diets are often low in calories because food choices are strictly limited, so they may cause short-term weight loss. But a reduced-calorie eating plan that includes recommended amounts of carbohydrate, protein, and fat will also allow you to lose weight. By following a balanced eating plan, you will not have to stop eating whole classes of foods, such as whole grains, fruits, and vegetables—and miss the key nutrients they contain. You may also find it easier to stick with a diet or eating plan that includes a greater variety of foods.

Myth: Starches are fattening and should be limited when trying to lose weight.

Fact: Many foods high in starch, like bread, rice, pasta, cereals, beans, fruits, and some vegetables (like potatoes and yams) are low in fat and calories. They become high in fat and calories when eaten in large portion sizes or when covered with high-fat toppings like butter, sour cream, or mayonnaise. Foods high in starch (also called complex carbohydrates) are an important source of energy for your body.

Tip: A healthy eating plan is one that emphasizes fruits, vegetables, whole grains, and fat-free or low-fat milk and milk products, includes lean meats, poultry, fish, beans, eggs, and nuts and is low in saturated fats, trans fat, cholesterol, salt (sodium), and added sugars.

Myth: Certain foods, like grapefruit, celery, or cabbage soup, can burn fat and make you lose weight.

Fact: No foods can burn fat. Some foods with caffeine may speed up your metabolism (the way your body uses energy, or calories) for a short time, but they do not cause weight loss.

Tip: The best way to lose weight is to cut back on the number of calories you eat and be more physically active.

Myth: Natural or herbal weight-loss products are safe and effective.

Fact: A weight-loss product that claims to be "natural" or "herbal" is not necessarily safe. These products are not usually scientifically tested to prove that they are safe or that they work. For example, herbal products containing ephedra (now banned by the U.S. government) have caused serious health problems and even death. Newer products that claim to be ephedra free are not necessarily danger-free, because they may contain ingredients similar to ephedra.

Tip: Talk with your health care provider before using any weight-loss product. Some natural or herbal weight-loss products can be harmful.

Meal Myths

Myth: "I can lose weight while eating whatever I want."

Fact: To lose weight, you need to use more calories than you eat. It is possible to eat any kind of food you want and lose weight. You need to limit the number of calories you eat every day and/or increase your daily physical activity. Portion control is the key. Try eating smaller amounts of food and choosing foods that are low in calories.

Tip: When trying to lose weight, you can still eat your favorite foods—as long as you pay attention to the total number of calories that you eat.

Myth: Low-fat or fat-free means no calories.

Fact: A low-fat or fat-free food is often lower in calories than the same size portion of the full-fat product. But many processed low-fat or fat-free foods have just as many calories as the full-fat versions of the same foods—or even more calories. They may contain added sugar, flour, or starch thickeners to improve flavor and texture after fat is removed. These ingredients add calories.

Tip: Read the Nutrition Facts on a food package to find out how many calories are in a serving. Check the serving size too—it may be less than you are used to eating.

Myth: Fast foods are always an unhealthy choice and you should not eat them when dieting.

Fact: Fast foods can be part of a healthy weight-loss program with a little bit of know-how.

Tip: Avoid supersized combo meals, or split one with a friend. Sip on water or fat-free milk instead of soda. Choose salads and grilled foods, like a grilled chicken breast sandwich or small hamburger. Try a "fresco" taco (with salsa instead of cheese or sauce) at taco stands. Fried foods, like french fries and fried chicken, are high in fat and calories, so order them only once in a while, order a small portion, or split an order with a friend. Also, use only small amounts of high-fat, high-calorie toppings, like regular mayonnaise, salad dressings, bacon, and cheese.

Myth: Skipping meals is a good way to lose weight.

Fact: Studies show that people who skip breakfast and eat fewer times during the day tend to be heavier than people who eat a healthy breakfast and eat four or five times a day. This may be because people who skip meals tend to feel hungrier later on, and eat more than they normally would. It may also be that eating many small meals throughout the day helps people control their appetites.

Tip: Eat small meals throughout the day that include a variety of healthy, low-fat, low-calorie foods.

Lifting Weights Can Actually Help You Maintain Weight

Lifting weights or doing strengthening activities like push-ups and crunches on a regular basis won't just bulk you up, but it can actually help you maintain or lose weight. These activities can help you build muscle, and muscle burns more calories than body fat. So if you have more muscle, you burn more calories—even sitting still. Doing strengthening activities two or three days a week will not "bulk you up." Only intense strength training, combined with a certain genetic background, can build very large muscles.

In addition to doing moderate-intensity physical activity (like walking two miles in 30 minutes) on most days of the week, try to do strengthening activities two to three days a week. You can lift weights, use large rubber bands (resistance bands), do push-ups or sit-ups, or do household or garden tasks that make you lift or dig. Strength training helps keep your bones strong while building muscle, which can help burn calories.

Myth: Eating after 8 p.m. causes weight gain.

Fact: It does not matter what time of day you eat. It is what and how much you eat and how much physical activity you do during the whole day that determines whether you gain, lose, or maintain your weight. No matter when you eat, your body will store extra calories as fat.

Tip: If you want to have a snack before bedtime, think first about how many calories you have eaten that day. And try to avoid snacking in front of the TV at night—it may be easier to overeat when you are distracted by the television.

Food Myths

Myth: Nuts are fattening and you should not eat them if you want to lose weight.

Fact: In small amounts, nuts can be part of a healthy weight-loss program. Nuts are high in calories and fat. However, most nuts contain healthy fats that do not clog arteries. Nuts are also good sources of protein, dietary fiber, and minerals including magnesium and copper.

Tip: Enjoy small portions of nuts. One-half ounce of mixed nuts has about 84 calories.

Myth: Eating red meat is bad for your health and makes it harder to lose weight.

Fact: Eating lean meat in small amounts can be part of a healthy weight-loss plan. Red meat, pork, chicken, and fish contain some cholesterol and saturated fat (the least healthy kind of fat). They also contain healthy nutrients like protein, iron, and zinc.

Tip: Choose cuts of meat that are lower in fat and trim all visible fat. Lower fat meats include pork tenderloin and beef round steak, tenderloin, sirloin tip, flank steak, and extra lean ground beef. Also, pay attention to portion size. Three ounces of meat or poultry is the size of a deck of cards.

Myth: Dairy products are fattening and unhealthy.

Fact: Low-fat and fat-free milk, yogurt, and cheese are just as nutritious as whole-milk dairy products, but they are lower in fat and calories. Dairy products have many nutrients your body needs. They offer protein to build muscles and help organs work properly, and calcium to strengthen bones. Most milk and some yogurt are fortified with vitamin D to help your body use calcium.

Tip: The 2010 *Dietary Guidelines for Americans* recommends consuming three cups per day of fat-free/low-fat milk or equivalent milk products (for adults and children and adolescents ages 9 to 18 years). If you cannot digest lactose (the sugar found in dairy products), choose low-lactose or lactose-free dairy products, or other foods and beverages that offer calcium and vitamin D.

Myth: "Going vegetarian" means you are sure to lose weight and be healthier.

Fact: Research shows that people who follow a vegetarian eating plan, on average, eat fewer calories and less fat than non-vegetarians. They also tend to have lower body weights relative to their heights than non-vegetarians. Choosing a vegetarian eating plan with a low fat content may be helpful for weight loss. But vegetarians—like non-vegetarians—can make food choices that contribute to weight gain, like eating large amounts of high-fat, high-calorie foods or foods with little or no nutritional value.

Vegetarian diets should be as carefully planned as non-vegetarian diets to make sure they are balanced. Nutrients that non-vegetarians normally get from animal products, but that are not always found in a vegetarian eating plan, are iron, calcium, vitamin D, vitamin B12, zinc, and protein.

Tip: Choose a vegetarian eating plan that is low in fat and that provides all of the nutrients your body needs. Food and beverage sources of nutrients that may be lacking in a vegetarian diet are listed below.

- Iron can be found in cashews, spinach, lentils, garbanzo beans, fortified bread or cereal

- Calcium can be found in dairy products, fortified soy-based beverages, tofu made with calcium sulfate, collard greens, kale, or broccoli

- Vitamin D can be found in fortified foods and beverages including milk, soy-based beverages, and cereal

- Vitamin B12 can be found in eggs, dairy products, fortified cereal or soy-based beverages, tempeh, and miso (tempeh and miso are foods made from soybeans)

- Zinc can be found in whole grains (especially the germ and bran of the grain), nuts, tofu, and leafy vegetables (spinach, cabbage, lettuce)

- Protein can be found in eggs, dairy products, beans, peas, nuts, seeds, tofu, tempeh, and soy-based burgers

If you do not know whether or not to believe a weight-loss or nutrition claim, check it out. The Federal Trade Commission has information on deceptive weight-loss advertising claims. You can find this online at http://www.ftc.com. You can also find out more about nutrition and weight loss by talking with a registered dietitian. To find a registered dietitian in your area, visit the American Dietetic Association online at http://www.eatright.org.

Chapter 40

Choosing A Safe And Successful Weight-Loss Program

Choosing a weight-loss program may be a difficult task. You may not know what to look for in a weight-loss program or what questions to ask. This chapter can help you talk to your health care professional about weight loss and get the best information before choosing a program.

Talk With Your Health Care Professional

If your health care provider tells you that you should lose weight and you want to find a weight-loss program to help you, look for one that is based on regular physical activity and an eating plan that is balanced, healthy, and easy to follow.

You may want to talk with your doctor or other health care professional about controlling your weight before you decide on a weight-loss program. Doctors do not always address issues such as healthy eating, physical activity, and weight management during general office visits. It is important for you to start the discussion in order to get the information you need. Even if you feel uncomfortable talking about your weight with your doctor, remember that he or she is there to help you improve your health. Take advantage of the following tips:

- Tell your health care professional that you would like to talk about your weight. Share your concerns about any medical conditions you have or medicines you are taking.

- Write down your questions in advance.

- Bring pen and paper to take notes.

About This Chapter: Excerpted from, "Choosing A Safe And Successful Weight-Loss Program," National Institute of Diabetes and Digestive and Kidney Diseases, April 2008.

- Bring a friend or family member along for support if this will make you feel more comfortable.

- Make sure you understand what your health care provider is saying. Do not be afraid to ask questions if there is something you do not understand.

- Ask for other sources of information like brochures or websites.

- If you want more support, ask for a referral to a registered dietitian, a support group, or a commercial weight-loss program.

- Call your health care professional after your visit if you have more questions or need help.

Ask Questions

Find out as much as you can about your health needs before joining a weight-loss program. Here are some questions you might want to ask your health care professional:

About Your Weight

- Do I need to lose weight? Or should I just avoid gaining more?

- Is my weight affecting my health?

- Could my extra weight be caused by a health problem such as hypothyroidism or by a medicine I am taking? (Hypothyroidism is when your thyroid gland does not produce enough thyroid hormone, a condition that can slow your metabolism—how your body creates and uses energy.)

About Weight Loss

- What should my weight-loss goal be?

- How will losing weight help me?

About Nutrition And Physical Activity

- How should I change my eating habits?

- What kinds of physical activity can I do?

- How much physical activity do I need?

About Treatment

- Should I take weight-loss drugs?

- What about weight-loss surgery?

- What are the risks of weight-loss drugs or surgery?

- Could a weight-loss program help me?

A Responsible And Safe Weight-Loss Program

If your health care provider tells you that you should lose weight and you want to find a weight-loss program to help you, look for one that is based on regular physical activity and an eating plan that is balanced, healthy, and easy to follow. Weight-loss programs should encourage healthy behaviors that help you lose weight and that you can stick with every day. Safe and effective weight-loss programs should include the following:

- Healthy eating plans that reduce calories but do not forbid specific foods or food groups.

- Tips to increase moderate-intensity physical activity.

- Tips on healthy habits that also keep your cultural needs in mind, such as lower-fat versions of your favorite foods.

- Slow and steady weight loss. Depending on your starting weight, experts recommend losing weight at a rate of a half-pound to two pounds per week. Weight loss may be faster at the start of a program.

- Medical care if you are planning to lose weight by following a special formula diet, such as a very low-calorie diet (a program that requires careful monitoring from a doctor).

- A plan to keep the weight off after you have lost it.

Get Familiar With The Program

Gather as much information as you can before deciding to join a program. Professionals working for weight-loss programs should be able to answer the questions listed below.

- What does the weight-loss program consist of?

- Does the program offer one-on-one counseling or group classes?

- Do you have to follow a specific meal plan or keep food records?

- Do you have to purchase special food, drugs, or supplements?

- If the program requires special foods, can you make changes based on your likes and dislikes and food allergies?

- Does the program help you be more physically active, follow a specific physical activity plan, or provide exercise instruction?

- Does the program teach you to make positive and healthy behavior changes?

- Is the program sensitive to your lifestyle and cultural needs?

- Does the program provide ways to keep the weight off? Will the program provide ways to deal with such issues as what to eat at social or holiday gatherings, changes to work schedules, lack of motivation, and injury or illness?

A "Stick-to-It" Diet Is More Important Than a Popular One

With over 1,000 diet books available on bookstore shelves, popular diets clearly have become increasingly prevalent. At the same time, they have also become increasingly controversial, because some depart substantially from mainstream medical advice or have been criticized by various medical authorities.

A comparison of several popular diets by Agricultural Research Service (ARS)-funded researchers showed that at the end of the day, or in this case at the end of the year, sticking with a diet—more than the type of a diet—is the key to losing weight.

The study was conducted by Michael L. Dansinger, Ernst J. Schaefer, and Joi A. Gleason of the Lipid Metabolism Laboratory at the Jean Mayer USDA Human Nutrition Research Center on Aging at Tufts University and Tufts-New England Medical Center in Boston.

Published last year in the *Journal of the American Medical Association*, the study compared the relative merits of four of the most popular weight-loss diets. These included the Atkins (carbohydrate restriction), Ornish (fat restriction), Weight Watchers (calorie and portion size restriction), and Zone (high-glycemic-load carbohydrate restriction and increased protein) diets.

The researchers randomly assigned 160 overweight or obese volunteers to use one of the four diets. All participants were provided with the diet book and four 1-hour instructional classes to help them assimilate the rules of their assigned diets. The 40 participants in each of the four diet groups were representative—in terms of age, race, sex, body mass index, and metabolic characteristics—of the overweight population in the United States.

The results in terms of both weight loss and reduction in heart disease risk factors were compared among "completers," or those who stayed with the study for an entire year.

Only about half the volunteers completed the program while on what the authors considered to be more extreme diet plans: Atkins and Ornish diets. In contrast, 65% were able to complete the more moderate diet plans: Weight Watchers and Zone. Still, those that stayed in the program tended to loosen their resolve by about six months, as determined by their self-reported food records.

"The bottom line was that it wasn't so much the type of diet followed that led to successful weight loss, but the ability of participants to stick with the program for the entire year's time," says Schaefer.

- What are the staff qualifications?

- Who supervises the program?

- What type of weight management training, experience, education, and certifications do the staff have?

- Does the product or program carry any risks?

- Could the program hurt you?

"The study showed that whether volunteers restricted carbohydrate calories or fat calories—whether they lowered intake overall, or balanced intake overall—everybody lost weight," says Schaefer. "Ultimately, it comes down to calorie restriction. The strongest predictor of weight loss was not the type of diet, but compliance with the diet plan that subjects were given."

The finding lends credence to the importance of adopting a caloric-restriction diet that doesn't conflict with one's natural affinities for specific allowable foods.

"Implementing a dietary regimen that can transition an individual into a healthful eating pattern after the diet ends is also very important," says ARS Human Nutrition National Program Leader Molly Kretsch. "Lifestyle practices that help people maintain a healthy body weight, incorporate the right balance of foods and appropriate portion sizes, and increase their physical activity are the keys to long-term weight management."

Among those who stayed in the program for the entire 12-month period, all four diet plans promoted a 10% improvement in the balance of "good" (HDL) and "bad" (LDL) cholesterol levels. "The particular diet plan the long-term dieter followed did not seem to matter that much," says Dansinger. "The long-term dieters reduced their ratio of good to bad cholesterol according to how much weight they lost."

Those who improved their cholesterol ratios by 10% improved their heart disease risk factors by 20%. "For every 1% of weight loss a dieter achieves, there will be a 2%, or twice as much, reduction in heart disease risk factors," says Dansinger.

In addition, all four diet plans promoted lower blood insulin levels as well as lower levels of C reactive protein (CRP). High levels of CRP in the blood have been linked to heart disease.

Future studies will focus on identifying practical techniques to increase dietary adherence—including ways to match individuals with the diets best suited to their food preferences and lifestyles. "We also plan to test different versions of the new USDA diet and look specifically at the results from a diet with higher and lower glycemic index values," says Schaefer.

Source: Excepted from "A "Stick-to-It" Diet Is More Important Than a Popular One," *Agricultural Research Magazine*, U.S. Department of Agriculture (www.usda.gov), March 2006, Vol. 54, No 3.

- Could the recommended drugs or supplements harm your health?

- Do participants talk with a doctor?

- Does a doctor run the program?

- Will the program's doctors work with your personal doctor if you have a medical condition such as high blood pressure or are taking prescribed drugs?

- Is there ongoing input and follow-up from a health care professional to ensure your safety while you participate in the program?

- How much does the program cost?

- What is the total cost of the program?

- Are there other costs, such as weekly attendance fees, food and supplement purchases, etc.?

- Are there fees for a follow-up program after you lose weight?

- Are there other fees for medical tests?

- What results do participants typically have?

- How much weight does an average participant lose and how long does he or she keep the weight off?

- Does the program offer publications or materials that describe what results participants typically have?

If you are interested in finding a weight-loss program near you, ask your health care provider for a referral or contact your local hospital.

Chapter 41

Diet Don'ts

Nutrition experts at the American Heart Association (AHA) recommend adopting healthy eating habits permanently, rather than impatiently pursuing crash diets in hopes of losing unwanted pounds in a few days.

Why does the AHA care about these diets?

AHA wants to inform the public about misleading weight-loss claims. Many of these diets—like the infamous Cabbage Soup Diet—can undermine your health, cause physical discomfort (abdominal discomfort and flatulence [gas]), and lead to disappointment when you regain weight soon after you lose it.

- Quick-weight-loss diets usually overemphasize one particular food or type of food. They violate the first principle of good nutrition: Eat a balanced diet that includes a variety of foods. If you are able to stay on such a diet for more than a few weeks, you may develop nutritional deficiencies, because no one type of food has all the nutrients you need for good health. The Cabbage Soup Diet mentioned above is an example. This so-called fat-burning soup is eaten mostly with fruits and vegetables. The diet supposedly helps heart patients lose 10–17 pounds in seven days before surgery. There are no "superfoods." That's why you should eat moderate amounts from all food groups, not large amounts of a few special foods.

- These diets also violate a second important principle of good nutrition: Eating should be enjoyable. These diets are so monotonous and boring that it's almost impossible to stay on them for long periods.

About This Chapter: "Quick-Weight-Loss or Fad Diets," reprinted with permission www.heart.org. © 2011 American Heart Association, Inc.

Let's set the record straight: Many of these diets falsely say they are endorsed by or authored by the American Heart Association. The public should know that the real American Heart Association diet and lifestyle recommendations emphasize flexibility in food selection and stress the importance of eating more nutrient-rich foods—that have vitamins, minerals, fiber, and other nutrients but are lower in calories—and fewer nutrient-poor foods.

Unlike an incomplete liquid protein diet or other fad diets, a good diet can be eaten for years to maintain desirable body weight and good health. Fad diets fail to provide ways to keep weight off.

- Some major medical centers prescribe extremely low-calorie, high-protein diets for selected patients who are carefully monitored by physicians.

In what other ways are quick-weight-loss diets flawed?

- Many don't encourage physical activity—for example, walking 30 minutes most or all days of the week. Being physically active helps you maintain weight loss over a long time. Physical inactivity is a major risk factor for heart disease and stroke.

- Because most quick-weight-loss diets require drastic changes in eating patterns, you can't stay on them for long. Following a regimen for a few weeks won't give you the chance to learn about how to permanently change your eating patterns.

- In addition, many fad diets are based on "food folklore," some dating back to the early 19th century. They have not been documented to be safe in the long term. Ideas about "fat-burning foods" and "food combining" are also classified by the American Heart Association as unsubstantiated myths.

Creating A Calorie Deficit To Reduce Weight

Knowing one's daily calorie needs may be a useful reference point for determining whether the calories that a person eats and drinks are appropriate in relation to the number of calories needed each day. The best way for people to assess whether they are eating the appropriate number of calories is to monitor body weight and adjust calorie intake and participation in physical activity based on changes in weight over time. A calorie deficit of 500 calories or more per day is a common initial goal for weight loss for adults. However, maintaining a smaller deficit can have a meaningful influence on body weight over time.

The effect of a calorie deficit on weight does not depend on how the deficit is produced—by reducing calorie intake, increasing expenditure, or both. Yet, in research studies, a greater proportion of the calorie deficit is often due to decreasing calorie intake with a relatively smaller fraction due to increased physical activity.

Source: Excerpted from *Dietary Guidelines for Americans 2010*, U.S. Department of Agriculture, December 2010.

Weight Management And Macronutrient Proportions

To manage body weight, Americans should consume a diet that has an appropriate total number of calories and that is within the Acceptable Macronutrient Distribution Ranges (AMDR). Strong evidence shows that there is no optimal proportion of macronutrients that can facilitate weight loss or assist with maintaining weight loss.

Although diets with a wide range of macronutrient proportions have been documented to promote weight loss and prevent weight regain after loss, evidence shows that the critical issue is not the relative proportion of macronutrients in the diet, but whether or not the eating pattern is reduced in calories and the individual is able to maintain a reduced-calorie intake over time.

The total number of calories consumed is the essential dietary factor relevant to body weight. In adults, moderate evidence suggests that diets that are less than 45 percent of total calories as carbohydrate or more than 35 percent of total calories as protein are generally no more effective than other calorie-controlled diets for long-term weight loss and weight maintenance. Therefore, individuals who wish to lose weight or maintain weight loss can select eating patterns that maintain appropriate calorie intake and have macronutrient proportions that are within the AMDR ranges recommended in the Dietary Reference Intakes.

Recommended Macronutrient Proportions By Age

Young Children (1–3 Years)

- Carbohydrate: 45–65%
- Protein: 5–20%
- Fat: 30–40%

Older Children And Adolescents (4–18 Years)

- Carbohydrate: 45–65%
- Protein: 10–30%
- Fat: 25–35%

Adults (19 Years And Older)

- Carbohydrate: 45–65%
- Protein: 10–35%
- Fat: 20–35%

Source of data: Institute of Medicine. Dietary Reference Intakes for Energy, Carbohydrate, Fiber, Fat, Fatty Acids, Cholesterol, Protein, and Amino Acids. Washington (DC): The National Academies Press; 2002.

Source of information: Excerpted from *Dietary Guidelines for Americans 2010*, U.S. Department of Agriculture, December 2010.

Despite what quick-weight-loss diet books may say, the only sensible way to lose weight and maintain a healthy weight permanently is to eat less and balance your food intake with physical activity.

What is the best way to lose weight?

A healthy diet rich in fresh fruits and vegetables, whole grains, and fat-free or low-fat dairy products, along with regular physical activity, can help most people manage and maintain weight loss for both cardiovascular health and appearance. The American Heart Association urges people to take a safe and proven route to losing and maintaining weight—by following AHA guidelines for healthy, nutritionally balanced weight loss for a lifetime of good health.

Chapter 42

Should I Gain Weight?

"I want to play hockey, like I did in middle school, but now that I'm in high school, the other guys have bulked up and I haven't. What can I do?"

"All of my friends have broad shoulders and look like they lift weights. No matter what I do, I just look scrawny. What can I do?"

"It's not like I want to gain a lot of weight, but I'd like to look like I have some curves, like the girls I see on TV. What can I do?"

A lot of teens think that they're too skinny, and wonder if they should do something about it.

Why Do People Want To Gain Weight?

Some of the reasons people give for wanting to gain weight are:

"I'm worried that there's something wrong with me." If you want to gain weight because you think you have a medical problem, talk to your doctor. Although certain health conditions can cause a person to be underweight, most of them have symptoms other than skinniness, like stomach pain or diarrhea. So it's likely that if some kind of medical problem is making you skinny, you probably wouldn't feel well.

"I'm worried because all of my friends have filled out and I haven't." Many guys and girls are skinny until they start to go through puberty. The changes that come with puberty include weight gain and, in guys, broader shoulders and increased muscle mass.

About This Chapter: "Should I Gain Weight?" October 2010, reprinted with permission from www.kidshealth .org. Copyright © 2010 The Nemours Foundation. This information was provided by KidsHealth, one of the largest resources online for medically reviewed health information written for parents, kids, and teens. For more articles like this one, visit www.KidsHealth.org, or www.TeensHealth.org.

Because everyone is on a different schedule, some of your friends may have started to fill out when they were as young as 8 (if they're girls) or 10 (if they're guys). But for some normal kids, puberty may not start until 12 or later for girls and 14 or later for guys. And whenever you start puberty, it may take three or four years for you to fully develop and gain all of the weight and muscle mass you will have as an adult.

Some people experience what's called delayed puberty. If you are one of these "late bloomers," you may find that some relatives of yours developed late, too. Most teens who have delayed puberty don't need to do anything; they'll eventually develop normally—and that includes gaining weight and muscle. If you are concerned about delayed puberty, though, talk to your doctor.

"I've always wanted to play a certain sport; now I don't know if I can." Lots of people come to love a sport in grade school or middle school—and then find themselves on the bench when their teammates develop faster. If you've always envisioned yourself playing football, it can be tough when your body doesn't seem to want to measure up. You may need to wait until your body goes through puberty before you can play football on the varsity squad.

Another option to consider is switching your ambitions to another sport. If you were the fastest defensive player on your middle school football team but now it seems that your body type is long and lean, maybe track and field is for you. Many adults find that the sports they love the most are those that fit their body types the best.

"I just hate the way I look." Developing can be tough enough without the pressure to be perfect. Your body changes (or doesn't change), your friends' bodies change (or don't), and you all spend a lot of time noticing. It's easy to judge both yourself and others based on appearances. Sometimes, it can feel like life is some kind of beauty contest.

Your body is your own, and as frustrating as it may seem to begin with, there are certain things you can't speed up or change. But there is one thing you can do to help: Work to keep your body healthy so that you can grow and develop properly. Self-esteem can play a part here, too. People who learn to love their bodies and accept them for what they are carry themselves well and project a type of self-confidence that helps them look attractive.

If you're having trouble with your body image, talk about how you feel with someone you like and trust who's been through it—maybe a parent, doctor, counselor, coach, or teacher.

It's The Growth, Not The Gain

No matter what your reason is for wanting to gain weight, here's a simple fact: The majority of teens have no reason—medical or otherwise—to try to gain weight. An effort like this will at best simply not work and at worst increase your body fat, putting you at risk for health problems.

So focus on growing strong, not gaining weight. Keeping your body healthy and fit so that it grows well is an important part of your job as a teen. Here are some things you can do to help this happen:

Make nutrition your mission: Your friends who want to slim down are eating more salads and fruit. Here's a surprise: So should you. You can do more for your body by eating a variety of healthier foods instead of trying to pack on weight by forcing yourself to eat a lot of unhealthy high-fat, high-sugar foods. Chances are, trying to force-feed yourself won't help you gain weight anyway, and if you do, you'll mostly just be gaining excess body fat.

Eating well at this point in your life is important for lots of reasons. Good nutrition is a key part of normal growth and development. It's also wise to learn good eating habits now—they'll become second nature, which will help you stay healthy and fit without even thinking about it.

Keep on moving: Another way to keep your body healthy is to incorporate exercise into your routine. This can include walking to school, playing Frisbee with your friends, or helping out with some household chores. Or you might choose to work out at a gym or with a sports team. A good rule of thumb for exercise amounts during the teen years: Try to get at least 60 minutes of moderate to vigorous physical activity every day.

Quick Nutrition Tips

Eating a variety of healthy foods, making time for regular meals and snacks, and eating only until you are full will give your body its best chance to stay healthy as it gets the fuel and nutrients it needs.

Good nutrition doesn't have to be complicated. Here are some simple tips:

- Eat lots of vegetables, and fruits
- Choose whole grains
- Eat breakfast every day
- Eat healthy snacks
- Limit less nutritious foods, like chips and soda

Strength training, when done safely, is a healthy way to exercise, but it won't necessarily bulk you up. Guys especially get more muscular during puberty, but puberty is no guarantee that you'll turn into a cover model for *Muscle & Fitness* in a couple of years—some people just don't have the kind of body type for this to happen. Our genes play an important role in determining our body type. Adult bodies come in all different shapes and sizes, and some people stay lean their entire lives, no matter what they do.

If you've hit puberty, the right amount of strength training will help your muscles become stronger and have more endurance. And, once a boy has reached puberty, proper weight training can help him bulk up, if that's the goal. Girls can benefit from strength training, too, but they won't bulk up like boys. Be sure to work with a certified trainer, who can show you how to do it without injuring yourself.

Get the skinny on supplements: Thinking about drinking something from a can or taking a pill to turn you buff overnight? Guess what: Supplements or pills that make promises like this are at best a waste of money and at worst potentially harmful to your health.

The best way to get the fuel you need to build muscle is by eating well. Before you take any kind of supplement at all, even if it's just a vitamin pill, talk to your doctor.

Sleep your way to stunning: Sleep is an important component of normal growth and development. If you get enough, you'll have the energy to fuel your growth. Your body is at work while it sleeps—oxygen moves to the brain, growth hormones are released, and your bones keep on developing, even while you're resting.

Focus on feeling good: It can help to know that your body is likely to change in the months and years ahead. Few of us look like we did at 15 when we're 25. But it's also important to realize that feeling good about yourself can make you more attractive to others, too.

Chapter 43

How To Spot Nutrition-Related Health Fraud

Tip-Offs To Rip-Offs: How To Spot Health Fraud

You don't have to look far to find a health product that's totally bogus—or a consumer who's totally unsuspecting. Promotions for fraudulent products show up daily in newspaper and magazine ads and TV "infomercials." They accompany products sold in stores, on the internet, and through mail-order catalogs. They're passed along by word-of-mouth.

And consumers respond, spending billions of dollars a year on fraudulent health products, according to Dr. Stephen Barrett, head of Quackwatch Inc., a nonprofit corporation that combats health fraud. Hoping to find a cure for what ails them, improve their well-being, or just look better, consumers often fall victim to products and devices that do nothing more than cheat them out of their money, steer them away from useful, proven treatments, and possibly do more bodily harm than good.

"There's a lot of money to be made," says Bob Gatling, director of the program operations staff in the Center for Devices and Radiological Health at the U.S. Food and Drug Administration (FDA). "People want to believe there's something that can cure them."

FDA describes health fraud as "articles of unproven effectiveness that are promoted to improve health, well being or appearance." The articles can be drugs, devices, foods, or cosmetics for human or animal use.

FDA shares federal oversight of health fraud products with the Federal Trade Commission (FTC). FDA regulates safety, manufacturing, and product labeling, including claims in labeling, such as package inserts and accompanying literature. FTC regulates advertising of these products.

About This Chapter: Excerpted from "How To Spot Health Fraud," U.S. Food and Drug Administration (www.fda .gov), February 2010.

Because of limited resources, says Joel Aronson, team leader for the nontraditional drug compliance team in FDA's Center for Drug Evaluation and Research, the agency's regulation of health fraud products is based on a priority system that depends on whether a fraudulent product poses a direct or indirect risk.

When the use of a fraudulent product results in injuries or adverse reactions, it's a direct risk. When the product itself does not cause harm but its use may keep someone away from proven, sometimes essential, medical treatment, the risk is indirect. For example, a fraudulent product touted as a cure for diabetes might lead someone to delay or discontinue insulin injections or other proven treatments.

While FDA remains vigilant against health fraud, many fraudulent products may escape regulatory scrutiny, maintaining their hold in the marketplace for some time to lure increasing numbers of consumers into their web of deceit.

How can you avoid being scammed by a worthless product? Though health fraud marketers have become more sophisticated about selling their products, Aronson says, these charlatans often use the same old phrases and gimmicks to gain consumers' attention—and trust. You can protect yourself by learning some of their techniques.

The following products typify three fraudulent products whose claims prompted FDA to issue warning letters to the products' marketers, notifying them that their products violated federal law. Two of the products also were added to FDA's import alert list of unapproved new drugs promoted in the United States. Products under import alert are barred from entry onto the U.S. market.

Take a look at these products' promotions. They are rife with the kind of red flags to look out for when deciding whether to try a health product unknown to you.

Product No. 1: Pure Emu Oil

FDA determined that a pure emu oil product marketed to treat or cure a wide range of diseases was an unapproved drug. Its marketer had never submitted to FDA data to support the product's safe and effective use.

One Product Does It All

Be suspicious of products that claim to cure a wide range of unrelated diseases—particularly serious diseases, such as cancer and diabetes. No product can treat every disease and condition, and for many serious diseases, there are no cures, only therapies to help manage them.

Cancer, AIDS, diabetes, and other serious diseases are big draws because people with these diseases are often desperate for a cure and willing to try just about anything.

Weighing The Evidence In Diet Ads

Flip through a magazine, scan a newspaper, or channel surf and you see them everywhere: Ads that promise quick and easy weight loss without diet or exercise. Wouldn't it be nice if—as the ads claim—you could lose weight simply by taking a pill, wearing a patch, or rubbing in a cream? Too bad claims like that are almost always false.

Doctors, dieticians, and other experts agree that the best way to lose weight is to eat fewer calories and increase your physical activity so you burn more energy. A reasonable goal is to lose about a pound a week. For most people, that means cutting about 500 calories a day from your diet, eating a variety of nutritious foods, and exercising regularly.

When it comes to evaluating claims for weight loss products, the Federal Trade Commission (FTC) recommends a healthy portion of skepticism. Before you spend money on products that promise fast and easy results, weigh the claims carefully. Think twice before wasting your money on products that make any of the following false claims:

"Lose weight without diet or exercise!" Achieving a healthy weight takes work. Take a pass on any product that promises miraculous results without the effort. Buy one and the only thing you'll lose is money.

"Lose weight no matter how much you eat of your favorite foods!" Beware of any product that claims that you can eat all you want of high-calorie foods and still lose weight. Losing weight requires sensible food choices. Filling up on healthy vegetables and fruits can make it easier to say no to fattening sweets and snacks.

"Lose weight permanently! Never diet again!" Even if you're successful in taking the weight off, permanent weight loss requires permanent lifestyle changes. Don't trust any product that promises once-and-for-all results without ongoing maintenance.

"Block the absorption of fat, carbs, or calories!" Doctors, dieticians, and other experts agree that there's simply no magic non-prescription pill that will allow you to block the absorption of fat, carbs, or calories. The key to curbing your craving for those "downfall foods" is portion control. Limit yourself to a smaller serving or a slimmer slice.

"Lose 30 pounds in 30 days!" Losing weight at the rate of a pound or two a week is the most effective way to take it off and keep it off. At best, products promising lightning-fast weight loss are false. At worst, they can ruin your health.

"Everybody will lose weight!" Your habits and health concerns are unique. There is simply no one-size-fits-all product guaranteed to work for everyone. Team up with your health care provider to design a personalized nutrition and exercise program suited to your lifestyle and metabolism.

"Lose weight with our miracle diet patch or cream!" You've seen the ads for diet patches or creams that claim to melt away the pounds. Don't believe them. There's nothing you can wear or apply to your skin that will cause you to lose weight.

Source: Excerpted from "Weighing the Evidence in Diet Ads," Federal Trade Commission, November 2004. Despite the older date of this document, the cautions about fraudulent advertising are still pertinent.

Personal Testimonials

Personal testimonies can tip you off to health fraud because they are difficult to prove. Often, says Reynaldo Rodriguez, a compliance officer and health fraud coordinator for FDA's Dallas district office, testimonials are personal case histories that have been passed on from person to person. Or, the testimony can be completely made up.

"This is the weakest form of scientific validity," Rodriguez says. "It's just compounded hearsay."

Some patients' favorable experiences with a fraudulent product may be due more to a remission in their disease or from earlier or concurrent use of approved medical treatments, rather than use of the fraudulent product itself.

Quick Fixes

Be wary of talk that suggests a product can bring quick relief or provide a quick cure, especially if the disease or condition is serious. Even with proven treatments, few diseases can be treated quickly. Note also that the words "in days" can really refer to any length of time. Fraud promoters like to use ambiguous language like this to make it easier to finagle their way out of any legal action that may result.

Product No. 2: Over-The-Counter Transdermal Weight-Loss Patch

FDA issued a warning letter to the marketer of the weight-loss product described here because it did not have an approved new drug application. Because of the newness of the dosage form—skin-delivery systems—FDA requires evidence of effectiveness, in the form of a new drug application, before the product can be marketed legally.

The product was marketed as "Natural" and as a "Healthy, simple and natural way to help you lose and control your weight."

Don't be fooled by the term "natural." It's often used in health fraud as an attention-grabber; it suggests a product is safer than conventional treatments. But the term doesn't necessarily equate to safety because some plants—for example, poisonous mushrooms—can kill when ingested. And among legitimate drug products, says Shelly Maifarth, a compliance officer and health fraud coordinator for FDA's Denver district office, 60% of over-the-counter drugs and 25% of prescription drugs are based on natural ingredients.

And, any product, synthetic or natural, potent enough to work like a drug is going to be potent enough to cause side effects.

Time-Tested Or Newfound Treatment

The product claimed, "This revolutionary innovation is formulated by using proven principles of natural health based upon 200 years of medical science." Usually it's one or the other, but this claim manages to suggest it's both a breakthrough and a decades-old remedy.

Claims of an "innovation," "miracle cure," "exclusive product," or "new discovery" or "magical" are highly suspect. If a product was a cure for a serious disease, it would be widely reported in the media and regularly prescribed by health professionals—not hidden in an obscure magazine or newspaper ad, late-night television show, or website promotion, where the marketers are of unknown, questionable or nonscientific backgrounds.

The same applies to products purported to be "ancient remedies" or based on "folklore" or "tradition." These claims suggest that these products' longevity proves they are safe and effective. But some herbs reportedly used in ancient times for medicinal purposes carry risks identified only recently.

Satisfaction Guaranteed

Another advertising ploy claims "...Guarantee: If after 30 days... you have not lost at least four pounds each week... your uncashed check will be returned to you..."

This is another red flag: money-back guarantees, no questions asked. Good luck getting your money back. Marketers of fraudulent products rarely stay in the same place for long. Because customers won't be able to find them, the marketers can afford to be generous with their guarantees.

Product No. 3: Unapproved Weight-Loss Product Marketed As An Alternative To A Prescription Drug Combination

FDA issued an import alert for a Canadian-made weight-loss product whose claims compared the product with two prescription weight-loss drugs taken off the market after FDA determined they posed a health hazard. The advertisements made these claims: "Promises of Easy Weight Loss: Finally, rapid weight loss without dieting!"

For most people, there is only one way to lose weight: Eat less food (or fewer high-calorie foods) and increase activity. Note the ambiguity of the term "rapid." A reasonable and healthy weight loss is about one to two pounds a week.

Paranoid Accusations

Claims included statements such as these: "Drug companies make it nearly impossible for doctors to resist prescribing their expensive pills for what ails you..." "It seems these billion dollar drug giants all have one relentless competitor in common they all constantly fear—natural remedies."

These claims suggest that health-care providers and legitimate manufacturers are in cahoots with each other, promoting only the drug companies' and medical device manufacturers' products for financial gain. The claims also suggest that the medical profession and legitimate drug and device makers strive to suppress unorthodox products because they threaten their financial standing.

"This [accusation] is an easy way to get consumers' attention," says Marjorie Powell, assistant general counsel for the Pharmaceutical Research and Manufacturers of America. "But I would ask the marketers of such claims, 'Where's the evidence?' It would seem to me that in this country, outside of a regulatory agency it would be difficult to stop someone from making a claim."

Think about this, too: Would the vast number of people in the health-care field block treatments that could help millions of sick, suffering patients, many of whom could be family and friends? "It flies in the face of logic," Barrett says on his Quackwatch website.

Meaningless Medical Jargon

Here are some examples: "...Hunger stimulation point (HSP)..." "...thermogenesis, which converts stored fats into soluble lipids..." "One of the many natural ingredients is inositol hexanicontinate."

Terms and scientific explanations such as these may sound impressive and may have an element of truth to them, but the public "has no way of discerning fact from fiction," Aronson says. Fanciful terms, he says, generally cover up a lack of scientific proof.

Sometimes, the terms or explanations are lifted from a study published in a reputable scientific journal, even though the study was on another subject altogether, says Martin Katz, a compliance officer and health fraud coordinator for FDA's Florida district office. And chances are, few people will check the original published study.

"Most people who are taken in by health fraud will grasp at anything," he says. "They're not going to do the research. They're looking for a miracle."

Truth Or Dare

The underlying rule when deciding whether a product is authentic or not is to ask yourself, "Does it sound too good to be true?" If it does, it probably isn't true.

If you're still not sure, check it out, "Look into it—before you put it in your body or on your skin," says Reynaldo Rodriguez, a compliance officer and health fraud coordinator for FDA's Dallas district office.

How To Verify Health Claims

To check a product out, U.S. Food and Drug Administration (FDA) health fraud coordinators suggest these steps:

- Talk to a doctor or another health professional. "If it's an unproven or little-known treatment, always get a second opinion from a medical specialist," Rodriguez says.

- Talk to family members and friends. Legitimate medical practitioners should not discourage you from discussing medical treatments with others. Be wary of treatments offered by people who tell you to avoid talking to others because "it's a secret treatment or cure."

- Check with the Better Business Bureau or local attorneys general's offices to see whether other consumers have lodged complaints about the product or the product's marketer.

- Check with the appropriate health professional group—for example, the American Heart Association or American Diabetes Association if the products are promoted for heart disease or diabetes. Many of these groups have local chapters that can provide you with various resource materials about your disease.

- Contact the FDA office closest to you. Look for the number and address in the blue pages of the phone book under U.S. Government, Health and Human Services, or go to http://www.fda.gov/AboutFDA/ContactFDA/FindanOfficeorStaffMember/FDAPublicAffairs Specialists/default.htm on the FDA website. FDA can tell you whether the agency has taken action against the product or its marketer. Your call also may alert FDA to a potentially illegal product and prevent others from falling victim to health fraud.

Source: U.S. Food and Drug Administration (www.fda.gov), February 2010.

Chapter 44

Physical Activity And Health

Regular physical activity is one of the most important things you can do for your health. It can help to do the following:

- Control your weight
- Reduce your risk of cardiovascular disease
- Reduce your risk for type 2 diabetes and metabolic syndrome
- Reduce your risk of some cancers
- Strengthen your bones and muscles
- Improve your mental health and mood
- Improve your ability to do daily activities and prevent falls, if you're an older adult
- Increase your chances of living longer

If you're not sure about becoming active or boosting your level of physical activity because you're afraid of getting hurt, the good news is that moderate-intensity aerobic activity, like brisk walking, is generally safe for most people.

Start slowly. Cardiac events, such as a heart attack, are rare during physical activity. But the risk does go up when you suddenly become much more active than usual. For example, you can put yourself at risk if you don't usually get much physical activity and then all of a sudden do vigorous-intensity aerobic activity, like shoveling snow. That's why it's important to start slowly and gradually increase your level of activity.

About This Chapter: Excerpted from "Physical Activity And Health," Centers for Disease Control and Prevention, June 2010.

If you have a chronic health condition such as arthritis, diabetes, or heart disease, talk with your doctor to find out if your condition limits, in any way, your ability to be active. Then, work with your doctor to come up with a physical activity plan that matches your abilities. If your condition stops you from meeting the minimum Guidelines, try to do as much as you can. What's important is that you avoid being inactive. Even 60 minutes a week of moderate-intensity aerobic activity is good for you.

The bottom line is this: The health benefits of physical activity far outweigh the risks of getting hurt.

Control Your Weight

Looking to get to or stay at a healthy weight? Both diet and physical activity play a critical role in controlling your weight. You gain weight when the calories you burn, including those burned during physical activity, are less than the calories you eat or drink. When it comes to weight management, people vary greatly in how much physical activity they need. You may need to be more active than others to achieve or maintain a healthy weight.

To maintain your weight work your way up to 150 minutes of moderate-intensity aerobic activity, 75 minutes of vigorous-intensity aerobic activity, or an equivalent mix of the two each week. Strong scientific evidence shows that physical activity can help you maintain your weight over time. However, the exact amount of physical activity needed to do this is not clear since it varies greatly from person to person. It's possible that you may need to do more than the equivalent of 150 minutes of moderate-intensity activity a week to maintain your weight.

To lose weight and keep it off you will need a high amount of physical activity unless you also adjust your diet and reduce the amount of calories you're eating and drinking. Getting to and staying at a healthy weight requires both regular physical activity and a healthy eating plan.

Tips On Moving More

Physical activity can be fun. Do things you enjoy. Here are some examples:

- Dancing
- In-line skating
- Fast walking
- Playing sports
- Bicycling
- Swimming
- Group fitness classes, such as dance or aerobics

If you can, be physically active with a friend or a group. That way, you can cheer each other on, have a good time while being active, and feel safer when you are outdoors. Find a local school track or park where you can walk or run with your friends, or join a recreation center so you can work out or take a fun fitness class together.

Source: Excerpted from "Celebrate the Beauty of Youth," National Institute of Diabetes and Digestive And Kidney Diseases, November 2008.

Reduce Your Risk Of Cardiovascular Disease

Heart disease and stroke are two of the leading causes of death in the United States. But following physical activity guidelines and getting at least 150 minutes a week (two hours and 30 minutes) of moderate-intensity aerobic activity can put you at a lower risk for these diseases. You can reduce your risk even further with more physical activity. Regular physical activity can also lower your blood pressure and improve your cholesterol levels.

Reduce Your Risk Of Type-2 Diabetes And Metabolic Syndrome

Regular physical activity can reduce your risk of developing type 2 diabetes and metabolic syndrome. Metabolic syndrome is a condition in which you have some combination of too much fat around the waist, high blood pressure, low HDL cholesterol, high triglycerides, or high blood sugar. Research shows that lower rates of these conditions are seen with 120 to 150 minutes (two hours to two hours and 30 minutes) a week of at least moderate-intensity aerobic activity. And the more physical activity you do, the lower your risk will be.

Reduce Your Risk Of Some Cancers

Being physically active lowers your risk for two types of cancer: colon and breast. Research shows that physically active people have a lower risk of colon cancer than do people who are not active. Also, that physically active women have a lower risk of breast cancer than do people who are not active

Reduce your risk of endometrial and lung cancer. Although the research is not yet final, some findings suggest that your risk of endometrial cancer and lung cancer may be lower if you get regular physical activity compared to people who are not active.

Improve your quality of life. If you are a cancer survivor, research shows that getting regular physical activity not only helps give you a better quality of life, but also improves your physical fitness.

Strengthen Your Bones And Muscles

As you age, it's important to protect your bones, joints and muscles. Not only do they support your body and help you move, but keeping bones, joints and muscles healthy can help ensure that you're able to do your daily activities and be physically active. Research shows that doing aerobic, muscle-strengthening and bone-strengthening physical activity of at least a moderately-intense level can slow the loss of bone density that comes with age.

Hip fracture is a serious health condition that can have life-changing negative effects, especially for older adults. But research shows that people who do 120 to 300 minutes of at least moderate-intensity aerobic activity each week have a lower risk of hip fracture.

Regular physical activity helps with arthritis and other conditions affecting the joints. If you have arthritis, research shows that doing 130 to 150 (two hours and 10 minutes to two hours and 30 minutes) a week of moderate-intensity, low-impact aerobic activity can not only improve your ability to manage pain and do everyday tasks, but it can also make your quality of life better.

Build strong, healthy muscles. Muscle-strengthening activities can help you increase or maintain your muscle mass and strength. Slowly increasing the amount of weight and number of repetitions you do will give you even more benefits, no matter your age.

Improve Your Mental Health And Mood

Regular physical activity can help keep your thinking, learning, and judgment skills sharp as you age. It can also reduce your risk of depression and may help you sleep better. Research has shown that doing aerobic or a mix of aerobic and muscle-strengthening activities three to five times a week for 30 to 60 minutes can give you these mental health benefits. Some scientific evidence has also shown that even lower levels of physical activity can be beneficial.

Tips On Finding Time To Move More

Think you do not have time for physical activity? The good news is that you can be active for short periods of time throughout the day and still benefit. When fitting in physical activity, remember that any activity is better than none. So try to move more by making the following small changes to your daily routine:

- Get off the bus or subway one stop early and walk the rest of the way (be sure the area is safe).
- Park your car farther away and walk to your destination.
- Walk to each end of the mall when you go shopping.
- Take the stairs rather than the elevator or escalator (make sure the stairs have working lights).
- Put physical activity on your to-do list for the day. For example, plan on exercising right after school or work, before you can get distracted by dinner or going out.

Source: Excerpted from "Celebrate the Beauty of Youth," National Institute of Diabetes and Digestive And Kidney Diseases, November 2008.

Improve Your Ability To Do Daily Activities And Prevent Falls

A functional limitation is a loss of the ability to do everyday activities such as climbing stairs or grocery shopping.

How does this relate to physical activity? Middle-aged and older adults who are physically active have a lower risk of functional limitations than people who are inactive. For those who already have trouble doing some everyday activities, aerobic and muscle-strengthening activities can help improve the ability to do these types of tasks.

Increase Your Chances Of Living Longer

Science shows that physical activity can reduce your risk of dying early from the leading causes of death, like heart disease and some cancers. This is remarkable in the following two ways:

- Only a few lifestyle choices have as large an impact on your health as physical activity. People who are physically active for about seven hours a week have a 40 percent lower risk of dying early than those who are active for less than 30 minutes a week.

- You don't have to do high amounts of activity or vigorous-intensity activity to reduce your risk of premature death. You can put yourself at lower risk of dying early by doing at least 150 minutes a week of moderate-intensity aerobic activity.

Everyone can gain the health benefits of physical activity—age, ethnicity, shape or size—do not matter.

Chapter 45

Screen Time

Limit Your Time On A Computer And Watching TV

For many of us, limiting our computer usage and getting away from all screens can be a challenge. That means television screens, computer monitors, and even the handheld devices we use for checking e-mail, listening to music, watching TV, and playing video games on the go.

Health experts say screen time at home should be limited to two hours or less a day, unless it's work or homework-related. The time we spend in front of the screen could be better spent being more physically active, and setting a good example for others.

When it comes to teens, parents and caregivers might need to set limits on teens' computer time, TV watching, and video game playing to reduce how much time is spent in front of a screen. Research by the Henry J. Kaiser Foundation has shown that setting rules about media use is a challenge for many parents/caregivers:

- 28% of 8 to 18-year-olds said their parents set TV-watching rules

- 30% of 8 to 18-year-olds said their parents set rules about video game use

- 36% of 8 to 18-year-olds said their parents set rules about computer use

However, the same study also demonstrated that when parents set any media rules, children's media use is almost three hours lower per day.

Other Screen-Time Statistics

Children and teens ages 8 to 18 spend the following amount of time in front of the screen, daily:

About This Chapter: Excerpted from "Reduce Screen Time," National Heart Lung and Blood Institute, 2010, and "Decreasing Screen Time," Centers for Disease Control and Prevention, August 2007.

- Approximately 7.5 hours using entertainment media

- Approximately 4.5 hours watching TV

- Approximately 1.5 hours on the computer

- Over an hour playing video games

These data lie in stark contrast to the 25 minutes per day that teens spend reading books. Today's youth also have the following media in their bedrooms:

- More than one third have a computer, and internet access

- Half have video game players

- More than two-thirds have TVs

- Those with bedroom TVs spend an hour more in front of the screen than those without TVs

How To Decrease Your Screen Time

Interrupt your regularly scheduled programming to give yourself a healthier start on life.

More Screen Time Equals Less Activity Time

Don't touch that dial. Every day, children ages 8 to 13 spend nearly six hours watching TV, playing video games or on the computer. Two-thirds of youth have a TV in their room, and those kids spend another one and a half hours watching TV than their peers. The more time children spend in front of the screen, the more likely they are to be overweight. And children just aren't getting the recommended 60 minutes of daily physical activity.

So what can you do? The National Institutes of Health has the following tips:

- Agree to limit screen time to no more than two hours a day.
- Don't put a TV in your bedroom.
- Turn screen time into active time, by doing simple exercises during commercial breaks.

Source: Excerpted from, "More Screen Time Equals Less Activity Time," National Heart Lung and Blood Institute, 2010.

With more electronic entertainment options than ever before (48% of families with children ages 2 to 17 have a TV, VCR, video game console, and computer), it is harder to get children up and moving. During the last 20 years, the number of children in the United States who are physically active has decreased while the number of children who are overweight has doubled. The average American child spends over four and a half hours in front of a screen each day (TV, video tapes, video games or a computer), and watching TV accounts for two and a half of those hours alone. This national epidemic of overweight and obesity can be partly attributed to the over-consumption of media by children.

Recent studies conclude that the amount of time children spend watching television has a direct relationship to their weight. Children who viewed the most number of hours of television per day had the highest prevalence of obesity (this held true regardless of age, race/

ethnicity and family income). Children that were limited to one hour or less of TV per day were far less likely to be overweight than those who watch more. Boys and girls who watched more than four hours of TV per day had more body fat than those who watched less than two hours. Moreover, children that watched more hours per day of TV and for longer periods of time were less likely to engage in physical activity.

The number of hours spent watching television is more of a concern for older teens (ages 11 to 13) and minorities. More children aged 11 to 13 years watch four or more hours of TV per day. Research shows that minority children watch more hours of television per week than Caucasian children. Therefore, it is important that children of color be encouraged to engage more in physical activities. This is especially true for the Asian American and Pacific Islander community. The National Heart, Lung and Blood Institute reports that Asian Americans and Pacific Islanders exercise less compared to the general population.

Switching Channels

The lack of physical activity, poor nutrition, and increased media consumption contribute to emerging health issues for children and teens, such as high cholesterol and high blood pressure, diabetes, gall bladder disease and sleep apnea. One of the best ways to combat inactivity begins with monitoring your entertainment habits.

Tips For Limiting Screen Time

The American Academy of Pediatrics suggests that you can make a big impact in your life by taking these simple steps:

- Remove TV sets from your bedroom. Teens who watch television in their rooms watch an average of 4.6 more hours a week and are more likely to be overweight.

- Limit your total media time (with entertainment media) to no more than one to two hours per day. Studies have shown that for each additional hour children spend watching TV a day, there is a 2% increase in the chance that they'll be overweight.

- Engage in alternative entertainment. Try activities that include both physical activities and pro-social involvement, such as joining school and community clubs, taking classes or being active with the family. In fact, physical activity can help control weight and lower blood pressure as well as reduce feelings of depression and anxiety.

Source: Centers for Disease Control and Prevention, August 2007.

Part Six
Eating And Disease

Chapter 46

Disease Prevention Through Good Eating Habits

There are nutritional and dietary elements that have proven relationships to certain diseases or conditions.

Calcium And Osteoporosis

Calcium is one of the most important minerals for human life. Your body uses it to form and maintain healthy bones and teeth. Calcium also plays a vital role in nerve conduction, muscle contraction, and blood clotting.

Osteoporosis is a disease in which the calcium content of bones is very low. In this disease, calcium and phosphorus, which are normally present in the bones, become reabsorbed back into the body. This process results in brittle, fragile bones that are easily broken.

Getting enough calcium in the diet throughout childhood and puberty is one key to preventing osteoporosis. A person who does not get enough calcium growing up will not have sturdy bones. An older person who consumes a low-calcium diet is also at great risk for osteoporosis.

The recommended dietary allowances (RDA) for calcium are based on age, gender, and hormonal factors. Many foods, such as some vegetables, contain calcium. However, milk and dairy products are some of the best food sources. Calcium may also be obtained by taking supplements.

Fiber And Cancer

Dietary fiber is found in plant foods, where it occurs in two forms: soluble and insoluble.

About This Chapter: "Diet and Disease," © 2011 A.D.A.M., Inc. Reprinted with permission.

Soluble fiber attracts water and turns to gel during digestion. This process slows digestion and the rate of nutrient absorption from the stomach and intestine.

Soluble fiber is found in oat bran, barley, nuts, seeds, dried beans and legumes, lentils, peas, and some fruits and vegetables. Insoluble fiber also adds bulk (fiber) to the stool. It is found in wheat bran, vegetables, and whole grains.

A diet high in fiber is thought to reduce the risk of cancers of the rectum and colon.

Fruits, Vegetables, And Cancer

Eating more fruits and vegetables helps provide a good supply of fiber, vitamin A, vitamin C, beta carotene and other carotenoids, and valuable substances called phytochemicals. Studies have shown that a diet high in these nutrients and fiber can reduce the risk of developing cancers of the stomach, colon rectum, esophagus, larynx, and lung.

Vitamin C and beta carotene, which forms vitamin A, are antioxidants. As such, they protect body cells from oxidation, a process that can lead to cell damage and may play a role in cancer.

In addition to nutrients that are needed for normal metabolism, plant foods also contain phytochemicals, plant chemicals that may affect human health. There are hundreds of phytochemicals, and their exact role in promoting health is still uncertain. However, a growing body of evidence indicates that phytochemicals may help protect against cancer.

To get these benefits, eat more fruits and vegetables that contain vitamins A and C and beta carotene. These include dark-green leafy vegetables such as spinach, kale, collards, and turnip greens. Citrus fruits, such as oranges, grapefruit, and tangerines are also high in antioxidants. Other red, yellow, and orange fruits and vegetables, or their juices are also healthful choices. (Note: Juicing removes the fiber.)

Fiber And Coronary Heart Disease

Some fiber, especially soluble fiber, binds to lipids such as cholesterol. The fiber then carries the lipids out of the body through the stool. This lowers the concentration of lipids in the blood and may reduce the risk of coronary heart disease.

Fat And Cancer

A diet high in fat has been shown to increase the risk of cancers of the breast, colon, and prostate. A high-fat diet does not necessarily cause cancer. Rather, it may promote the development of cancer in people who are exposed to cancer-causing agents.

A diet high in fat may promote cancer by causing the body to secrete more of certain hormones that create a favorable environment for certain types of cancer. Breast cancer is one of these hormone-influenced cancers. High-fat diets also may change the characteristics of the cells to make them more vulnerable to cancer-causing agents.

To reduce fat in the diet, choose lean cuts of beef, lamb, and pork as well as skinless poultry and fish. Baking, broiling, poaching, and steaming are recommended cooking methods. Choose skim or low-fat milk and dairy products, as well as low-fat salad dressings.

Saturated Fat, Cholesterol, And Coronary Heart Disease

Eating too much saturated fat is one of the major risk factors for heart disease. A diet high in saturated fat causes cholesterol, a soft, waxy substance, to build up in the arteries. Eventually, the arteries harden and narrow. The result is an increased pressure in the arteries as well as strain on the heart to maintain adequate blood flow throughout the body.

Because of its high calorie content, too much dietary fat also increases the risk of heart disease in that it increases the likelihood that a person will become obese. Obesity is another risk factor for heart disease.

Sodium And Hypertension

Sodium is a mineral that helps the body regulate blood pressure. Sodium is also commonly known as salt. It also plays a role in the proper functioning of cell membranes, muscles, and nerves. Sodium concentration in the body is mainly controlled by the kidneys, adrenal glands, and the pituitary gland near the brain.

The balance between dietary intake and kidney excretion through urine determines how much salt you have in your body. Only a small amount of salt is lost through your stools or sweat. The more salt your body holds, the more fluid the body keeps, and vice versa.

Sodium-sensitive individuals may experience high blood pressure from too much sodium in the diet. The American Heart Association has developed specific guidelines for sodium intake. Dietary changes may help control high blood pressure. Salt intake may have little effect in persons without high blood pressure, but it may have a profound effect in sodium-sensitive individuals. Blood pressure is often controlled by diuretics that cause sodium excretion in the urine.

Alcohol

Alcohol use increases the risk of liver cancer. When combined with smoking, alcohol intake also increases the risk of cancers of the mouth, throat, larynx, and esophagus. In addition, alcohol intake is associated with an increased risk of breast cancer in women.

Alcohol is processed by the liver into energy for the body. Continued and excessive use of alcohol can damage the liver in various ways, including the development of a fatty liver. A fatty liver can lead to cirrhosis of the liver.

Alcohol can damage the lining of the small intestine and stomach, where most nutrients are digested. As a result, alcohol can impair the absorption of essential nutrients. Alcohol also increases the body's need for some nutrients, and interferes with the absorption and storage of other nutrients.

Continued and excessive use of alcohol can result in an increase in blood pressure. Chronic heavy drinking also can cause damage to the heart muscle (cardiomyopathy). In addition, stroke is associated with both chronic heavy drinking and binge drinking.

Nitrates And Cancer

Countries in which people eat a lot of salt-cured, smoked, and nitrite-cured foods have a high rate of cancer of the stomach and esophagus. Examples of such foods include bacon, ham, hot dogs, and salt-cured fish. Eat salted, smoked, or cured foods only on occasion.

Chapter 47

Eating And Oral Health

How does what I eat affect my oral health?

You may be able to prevent two of the most common diseases of modern civilization, tooth decay (caries) and periodontal (gum) disease, simply by improving your diet. Decay results when acid products from oral bacteria destroy the teeth and other hard tissues of the mouth. Certain foods and food combinations are linked to higher levels of cavity-causing bacteria. Although poor nutrition does not directly cause periodontal disease, many researchers believe that the disease progresses faster and is more severe in patients whose diet does not supply the necessary nutrients.

Poor nutrition affects the entire immune system, thereby increasing susceptibility to many disorders. People with lowered immune systems have been shown to be at higher risk for periodontal disease. Additionally, research shows a link between oral health and systemic conditions, such as diabetes and cardiovascular disease. So eating a variety of foods as part of a well-balanced diet may not only improve your dental health, but increasing fiber and vitamin intake may also reduce the risk of other diseases.

How can I plan my meals and snacks to promote better oral health?

Eat a well-balanced diet characterized by moderation and variety. Develop eating habits that follow the recommendations from reputable health organizations such as the American Dietetic Association and the National Institutes of Health. Choose foods from the five major

About This Chapter: "How Does What I Eat Affect My Oral Health?" © 2007 Academy of General Dentistry (www .knowyourteeth.com). Reprinted with copyright permission from the Academy of General Dentistry.

food groups: fruits, vegetables, breads and cereals, milk and dairy products and meat, chicken, fish or beans. Avoid fad diets that limit or eliminate entire food groups, which usually result in vitamin or mineral deficiencies.

Foods that cling to your teeth promote tooth decay. So when you snack, avoid soft, sweet, sticky foods such as cakes, candy and dried fruits. Instead, choose dentally healthy foods such as nuts, raw vegetables, plain yogurt, cheese, and sugarless gum or candy.

When you eat fermentable carbohydrates, such as crackers, cookies and chips, eat them as part of your meal, instead of by themselves. Combinations of foods neutralize acids in the mouth and inhibit tooth decay. For example, enjoy cheese with your crackers. Your snack will be just as satisfying and better for your dental health. One caution: malnutrition (bad nutrition) can result from too much nourishment as easily as too little. Each time you eat, you create an environment for oral bacteria to develop. Additionally, studies are showing that dental disease is just as related to overeating as heart disease, obesity, diabetes and hypertension. So making a habit of eating too much of just about anything, too frequently, should be avoided.

When should I consult my dentist about my nutritional status?

Always ask your dentist if you're not sure how your diet may affect your oral health. Conditions such as tooth loss, pain or joint dysfunction can impair chewing and are often found in elderly people, those on restrictive diets, and those who are undergoing medical treatment. People experiencing these problems may be too isolated or weakened to eat nutritionally balanced meals at a time when it is particularly critical. Talk to your dental health professional about what you can do for yourself or someone you know in these circumstances.

Saliva Helps Protect Oral Health

Always keep your mouth moist by drinking lots of water. Saliva protects both hard and soft oral tissues. If you have a dry mouth, supplement your diet with sugarless candy or gum to stimulate saliva.

Chapter 48

Heart Healthy Eating

Making healthy food choices is one important thing you can do to reduce your risk of heart disease—the leading cause of death of men and women in the United States.

According to the American Heart Association, about 80 million adults in the U.S. have at least one form of heart disease—disorders that prevent the heart from functioning normally—including coronary artery disease, heart rhythm problems, heart defects, infections, and cardiomyopathy (thickening or enlargement of the heart muscle).

Experts say you can reduce the risk of developing these problems with lifestyle changes that include eating a healthy diet. But with racks full of books and magazines about food and recipes, what is the best diet for a healthy heart?

U.S. Food and Drug Administration (FDA) nutrition expert Barbara Schneeman says to use the following simple guidelines when preparing meals:

- Balance calories to manage body weight

- Eat at least four and a half cups of fruits and vegetables a day, including a variety of dark green, red, and orange vegetables, beans, and peas

- Eat seafood (including oily fish) in place of some meat and poultry

- Eat whole grains—the equivalent of at least three single ounce servings a day

- Use oils to replace solid fats

- Use fat-free or low-fat versions of dairy products

About This Chapter: Excerpted from "Eat for a Healthy Heart," U.S. Food and Drug Administration (www.fda.gov), February 2011.

The government's *Dietary Guidelines for Americans 2010* also says Americans should reduce their sodium intake. The general recommendation is to eat less than 2,300 mg. of sodium a day. But Americans 51 years old or older, African-Americans of any age, and people with high blood pressure, diabetes, or chronic kidney disease should restrict their intake to 1,500 mg. The government estimates that about half the U.S. population is in one of those three categories.

What's It Mean?

Cardiovascular Disease: Diseases of the heart and diseases of the blood vessel system (arteries, capillaries, veins) within a person's entire body.

Diabetes: A disorder of metabolism—the way the body uses digested food for growth and energy. In diabetes, the pancreas either produces little or no insulin (a hormone that helps glucose, the body's main source of fuel, get into cells), or the cells do not respond appropriately to the insulin that is produced. The three main types of diabetes are type 1, type 2, and gestational diabetes. About 90 to 95 percent of people with diabetes have type 2. This form of diabetes is most often associated with older age, obesity, family history of diabetes, previous history of gestational diabetes, physical inactivity, and certain ethnicities. About 80 percent of people with type 2 diabetes are overweight. Prediabetes, also called impaired fasting glucose or impaired glucose tolerance, is a state in which blood glucose levels are higher than normal but not high enough to be called diabetes.

Hypertension: A condition, also known as high blood pressure, in which blood pressure remains elevated over time. Hypertension makes the heart work too hard, and the high force of the blood flow can harm arteries and organs, such as the heart, kidneys, brain, and eyes. Uncontrolled hypertension can lead to heart attacks, heart failure, kidney disease, stroke, and blindness. Prehypertension is defined as blood pressure that is higher than normal but not high enough to be defined as hypertension.

Source: Excerpted from *Dietary Guidelines for Americans 2010*, U.S. Department of Agriculture, December 2010.

Packaged And Restaurant Food

Schneeman, who heads FDA's Office of Nutrition, Labeling, and Dietary Supplements, says one way to make sure you're adhering to healthy guidelines is by using the nutrition labels on the packaged foods you buy.

"Product labels give consumers the power to compare foods quickly and easily so they can judge which products best fit into a heart healthy diet or meet other dietary needs," Schneeman says. "Remember, when you see a percent DV (daily value of key nutrients) on the label, 5% or less is low and 20% or more is high."

Use the following guidelines when choosing processed foods or eating in restaurants:

• Choose lean meats and poultry and bake it, broil it, or grill it.

Diet-Related Heart Risks

Cardiovascular Disease

- 81.1 million Americans—37 percent of the population—have cardiovascular disease. Major risk factors include high levels of blood cholesterol and other lipids, type 2 diabetes, hypertension (high blood pressure), metabolic syndrome, overweight and obesity, physical inactivity, and tobacco use.

- 16 percent of the U.S. adult population has high total blood cholesterol.

Hypertension

- 74.5 million Americans—34 percent of U.S. adults—have hypertension.

- Hypertension is a major risk factor for heart disease, stroke, congestive heart failure, and kidney disease.

- Dietary factors that increase blood pressure include excessive sodium and insufficient potassium intake, overweight and obesity, and excess alcohol consumption.

- 36 percent of American adults have prehypertension—blood pressure numbers that are higher than normal, but not yet in the hypertension range.

Diabetes

- Nearly 24 million people—almost 11 percent the population ages 20 years and older have diabetes. The vast majority of cases are type 2 diabetes, which is heavily influenced by diet and physical activity.

- About 78 million Americans—35 percent of the U.S. adult population ages 20 years or 18 older—have pre-diabetes. Pre-diabetes (also called impaired glucose tolerance or impaired fasting glucose) means that blood glucose levels are higher than normal, but not high enough to be called diabetes.

Source: Excerpted from *Dietary Guidelines for Americans 2010*, U.S. Department of Agriculture, December 2010.

- In a restaurant, opt for steamed, grilled, or broiled dishes instead of those that are sautéed or fried.

- Look on product labels for foods low in saturated fats, trans fats, and cholesterol. Most of the fats you eat should come from polyunsaturated and monounsaturated fats, such as those found in some types of fish, nuts, and vegetable oils.

- Check product labels for foods high in potassium (unless you've been advised to restrict the amount of potassium you eat). Potassium counteracts some of the effects of salt on blood pressure.

- Choose foods and beverages low in added sugars. Read the ingredient list to make sure that added sugars are not among the first ingredients. Ingredients in the largest amounts are listed first. Some names for added sugars include sucrose, glucose, high fructose corn syrup, corn syrup, maple syrup, and fructose. The nutrition facts on the product label give the total sugar content.

- Pick foods that provide dietary fiber, like fruits, beans, vegetables, and whole grains.

Chapter 49

The Childhood Obesity Problem

The Scope Of The Childhood Obesity Problem

Obesity rates have increased sharply in the United States over the past 30 years, and today, nearly one third of children and adolescents are overweight or obese. These children are developing "adult" diseases, such as type 2 diabetes and hypertension, and are at increased risk for heart disease, stroke, certain types of cancer and other serious chronic conditions.

The medical expenses and indirect costs associated with obesity place a significant burden on a health care system that already is overwhelmed and threaten our unstable economy. If something is not done to reverse the childhood obesity epidemic, our next generation can expect even larger medical bills and a health care system less capable of meeting its needs.

A clear picture of the epidemic can be seen in the hard numbers. Data from the National Health and Nutrition Examination Survey (NHANES) show that 16.9% of children and adolescents ages 2 to 19 were obese and 31.7% were obese or overweight in 2007–2008. These rates have soared over the past few decades:

- The obesity rate among children ages 2 to 5 has more than doubled (from 5% to 10.4%) during the past three decades.

- The obesity rate for children ages 6 to 11 has more than quadrupled (from 4.2% to 19.6%).

- The obesity rate for adolescents ages 12 to 19 has more than tripled (from 4.6 to 18.1%) during the past four decades.

About This Chapter: The information in this chapter is reprinted with permission from The Robert Wood Johnson Center to Prevent Childhood Obesity, © 2011. For additional information, visit www.reversechildhoodobesity.org.

The Cause

At the simplest level, childhood obesity is caused by an energy imbalance—children consuming more energy (calories) through foods and beverages than they expend through normal growth, physical activity, and daily living.

Developing research suggests that the environments our children live in have a profound impact on the foods they eat and the amount of activity they get. For example, most students have little or no time to be active at school, while junk foods and sugary drinks are readily available. Many families live in communities that offer limited access to affordable healthy foods, have few safe places for kids to play, or do not support walking or biking.

To reverse the childhood obesity epidemic, we must help kids balance the number of calories they're consuming and burning each day. This means making changes to the environments in which our children live, learn, and play that support healthy eating and physical activity. The Robert Wood Johnson Center to Prevent Childhood Obesity has suggested policy strategies at the federal, state, and local government levels as well as strategies for businesses, schools, community, and faith based organizations can begin to employ.

Facts And Definitions

The following facts and statistics present the best available evidence about factors that are contributing to the energy imbalance on both sides of the equation: energy in and energy out.

Energy In

One part of the solution to reversing the obesity epidemic is making healthy, nutritious foods and beverages more affordable and accessible; discouraging the consumption of unhealthy foods and beverages; and achieving an appropriate caloric intake are all important strategies for preventing childhood obesity. Achieving progress in these areas will require changes in communities, homes, schools, food availability and distribution, marketing and advertising practices and the information environment.

What's It Mean?

Energy Balance: How much energy is consumed through foods and beverages (calories) versus how much energy is burned (physical activity). A child's energy balance is affected by the energy (calories) consumed and the energy expended to support normal growth, physical activity, and daily living. What children eat and drink, and how much physical activity they get, are influenced by key features of their social, built, natural, and food environments.

Food Sources In The Home: In many neighborhoods—especially in low-income communities and communities of color—there is a lack of access to supermarkets, farmers' markets, or other sources of affordable, nutritious foods. Yet, research indicates that when people have access to healthy food options, they consume more fruits and vegetables.

Food Sources Outside Of The Home: Children today consume a significant amount of their daily calories away from home—either in school, at neighborhood stores, or at fast-food restaurants. Restaurant meals can add twice as many calories and three times more fat than home-prepared meals. Many schools offer "competitive foods" (those sold outside of the federally reimbursed school breakfast, lunch, and after-school snack programs), which are often low in nutritional value and high in calories, fat, and sodium. The most popular competitive food choices include cookies, candy, sweetened juice drinks, and carbonated soft drinks.

Food Types: Eating fast food and drinking sweetened beverages can lead to an overall greater intake of calories and fat, which can have a major impact on a child's weight and health. Added calories from consuming fast foods can result in a child gaining an extra six pounds per year. Consistent consumption of sugar-sweetened beverages can have similar consequences. In addition, a study of a school district in southeast Texas found that when children gain access to high-calorie, high-fat food there is a decrease in the consumption of fruits, vegetables, and milk.

Marketing/Advertising: In 2006, the Federal Trade Commission estimated that food and beverage companies spent more than $1.6 billion to market their products to children. More than 89% of food advertisements viewed by adolescents on TV are for unhealthy foods. This overabundance of unhealthy food advertising influences food and beverage preferences, as well as short-term caloric intake among children as young as two years old.

Energy Out

Lack of physical activity is a contributing factor in many illnesses and diseases, especially obesity. Today, many children do not have safe places to play in the communities where they live, and few schools provide quality physical education or other forms of physical activity on a daily basis. Reduced physical activity also has been linked to a lack of recreational programming, poor air quality, and safety concerns.

- More than half of children and adolescents are not getting the recommended minimum of 60 minutes or more of physical activity each day.

- Sedentary activities, such as watching TV, surfing the internet, or playing traditional video games are taking time away from physical activity. The more time adolescents spend watching television, the more likely they will become overweight or obese.

- Children also are losing opportunities to be physically active during school hours. Due to shrinking educational budgets and competing academic pressures, many schools have cut recess and physical education. Fewer than 4% of elementary schools provide daily physical education.

Body Mass Index

Body mass index (BMI) is a ratio of weight and height, and is a better assessment of obesity than weight alone. Using an accurate weight and height, BMI is calculated using the BMI formula.

Boys and girls grow and develop at different rates. Based upon Centers for Disease Control and Prevention (CDC) recommendations, a BMI percentile for children is calculated individually based on a child's sex, age, height, and weight. BMI percentiles are then used to categorize children according to whether they are underweight, healthy weight, overweight, or obese. A higher BMI percentile indicates greater risk for having or developing obesity-related health problems. Health care professionals group BMI percentiles to categorize children as follows:

- **Obese:** BMI-for-age and sex greater than or equal to 95th percentile
- **Overweight:** BMI-for-age and sex between 85th and less than 95th percentiles
- **Healthy weight:** BMI-for-age and sex between 5th and less than 85th percentiles
- **Underweight:** BMI-for-age and sex less than 5th percentile

A BMI assessment is only a screening tool, and an individual child's BMI should not be considered a definitive assessment of whether or not a child has a weight problem requiring attention. If parents have questions about the BMI assessment and their child's weight, or want to screen for other conditions commonly associated with obesity, they should consider talking to a health professional. BMI is the most widely accepted measurement to screen for weight-related health problems. In a 2003 policy statement, the American Academy of Pediatrics recommended that physicians regularly calculate BMI. The Institute of Medicine in its 2007 report also recommended that schools conduct annual BMI assessments and make this information available to parents.

Body Mass Index To Screen For Weight Category

BMI is the most widely accepted measurement to screen for weight-related health problems. In a 2003 policy statement, the American Academy of Pediatrics recommended that physicians regularly calculate BMI. The Institute of Medicine in its 2007 report also recommended that schools conduct annual BMI assessments and make this information available to parents.

Health Consequences

The ultimate cost of obesity is a drastically reduced quality of life and a shorter life span. Being overweight or obese puts children at risk for an array of associated health problems:

- Obesity increases the lifelong risk for type 2 diabetes, high blood pressure, osteoarthritis, stroke, certain kinds of cancer, and many other debilitating diseases.

- Researchers estimate that one out of every three males and two out of every five females born in the United States in the year 2000 will be diagnosed with diabetes.

- More than 100,000 children ages 5 to 14 suffer from asthma each year because of over-weight and obesity.

- Researchers predict that if current adolescent obesity rates continue, by 2035 there will be more than 100,000 additional cases of coronary heart disease attributable to obesity.

Economic Consequences

Obesity places an enormous burden on the health care system and the economy as a whole. Obese children cost the health care system roughly three times more than the average child. Those who also lack insurance or access to health care place an even greater burden on the health care system.

Childhood obesity is estimated to cost $14 billion annually in direct health expenses, and children covered by Medicaid account for $3 billion of those expenses.

The average total health expenses for a child treated for obesity under private insurance is $3,743 annually, while the average health cost for all children covered by private insurance is about $1,108.30.

Annually, the average total health expenses for a child treated for obesity under Medicaid is $6,730, while the average health cost for all children on Medicaid is $2,446.

Among adults, the increased prevalence of obesity was responsible for almost $40 billion of increased medical spending through 2006, including $7 billion in Medicare prescription drug costs. The medical costs of adult obesity were estimated at $147 billion per year by 2008.

Between 1999 and 2005 there was a near-doubling in hospitalizations of children with a diagnosis of obesity and an increase in costs from $125.9 million to $237.6 million (in 2005 dollars) between 2001 and 2005.

Disparities

Health disparities refer to the rates at which different populations bear the burden of disease. The obesity epidemic impacts all races and ethnicities but some populations are disproportionately affected. As one study summarized, "Health, disease, and death are not randomly distributed…illness concentrates among low-income people and people of color residing in certain geographical places."

Income

Six states (Mississippi, Louisiana, Kentucky, Arkansas, West Virginia, and Tennessee) have both poverty and adult obesity rates that are among the top ten in the nation.

Residents of communities with high levels of poverty have less access to places where they can be physically active, such as parks, green spaces, bike paths, and lanes. In some communities, parents cannot provide their children with healthy foods because they don't have access to quality, full-service supermarkets. In fact, low-income areas have access to half as many supermarkets as wealthy areas.

Racial/Ethnic

Within equivalent levels of socioeconomic status, race still serves as a determinant of health. Children, as a subgroup, are more racially and ethnically diverse than the nation's population as a whole, and obesity prevalence rates are highest among children and adolescents of color.

Mexican American and African American children ages 6 to 11 are more likely to be obese or overweight than white children. Almost 43% of Mexican American children and almost 37% of African American children are obese or overweight, compared with "only" about 32% of white children.

Data on Native American children is limited and rates vary across tribes and regions, making it difficult to generalize the severity of obesity levels among this population. However, in the Aberdeen Area, which includes tribes in North Dakota, South Dakota, Nebraska, and Iowa, a study of youths ages 5 to 17 found that 48% of American Indian males and 46% of American Indian females were obese or overweight.

Hispanic and African American children are more likely to develop diabetes than white children. White males born in 2000 have a 27% risk of being diagnosed with diabetes during their lifetimes, while Hispanic and African American males have a 45% and 40% lifetime risk, respectively. White females born in 2000 have a 31% risk of being diagnosed with diabetes during their lifetimes, while Hispanic and African American females have a 53% and 49% lifetime risk, respectively.

Regional

Eight of the ten states with the highest childhood obesity rates in the nation are in the South, leaving this region with a disproportionate number of obese children and adolescents.

Among the states, West Virginia had the highest rate of childhood obesity at almost 21%, while Utah had the lowest rate at almost 9%.

Chapter 50

Dealing With Celiac Disease

Celiac disease is a digestive disease that damages the small intestine and interferes with absorption of nutrients from food. People who have celiac disease cannot tolerate gluten, a protein in wheat, rye, and barley. Gluten is found mainly in foods but may also be found in everyday products such as medicines, vitamins, and lip balms.

When people with celiac disease eat foods or use products containing gluten, their immune system responds by damaging or destroying villi—the tiny, fingerlike protrusions lining the small intestine. Villi normally allow nutrients from food to be absorbed through the walls of the small intestine into the bloodstream. Without healthy villi, a person becomes malnourished, no matter how much food one eats.

Celiac disease is both a disease of malabsorption—meaning nutrients are not absorbed properly—and an abnormal immune reaction to gluten. Celiac disease is also known as celiac sprue, nontropical sprue, and gluten-sensitive enteropathy. Celiac disease is genetic, meaning it runs in families. Sometimes the disease is triggered—or becomes active for the first time—after surgery, pregnancy, childbirth, viral infection, or severe emotional stress.

Symptoms Of Celiac Disease

Symptoms of celiac disease vary from person to person. Symptoms may occur in the digestive system or in other parts of the body. Digestive symptoms are more common in infants and young children and may include the following:

- Abdominal bloating and pain

About This Chapter: Excerpted from "Celiac Disease," National Institute of Diabetes and Digestive and Kidney Diseases (www.nih.niddk.gov), September 2008.

- Chronic diarrhea
- Vomiting
- Constipation
- Pale, foul-smelling, or fatty stool
- Weight loss

Irritability is another common symptom in children. Malabsorption of nutrients during the years when nutrition is critical to a child's normal growth and development can result in other problems such as failure to thrive in infants, delayed growth and short stature, delayed puberty, and dental enamel defects of the permanent teeth.

Adults are less likely to have digestive symptoms and may instead have one or more of the following:

- Unexplained iron-deficiency anemia
- Fatigue
- Bone or joint pain
- Arthritis
- Bone loss or osteoporosis
- Depression or anxiety
- Tingling numbness in the hands and feet
- Seizures
- Missed menstrual periods
- Infertility or recurrent miscarriage
- Canker sores inside the mouth
- An itchy skin rash called dermatitis herpetiformis

People with celiac disease may have no symptoms but can still develop complications of the disease over time. Long-term complications include malnutrition—which can lead to anemia, osteoporosis, and miscarriage, among other problems—liver diseases, and cancers of the intestine.

Varied Celiac Disease Symptoms

Researchers are studying the reasons celiac disease affects people differently. The length of time a person was breastfed, the age a person started eating gluten-containing foods, and the amount of gluten-containing foods one eats are three factors thought to play a role in when and how celiac disease appears. Some studies have shown, for example, that the longer a person was breastfed, the later the symptoms of celiac disease appear.

Symptoms also vary depending on a person's age and the degree of damage to the small intestine. Many adults have the disease for a decade or more before they are diagnosed. The longer a person goes undiagnosed and untreated, the greater the chance of developing long-term complications.

Other Health Problems People With Celiac Disease Have

People with celiac disease tend to have other diseases in which the immune system attacks the body's healthy cells and tissues. The connection between celiac disease and these diseases may be genetic. They include the following:

- Type 1 diabetes
- Autoimmune thyroid disease
- Autoimmune liver disease
- Rheumatoid arthritis
- Addison disease, a condition in which the glands that produce critical hormones are damaged
- Sjögren syndrome, a condition in which the glands that produce tears and saliva are destroyed

Diagnosing Celiac Disease

Recognizing celiac disease can be difficult because some of its symptoms are similar to those of other diseases. Celiac disease can be confused with irritable bowel syndrome, iron-deficiency anemia caused by menstrual blood loss, inflammatory bowel disease, diverticulitis, intestinal infections, and chronic fatigue syndrome. As a result, celiac disease has long been underdiagnosed or misdiagnosed. As doctors become more aware of the many varied symptoms of the disease and reliable blood tests become more available, diagnosis rates are increasing.

Celiac Disease More Common Than Originally Believed

Celiac disease affects people in all parts of the world. Originally thought to be a rare childhood syndrome, celiac disease is now known to be a common genetic disorder. More than two million people in the United States have the disease, or about one in 133 people. Among people who have a first-degree relative—a parent, sibling, or child—diagnosed with celiac disease, as many as one in 22 people may have the disease.

Celiac disease is also more common among people with other genetic disorders including Down syndrome and Turner syndrome, a condition that affects girls' development.

Blood Tests

People with celiac disease have higher than normal levels of certain autoantibodies—proteins that react against the body's own cells or tissues—in their blood. To diagnose celiac disease, doctors will test blood for high levels of anti-tissue transglutaminase antibodies (tTGA) or anti-endomysium antibodies (EMA). If test results are negative but celiac disease is still suspected, additional blood tests may be needed.

Before being tested, one should continue to eat a diet that includes foods with gluten, such as breads and pastas. If a person stops eating foods with gluten before being tested, the results may be negative for celiac disease even if the disease is present.

Intestinal Biopsy

If blood tests and symptoms suggest celiac disease, a biopsy of the small intestine is performed to confirm the diagnosis. During the biopsy, the doctor removes tiny pieces of tissue from the small intestine to check for damage to the villi. To obtain the tissue sample, the doctor eases a long, thin tube called an endoscope through the patient's mouth and stomach into the small intestine. The doctor then takes the samples using instruments passed through the endoscope.

Dermatitis Herpetiformis

Dermatitis herpetiformis (DH) is an intensely itchy, blistering skin rash that affects 15% to 25% of people with celiac disease. The rash usually occurs on the elbows, knees, and buttocks. Most people with DH have no digestive symptoms of celiac disease.

DH is diagnosed through blood tests and a skin biopsy. If the antibody tests are positive and the skin biopsy has the typical findings of DH, patients do not need to have an intestinal biopsy. Both the skin disease and the intestinal disease respond to a gluten-free diet and recur if gluten is added back into the diet. The rash symptoms can be controlled with antibiotics such as dapsone. Because dapsone does not treat the intestinal condition, people with DH must maintain a gluten-free diet.

Screening

Screening for celiac disease means testing for the presence of autoantibodies in the blood in people without symptoms. Americans are not routinely screened for celiac disease. However, because celiac disease is hereditary, family members of a person with the disease may wish to be tested. About 4% to 12% of an affected person's first-degree relatives will also have the disease.

Celiac Disease Treatment

The only treatment for celiac disease is a gluten-free diet. Doctors may ask a newly diagnosed person to work with a dietitian on a gluten-free diet plan. A dietitian is a health care professional who specializes in food and nutrition. Someone with celiac disease can learn from a dietitian how to read ingredient lists and identify foods that contain gluten in order to make informed decisions at the grocery store and when eating out.

For most people, following this diet will stop symptoms, heal existing intestinal damage, and prevent further damage. Improvement begins within days of starting the diet. The small intestine usually heals in three to six months in children but may take several years in adults. A healed intestine means a person now has villi that can absorb nutrients from food into the bloodstream.

To stay well, people with celiac disease must avoid gluten for the rest of their lives. Eating even a small amount of gluten can damage the small intestine. The damage will occur in anyone with the disease, including people without noticeable symptoms. Depending on a person's age at diagnosis, some problems will not improve, such as short stature and dental enamel defects.

Some people with celiac disease show no improvement on the gluten-free diet. The most common reason for poor response to the diet is that small amounts of gluten are still being consumed. Hidden sources of gluten include additives such as modified food starch, preservatives, and stabilizers made with wheat. And because many corn and rice products are produced in factories that also manufacture wheat products, they can be contaminated with wheat gluten.

Rarely, the intestinal injury will continue despite a strictly gluten-free diet. People with this condition, known as refractory celiac disease, have severely damaged intestines that cannot heal. Because their intestines are not absorbing enough nutrients, they may need to receive nutrients directly into their bloodstream through a vein, or intravenously. Researchers are evaluating drug treatments for refractory celiac disease.

The Gluten-Free Diet

A gluten-free diet means not eating foods that contain wheat, rye, and barley. The foods and products made from these grains should also be avoided. In other words, a person with celiac disease should not eat most grain, pasta, cereal, and many processed foods.

Despite these restrictions, people with celiac disease can eat a well-balanced diet with a variety of foods. They can use potato, rice, soy, amaranth, quinoa, buckwheat, or bean flour instead of wheat flour. They can buy gluten-free bread, pasta, and other products from stores that carry organic foods, or order products from special food companies. Gluten-free products are increasingly available from mainstream stores.

"Plain" meat, fish, rice, fruits, and vegetables do not contain gluten, so people with celiac disease can freely eat these foods. In the past, people with celiac disease were advised not to eat oats. New evidence suggests that most people can safely eat small amounts of oats, as long as the oats are not contaminated with wheat gluten during processing. People with celiac disease should work closely with their health care team when deciding whether to include oats in their diet.

The gluten-free diet requires a completely new approach to eating. Newly diagnosed people and their families may find support groups helpful as they learn to adjust to a new way of life. People with celiac disease must be cautious about what they buy for lunch at school or work, what they purchase at the grocery store, what they eat at restaurants or parties, and what they grab for a snack. Eating out can be a challenge. When in doubt about a menu item, a person with celiac disease should ask the waiter or chef about ingredients and preparation or if a gluten-free menu is available.

Gluten is also used in some medications. People with celiac disease should ask a pharmacist if prescribed medications contain wheat. Because gluten is sometimes used as an additive in unexpected products—such as lipstick and play dough—reading product labels is important. If the ingredients are not listed on the label, the manufacturer should provide a list upon request. With practice, screening for gluten becomes second nature.

The Gluten-Free Diet: Some Examples

In 2006, the American Dietetic Association updated its recommendations for a gluten-free diet. The following information is based on the 2006 recommendations. This list is not complete, so people with celiac disease should discuss gluten-free food choices with a dietitian or physician who specializes in celiac disease. People with celiac disease should always read food ingredient lists carefully to make sure the food does not contain gluten.

Allowed Foods

- Amaranth
- Arrowroot
- Buckwheat
- Cassava
- Corn
- Flax
- Indian rice grass
- Job's tears
- Legumes
- Millet

Allergen Labeling

The Food Allergen Labeling and Consumer Protection Act, which took effect on January 1, 2006, requires food labels to clearly identify wheat and other common food allergens in the list of ingredients.

- Nuts
- Sago
- Tapioca
- Potatoes
- Seeds
- Teff
- Quinoa
- Sorghum
- Wild rice
- Rice
- Soy
- Yucca

Foods To Avoid

Wheat

- Including einkorn, emmer, spelt, kamut
- Wheat starch, wheat bran, wheat germ, cracked wheat, hydrolyzed wheat protein
- Barley
- Rye
- Triticale (a cross between wheat and rye)

Other Wheat Products

- Bromated flour
- Graham flour
- Semolina
- Durum flour
- Phosphated flour
- White flour
- Enriched flour
- Plain flour
- Farina
- Self-rising flour

Processed Foods That May Contain Wheat, Barley, Or Rye

Most of these foods can be found gluten-free. When in doubt, check with the food manufacturer.

- Bouillon cubes
- Syrup
- Chips/potato chips
- Communion wafers
- Gravy
- Matzo
- Sauces
- Self-basting turkey
- Soy sauce
- Brown rice
- Candy
- Cold cuts, hot dogs, salami, sausage
- French fries
- Imitation fish
- Rice mixes
- Seasoned tortilla chips
- Soups
- Vegetables in sauce

Source for food examples: Thompson T. *Celiac Disease Nutrition Guide, 2nd ed.* Chicago: American Dietetic Association; 2006. © American Dietetic Association. Adapted with permission. For a complete copy of the Celiac Disease Nutrition Guide, please visit www.eatright.org.

Hope Through Research

The National Institute of Diabetes and Digestive and Kidney Diseases conducts and supports research on celiac disease. Researchers are studying new options for diagnosing celiac disease, including capsule endoscopy. In this technique, patients swallow a capsule containing a tiny video camera that records images of the small intestine.

Several drug treatments for celiac disease are under evaluation. Researchers are also studying a combination of enzymes—proteins that aid chemical reactions in the body—that detoxify gluten before it enters the small intestine.

Scientists are also developing educational materials for standardized medical training to raise awareness among health care providers. The hope is that increased understanding and awareness will lead to earlier diagnosis and treatment of celiac disease.

Participants in clinical trials can play a more active role in their own health care, gain access to new research treatments before they are widely available, and help others by contributing to medical research.

Points To Remember

- People with celiac disease cannot tolerate gluten, a protein in wheat, rye, and barley.
- Untreated celiac disease damages the small intestine and interferes with nutrient absorption.
- Without treatment, people with celiac disease can develop complications such as osteoporosis, anemia, and cancer.
- A person with celiac disease may or may not have symptoms.
- Diagnosis involves blood tests and, in most cases, a biopsy of the small intestine.
- Since celiac disease is hereditary, family members of a person with celiac disease may wish to be tested.
- Celiac disease is treated by eliminating all gluten from the diet. The gluten-free diet is a lifetime requirement.
- A dietitian can teach a person with celiac disease about food selection, label reading, and other strategies to help manage the disease.

Chapter 51

Dealing With Diabetes

What is diabetes?

Diabetes means that your blood glucose, also called blood sugar, is too high. Glucose comes from the food you eat and is needed to fuel our bodies. Glucose is also stored in our liver and muscles. Your blood always has some glucose in it because your body needs glucose for energy. But having too much glucose in your blood is not healthy.

An organ called the pancreas makes insulin. Insulin helps glucose get from your blood into your cells. Cells take the glucose and turn it into energy.

If you have diabetes, the pancreas makes little or no insulin or your cells cannot use insulin very well. Glucose builds up in your blood and cannot get into your cells. If your blood glucose stays too high, it can damage many parts of the body such as the heart, eyes, kidneys, and nerves.

Are there different types of diabetes?

Yes. There are three main types of diabetes. In type 1 diabetes, the cells in the pancreas that make insulin are destroyed. If you have type 1 diabetes, you need to get insulin from shots or a pump everyday. Most teens can learn to adjust the amount of insulin they take according to their physical activity and eating patterns. This makes it easier to manage your diabetes when you have a busy schedule. Type 1 used to be called "insulin-dependent" or "juvenile" diabetes.

In type 2 diabetes, the pancreas still makes some insulin but cells cannot use it very well. If you have type 2 diabetes, you may need to take insulin or pills to help your body's supply of

About This Chapter: This chapter begins with excerpts "What Is Diabetes?" National Diabetes Education Program, November 2007; it continues with excerpts from "What I Need To Know About Eating and Diabetes," National Diabetes Information Clearinghouse, October 2007.

insulin work better. Type 2 used to be called "adult-onset diabetes." Now more teens are getting type 2, especially if they are overweight.

Gestational diabetes is a type of diabetes that occurs when women are pregnant. Having it raises their risk for getting diabetes, mostly type 2, for the rest of their lives. It also raises their child's risk for being overweight and for getting type 2 diabetes.

What do I need to do to take care of my diabetes?

The key to taking care of your diabetes is to keep your blood glucose as close to normal as possible. The best way to do this is to do the following:

- Make healthy food choices

- Eat the right amounts of food

- Be active everyday

- Stay at a healthy weight

- Take your medicines

- Check your blood glucose as planned with your health care team

Your doctor will tell you what blood glucose level is right for you. Your goal is to keep your blood glucose as close to this level as you can. Your doctor or diabetes educator will teach you how to check your blood glucose with a glucose meter.

Why do teens get diabetes?

Both genes and things like viruses and toxins may cause a person to get type 1 diabetes. Studies are being done to identify the causes of type 1 diabetes and to stop the process that destroys the pancreas. Researchers can now predict who is at risk for developing type 1 diabetes and in the future may be able to prevent or delay the onset of the disease.

Being overweight increases the risk for type 2 diabetes. Teens who make unhealthy food choices, are not physically active, or who have a family member with diabetes are more likely to get type 2 diabetes. Some racial groups have a greater chance of getting diabetes—American Indians, Alaska Natives, African Americans, Hispanics/Latinos, Asian Americans, and Pacific Islanders.

It is not true that eating too much sugar causes diabetes.

Source: National Diabetes Education Program, November 2007.

It helps to know what affects your blood glucose level. Food, illness, and stress raise your blood glucose. Insulin or pills and being physically active lower your blood glucose. Talk with your doctor or diabetes educator about how these things change your blood glucose levels and how you can make changes in your diabetes plan.

Carbohydrates, or carbs for short, are a good source of energy for our bodies. But if you eat too many carbs at one time, your blood glucose can get too high. Many foods contain carbs. Great carb choices include whole grain foods, nonfat or low-fat milk, and fresh fruits and vegetables. Eat more of them rather than white bread, whole milk, sweetened fruit drinks, regular soda, potato chips, sweets, and desserts.

Why do I need to take care of my diabetes?

If you take care of your diabetes you can lower your risk for other health problems. High blood glucose can harm blood vessels and cause heart attacks or strokes. It can also damage organs in the body and cause blindness, kidney failure, loss of toes or feet, gum problems, or loss of teeth.

The good news is that when you take care of your diabetes, you can reduce or avoid these problems.

Do not let diabetes stop you. You can do all the things your friends do and live a long and healthy life.

Eating And Diabetes

Making wise food choices can help you feel good every day, lose weight if you need to, and lower your risk for heart disease, stroke, and other problems caused by diabetes.

Healthful eating helps keep your blood glucose, also called blood sugar, in your target range. Physical activity and, if needed, diabetes medicines also help. The diabetes target range is the blood glucose level suggested by diabetes experts for good health. You can help prevent health problems by keeping your blood glucose levels on target.

What should my blood glucose levels be?

Talk with your health care provider about your blood glucose target levels and write them down.

Ask your doctor how often you should check your blood glucose on your own. Also ask your doctor for an A1C test at least twice a year. Your A1C number gives your average blood glucose for the past three months. The results from your blood glucose checks and your A1C test will tell you whether your diabetes care plan is working.

For people taking certain diabetes medicines, following a schedule for meals, snacks, and physical activity is best. However, some diabetes medicines allow for more flexibility. You'll work with your health care team to create a diabetes plan that's best for you. Talk with your doctor or diabetes teacher about how many meals and snacks to eat each day.

Table 51.1. Target Blood Glucose Levels For People With Diabetes

Before meals	70 to 130
1 to 2 hours after the start of a meal	less than 180

How does physical activity affect food choices?

What you eat and when also depend on how much you exercise. Physical activity is an important part of staying healthy and controlling your blood glucose. Keep the following points in mind:

- Talk with your doctor about what types of exercise are safe for you.

- Make sure your shoes fit well and your socks stay clean and dry (check your feet for redness or sores after exercising and call your doctor if you have sores that do not heal).

- Warm up and stretch for five to ten minutes before you exercise then cool down for several minutes after you exercise (for example, walk slowly at first, stretch, walk faster, and then finish up by walking slowly again).

- Ask your doctor whether you should exercise if your blood glucose level is high.

- Ask your doctor whether you should have a snack before you exercise.

- Know the signs of low blood glucose, also called hypoglycemia (always carry food or glucose tablets to treat low blood glucose).

- Always wear your medical identification or other ID.

- Find an exercise buddy (many people find they are more likely to do something active if a friend joins them).

Remember

What you eat and when you eat affect how your diabetes medicines work. Talk with your doctor or diabetes teacher about when to take your diabetes medicines. Write down in the names of your diabetes medicines, when to take them, and how much to take.

Source: National Diabetes Information Clearinghouse, October 2007.

What if my blood sugar gets too low?

Low blood glucose (called hypoglycemia) can make you feel shaky, weak, confused, irritable, hungry, or tired. You may sweat a lot or get a headache. If you have these symptoms, check your blood glucose. If it is below 70, have one of the following right away:

- Three or four glucose tablets

- One serving of glucose gel—the amount equal to 15 grams of carbohydrate

- Half a cup (four ounces) of any fruit juice

- Half a cup (four ounces) of a regular (not diet) soft drink

- One cup (eight ounces) of milk

- Five or six pieces of hard candy

- One tablespoon of sugar or honey

After 15 minutes, check your blood glucose again. If it's still too low, have another serving. Repeat these steps until your blood glucose level is 70 or higher. If it will be an hour or more before your next meal, have a snack as well.

What is the diabetes food pyramid

The diabetes food pyramid can help you make wise food choices. It divides foods into groups, based on what they contain. Eat more from the groups at the bottom of the pyramid and less from the groups at the top. Foods from the starches, fruits, vegetables, and milk groups are highest in carbohydrate. They affect your blood glucose levels the most.

How much should I eat each day?

Have about 1,200 to 1,600 calories a day if you are the following:

- Small woman who exercises

- Small or medium-sized woman who wants to lose weight

- Medium-sized woman who does not exercise much

Choose the following servings from these food groups to have 1,200 to 1,600 calories a day:

- Six starches

- Two milks

341

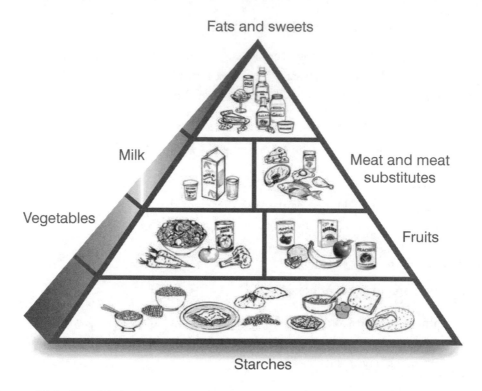

Figure 51.1. The Diabetes Food Pyramid (Source: National Diabetes Information Clearinghouse).

- Three vegetables

- Four to six ounces meat and meat substitutes

- Two fruits

- Up to three fats

Have about 1,600 to 2,000 calories a day if you are the following:

- Large woman who wants to lose weight

- Small man at a healthy weight

- Medium-sized man who does not exercise much

- Medium-sized or large man who wants to lose weight

Choose the following servings from these food groups to have 1,600 to 2,000 calories a day:

- Eight starches
- Two milks
- Four vegetables
- Four to six ounces meat and meat substitutes
- Three fruits
- Up to four fats

Have about 2,000 to 2,400 calories a day if you are the following:

- Medium-sized or large man who exercises a lot or has a physically active job
- Large man at a healthy weight
- Medium-sized or large woman who exercises a lot or has a physically active job

Choose the following servings from these food groups to have 2,000 to 2,400 calories a day:

- Ten starches
- Two milks
- Four vegetables
- Five to seven ounces meat and meat substitutes
- Four fruits
- Up to five fats

Talk with your diabetes teacher about how to make a meal plan that fits the way you usually eat, your daily routine, and your diabetes medicines. Then make your own plan.

What are healthy ways to eat starches?

Starches are bread, grains, cereal, pasta, and starchy vegetables like corn and potatoes. They provide carbohydrate, vitamins, minerals, and fiber. Whole grain starches are healthier because they have more vitamins, minerals, and fiber.

Eat some starches at each meal. Eating starches is healthy for everyone, including people with diabetes. Examples of starches include bread, pasta, corn, pretzels, potatoes, rice, crackers, cereal, tortillas, beans, yams, and lentils.

- Buy whole grain breads and cereals.

- Eat fewer fried and high-fat starches such as regular tortilla chips and potato chips, french fries, pastries, or biscuits. Try pretzels, fat-free popcorn, baked tortilla chips or potato chips, baked potatoes, or low-fat muffins.

- Use low-fat or fat-free plain yogurt or fat-free sour cream instead of regular sour cream on a baked potato.

- Use mustard instead of mayonnaise on a sandwich.

- Use low-fat or fat-free substitutes such as low-fat mayonnaise or light margarine on bread, rolls, or toast.

- Eat cereal with fat-free (skim) or low-fat (1%) milk.

What are healthy ways to eat vegetables?

Vegetables provide vitamins, minerals, and fiber. They are low in carbohydrate. Examples of vegetables include lettuce, broccoli, vegetable juice, spinach, peppers, carrots, green beans, tomatoes, celery, chilies, greens, and cabbage. If your plan includes more than one serving at a meal, you can choose several types of vegetables or have two or three servings of one vegetable.

- Eat raw and cooked vegetables with little or no fat, sauces, or dressings.

- Try low-fat or fat-free salad dressing on raw vegetables or salads.

- Steam vegetables using water or low-fat broth.

- Mix in some chopped onion or garlic.

- Use a little vinegar or some lemon or lime juice.

- Add a small piece of lean ham or smoked turkey instead of fat to vegetables when cooking.

- Sprinkle with herbs and spices.

- If you do use a small amount of fat, use canola oil, olive oil, or soft margarines (liquid or tub types) instead of fat from meat, butter, or shortening.

What are healthy ways to eat fruits?

Fruits provide carbohydrate, vitamins, minerals, and fiber. Examples of fruits include apples, fruit juice, strawberries, dried fruit, grapefruit, bananas, raisins, oranges, watermelon, peaches, mango, guava, papaya, berries, and canned fruit.

- Eat fruits raw or cooked, as juice with no sugar added, canned in their own juice, or dried.

- Buy smaller pieces of fruit.

- Choose pieces of fruit more often than fruit juice. Whole fruit is more filling and has more fiber.

- Save high-sugar and high-fat fruit desserts such as peach cobbler or cherry pie for special occasions.

What are healthy ways to have milk?

Milk provides carbohydrate, protein, calcium, vitamins, and minerals.

- Drink fat-free (skim) or low-fat (1%) milk.

- Eat low-fat or fat-free fruit yogurt sweetened with a low-calorie sweetener.

- Use low-fat plain yogurt as a substitute for sour cream.

What are healthy ways to eat meat and meat substitutes?

The meat and meat substitutes group includes meat, poultry, eggs, cheese, fish, and tofu. Eat small amounts of some of these foods each day. Meat and meat substitutes provide protein, vitamins, and minerals. Examples of meat and meat substitutes include chicken, beef, fish, canned tuna or other fish, eggs, peanut butter, tofu, cottage cheese, cheese, pork, lamb, and turkey.

- Buy cuts of beef, pork, ham, and lamb that have only a little fat on them. Trim off the extra fat.

- Eat chicken or turkey without the skin.

- Cook meat and meat substitutes in low-fat ways (broil, grill, stir-fry, roast, steam or microwave).

- To add more flavor, use vinegars, lemon juice, soy sauce, salsa, ketchup, barbecue sauce, herbs, and spices.

- Cook eggs using cooking spray or a non-stick pan.

- Limit the amount of nuts, peanut butter, and fried foods you eat because they are high in fat.

- Check food labels and choose low-fat or fat-free cheese.

What are healthy ways to eat fats and sweets?

Limit the amount of fats and sweets you eat. Fats and sweets are not as nutritious as other foods. Fats have a lot of calories. Sweets can be high in carbohydrate and fat. Some contain saturated fats, trans fats, and cholesterol that increase your risk of heart disease. Limiting these foods will help you lose weight and keep your blood glucose and blood fats under control. Examples of fats include salad dressing, oil, cream cheese, butter, margarine, mayonnaise, avocado, olives, and bacon. Examples of sweets include cake, ice cream, pie, syrup, cookies, and doughnuts.

- Try having sugar-free popsicles, diet soda, fat-free ice cream or frozen yogurt, or sugar-free hot cocoa mix.

- Share desserts in restaurants.

- Order small or child-size servings of ice cream or frozen yogurt.

- Divide homemade desserts into small servings, wrap each individually, and freeze extra servings.

- Remember, fat-free and low-sugar foods still have calories (talk with your diabetes teacher about how to fit sweets into your meal plan).

Chapter 52

Dealing With Food Allergies

What is food allergy?

Food allergy is an abnormal response to a food triggered by the body's immune system. There are several types of immune responses to food. This chapter focuses on one type of adverse reaction to food—that in which the body produces a specific type of antibody called immunoglobulin E (IgE).

The binding of IgE to specific molecules present in a food triggers the immune response. The response may be mild or in rare cases it can be associated with the severe and life-threatening reaction called anaphylaxis, which is described in a later section of this chapter. Therefore, if you have a food allergy, it is extremely important for you to work with your healthcare professional to learn what foods cause your allergic reaction.

What is an allergic reaction to food?

A food allergy occurs when the immune system responds to a harmless food as if it were a threat. The first time a person with food allergy is exposed to the food, no symptoms occur; but the first exposure primes the body to respond the next time. When the person eats the food again, an allergic response can occur.

Usually, the way you are first exposed to a food is when you eat it. But sometimes a first exposure or subsequent exposure can occur without your knowledge. This may be true in the case of peanut allergy. A person who experiences anaphylaxis on the first known exposure to peanut may have previously touched peanuts, used a peanut-containing skin care product, or breathed in peanut dust in the home or when close to other people eating peanuts.

About This Chapter: Excerpted from "Food Allergy: An Overview," National Institute of Allergy and Infectious Diseases (www.nih.niaid.gov), November 2010.

Generally, you are at greater risk for developing a food allergy if you come from a family in which allergies are common. These allergies are not necessarily food allergies but perhaps other allergic diseases, such as asthma or eczema (atopic dermatitis). If you have two parents who have allergies, you are more likely to develop food allergy than someone with one parent who has allergies.

An allergic reaction to food usually takes place within a few minutes to several hours after exposure to the allergen. The process of eating and digesting food and the location of mast cells both affect the timing and location of the reaction.

What is the allergic reaction process?

An allergic reaction to food is a two-step process.

- **Step 1:** The first time you are exposed to a food allergen, your immune system reacts as if the food were harmful and makes specific IgE antibodies to that allergen. The antibodies circulate through your blood and attach to mast cells and basophils. Mast cells are found in all body tissues, especially in areas of your body that are typical sites of allergic reactions. Those sites include your nose, throat, lungs, skin, and gastrointestinal (GI) tract. Basophils are found in your blood and also in tissues that have become inflamed due to an allergic reaction.

What's It Mean?

Allergen: A substance that causes an allergic reaction.

Anaphylaxis: A severe reaction to an allergen that may lead to death.

Antibody: A protein molecule tailor-made by the immune system to detect and help destroy invaders, such as bacteria, viruses, and toxins.

Basophils: White blood cells that contribute to allergic inflammatory reactions.

Epinephrine: A hormone, also called adrenaline, that works rapidly to contract blood vessels, preventing them from leaking fluid. It also relaxes airways, relieves cramping in the gastrointestinal tract, decreases swelling, and blocks itching and hives. Epinephrine is the drug in an EpiPen used to counter an anaphylactic reaction.

Histamine: A chemical stored in the granules of mast cells and basophil granules prior to release.

Mast Cells: Large granule-containing cells that are found in body tissues where typical allergic reactions occur.

Source: National Institute of Allergy and Infectious Diseases, November 2010.

Eosinophilic Esophagitis

Eosinophilic esophagitis (EoE) is a newly recognized chronic disease that can be associated with food allergies. It is increasingly being diagnosed in children and adults.

Symptoms of EoE include nausea, vomiting, and abdominal pain after eating. A person may also have symptoms that resemble acid reflux from the stomach. In older children and adults, it can cause more severe symptoms, such as difficulty swallowing solid food or solid food sticking in the esophagus for more than a few minutes. In infants, this disease may be associated with failure to thrive.

If you are diagnosed with EoE, you will probably be tested for allergies. In some situations, avoiding certain food allergens will be an effective treatment for EoE.

Source: National Institute of Allergy and Infectious Diseases, November 2010.

- **Step 2:** The next time you are exposed to the same food allergen, it binds to the IgE antibodies that are attached to the mast cells and basophils. The binding signals the cells to release massive amounts of chemicals such as histamine. Depending on the tissue in which they are released, these chemicals will cause you to have various symptoms of food allergy. The symptoms can range from mild to severe. A severe allergic reaction can include a potentially life-threatening reaction called anaphylaxis.

What are the symptoms of food allergy?

If you are allergic to a particular food, you may experience all or some of the following symptoms:

- Itching in your mouth
- Swelling of lips and tongue
- GI symptoms, such as vomiting, diarrhea, or abdominal cramps and pain
- Hives
- Worsening of eczema
- Tightening of the throat or trouble breathing
- Drop in blood pressure

What is anaphylaxis?

If you have a food allergy, there is a chance that you may experience a severe form of allergic reaction known as anaphylaxis. Anaphylaxis may begin suddenly and may lead to death if not immediately treated.

Anaphylaxis includes a wide range of symptoms that can occur in many combinations. Some symptoms are not life-threatening, but the most severe restrict breathing and blood circulation. Many different parts of your body can be affected:

- **Skin:** Itching, hives, redness, swelling
- **Nose:** Sneezing, stuffy nose, runny nose
- **Mouth:** Itching, swelling of lips or tongue
- **Throat:** Itching, tightness, difficulty swallowing, hoarseness
- **Chest:** Shortness of breath, cough, wheeze, chest pain, tightness
- **Heart:** Weak pulse, passing out, shock
- **Gastrointestinal (GI) Tract:** Vomiting, diarrhea, cramps
- **Nervous System:** Dizziness or fainting

Symptoms may begin within several minutes to several hours after exposure to the food. Sometimes the symptoms go away, only to return two to four hours later or even as many as eight hours later. When you begin to experience symptoms, you must seek immediate medical attention because anaphylaxis can be life-threatening.

Anaphylaxis caused by an allergic reaction to a certain food is highly unpredictable. The severity of a given attack does not predict the severity of subsequent attacks. The response will vary depending on several factors, such as tour sensitivity to the food, how much of the food you are exposed to, and how the food entered your body.

Any anaphylactic reaction may become dangerous and must be evaluated by a healthcare professional. Food allergy is the leading cause of anaphylaxis. However, medications, insect stings, and latex can also cause an allergic reaction that leads to anaphylaxis.

Cross-Reactive Food Allergies

If you have a life-threatening reaction to a certain food, your healthcare professional will show you how to avoid similar foods that may trigger this reaction. For example, if you have a history of allergy to shrimp, allergy testing will usually show that you are also allergic to other shellfish, such as crab, lobster, and crayfish. This is called cross-reactivity.

Source: National Institute of Allergy and Infectious Diseases, November 2010.

What are the most common food allergies in infants, children, and adults?

In infants and children, the most common foods that cause allergic reactions are the following:

- Egg
- Peanut
- Soy (primarily in infants)
- Milk
- Tree nuts such as walnuts
- Wheat

Allergy to cow's milk is common in infants and young children and can develop within days to months of birth. In children, allergy to cow's milk can cause abdominal pain, hives, and eczema. These symptoms are typically associated with IgE antibodies to milk. Abdominal pain is also a symptom of lactose intolerance, so only a healthcare professional can determine whether symptoms are caused by an allergic reaction to cow's milk. In other children, cow's milk can lead to a different type of reaction to milk, resulting in colic and sleeplessness, as well as blood in the stool and poor growth. This type of reaction to milk is associated with immune responses that are not related to IgE antibody.

In adults, the most common foods that cause allergic reactions are the following:

- Shellfish such as shrimp, crayfish, lobster, and crab
- Peanut
- Tree nuts
- Fish such as salmon

Food allergies generally develop early in life but can develop at any age. For example, milk allergy tends to develop early in life, whereas shrimp allergy generally develops later in life.

Children usually outgrow their egg, milk, and soy allergies, but people who develop allergies as adults usually have their allergies for life. Children generally do not outgrow their allergy to peanut.

Finally, foods that are eaten routinely increase the likelihood that a person will develop allergies to that food. In Japan, for example, rice allergy is more frequent than in the United States, and in Scandinavia, codfish allergy is more common than in the United States.

What is oral allergy syndrome?

Oral allergy syndrome (OAS) is an allergy to certain raw fruits and vegetables, such as apples, cherries, kiwis, celery, tomatoes, and green peppers. OAS occurs mostly in people with

351

hay fever, especially spring hay fever due to birch pollen and late summer hay fever due to ragweed pollen.

Eating the raw food causes an itchy, tingling sensation in the mouth, lips, and throat. It can also cause swelling of the lips, tongue, and throat; watery, itchy eyes; runny nose; and sneezing. Just handling the raw fruit or vegetable may cause a rash, itching, or swelling where the juice touches the skin.

Cooking or processing easily breaks down the proteins in the fruits and vegetables that cause OAS. Therefore, OAS typically does not occur with cooked or baked fruits and vegetables or processed fruits, such as in applesauce.

What is exercise-induced food allergy?

Exercise-induced food allergy is one situation that requires more than simply eating food to start a reaction. This type of reaction occurs after someone eats a specific food before exercising. As exercise increases and body temperature rises these symptoms may develop:

- Itching and light-headedness start
- Hives may appear
- Anaphylaxis may develop

Some people have this reaction from many foods, and others have it only after eating a specific food.

Treating exercised-induced food allergy is simple—avoid eating for a couple of hours before exercising. Crustacean shellfish, alcohol, tomatoes, cheese, and celery are common causes of exercise-induced food allergy reactions.

Is it food allergy or food intolerance?

Food allergy is sometimes confused with food intolerance. To find out the difference between food allergy and food intolerance, your healthcare professional will go through a list of possible causes for your symptoms.

There are several types of food intolerance:

Lactose Intolerance: Lactose is a sugar found in milk and most milk products. Lactase is an enzyme in the lining of the gut that breaks down or digests lactose. Lactose intolerance occurs when lactase is missing. Instead of the enzyme breaking down the sugar, bacteria in the gut break it down, which forms gas, which in turn causes symptoms of bloating, abdominal pain, and sometimes diarrhea.

Lactose intolerance is uncommon in babies and young children under the age of 5 years. Because lactase levels decline as people get older, lactose intolerance becomes more common with age. Lactose intolerance also varies widely based on racial and ethnic background. Your healthcare professional can use laboratory tests to find out whether your body can digest lactose.

Food Additives: Another type of food intolerance is a reaction to certain products that are added to food to enhance taste, add color, or protect against the growth of microbes. Several compounds such as MSG (monosodium glutamate) and sulfites are tied to reactions that can be confused with food allergy.

- MSG is a flavor enhancer. When taken in large amounts, it can cause some of the following symptoms: flushing, sensations of warmth, headache, and chest discomfort. These passing reactions occur rapidly after eating large amounts of food to which MSG has been added.

- Sulfites are found in food for several reasons: They have been added to increase crispness or prevent mold growth; they occur naturally in the food; they have been generated during the winemaking process. Sulfites can cause breathing problems in people with asthma. The Food and Drug Administration (FDA) has banned sulfites as spray-on preservatives for fresh fruits and vegetables. When sulfites are present in foods, they are listed on ingredient labels.

Gluten Intolerance: Gluten is a part of wheat, barley, and rye. Gluten intolerance is associated with celiac disease, also called gluten-sensitive enteropathy. This disease develops when the immune system responds abnormally to gluten. This abnormal response does not involve IgE antibody and is not considered a food allergy.

Food Poisoning: Some of the symptoms of food allergy, such as abdominal cramping, are common to food poisoning. However, food poisoning is caused by microbes, such as bacteria, and bacterial products, such as toxins, that can contaminate meats and dairy products.

Histamine Toxicity: Fish, such as tuna and mackerel that are not refrigerated properly and become contaminated by bacteria, may contain very high levels of histamine. A person who eats such fish may show symptoms that are similar to food allergy. However, this reaction is not a true allergic reaction. Instead, the reaction is called histamine toxicity or scombroid food poisoning.

Other: Several other conditions, such as ulcers and cancers of the GI tract, cause some of the same symptoms as food allergy. These symptoms, which include vomiting, diarrhea, and cramping abdominal pain, become worse when you eat.

How are food allergies diagnosed?

Your healthcare professional will begin by taking a detailed medical history to find out whether your symptoms are caused by an allergy to specific foods, a food intolerance, or other health problems.

A detailed history is the most valuable tool for diagnosing food allergy. Your healthcare professional will ask you several questions and listen to your history of food reactions to decide whether the facts fit a diagnosis of food allergy.

Your healthcare professional is likely to ask some of the following questions:

- Did your reaction come on quickly, usually within minutes to several hours after eating the food?

- Is your reaction always associated with a certain food?

- How much of this potentially allergenic food did you eat before you had a reaction?

- Have you eaten this food before and had a reaction?

- Did anyone else who ate the same food get sick?

- Did you take allergy medicines, and if so, did they help? (Antihistamines should relieve hives, for example.)

Diet Diary: Sometimes your healthcare professional can't make a diagnosis based only on your history. In that case, you may be asked to keep a record of what you eat and whether you have a reaction. This diet diary contains more details about the foods you eat than your history. From the diary, you and your healthcare professional may be able to identify a consistent pattern in your reactions.

Elimination Diet: The next step some healthcare professionals use is a limited elimination diet, in which the food that is suspected of causing an allergic reaction is removed from your diet. For example, if you suspect you are allergic to egg, your healthcare professional will instruct you to eliminate this one food from your diet. The limited elimination diet is done under the direction of your healthcare professional.

Skin Prick Test: If your history, diet diary, or elimination diet suggests a specific food allergy is likely, then your healthcare professional will use the skin prick test to confirm the diagnosis.

With a skin prick test, your healthcare professional uses a needle to place a tiny amount of food extract just below the surface of the skin on your lower arm or back. If you are allergic, there will be swelling or redness at the test site. This is a positive result. It means that there are IgE molecules on the skin's mast cells that are specific to the food being tested.

The skin prick test is simple and relatively safe, and results are ready in minutes. You can have a positive skin prick test to a food, however, without having an allergic reaction to that food. A healthcare professional often makes a diagnosis of food allergy when someone has both a positive skin prick test to a specific food and a history of reactions that suggests an allergy to the same food.

Blood Test: Instead of the skin prick test, your healthcare professional can take a blood sample to measure the levels of food-specific IgE antibodies. As with skin prick testing, positive blood tests do not necessarily mean that you have a food allergy. Your healthcare professional must combine these test results with information about your history of reactions to food to make an accurate diagnosis of food allergy.

Oral Food Challenge: Caution: Because an oral food challenge can cause a severe allergic reaction, it should always be conducted by a healthcare professional who has experience performing them.

An oral food challenge is the final method healthcare professionals use to diagnose food allergy. This method includes the following steps:

- Your healthcare professional gives you individual doses of various foods (masked so you do not know what food is present), some of which are suspected of starting an allergic reaction.

- Initially, the dose of food is very small, but the amount is gradually increased during the challenge.

- You swallow the individual dose.

- Your healthcare professional watches you to see whether a reaction occurs.

To prevent bias, oral food challenges are often done double blinded. In a true double-blind challenge, neither you nor your healthcare professional knows whether the substance you eat contains the likely allergen. Another medical professional has made up the individual doses. In a single-blind challenge, your healthcare professional knows what you are eating but you do not. A reaction only to suspected foods and not to the other foods tested confirms the diagnosis of a food allergy.

Can food allergies be cured or prevented?

There is currently no cure for food allergies. You can only prevent the symptoms of food allergy by avoiding the allergenic food. After you and your healthcare professional have identified the food(s) to which you are sensitive, you must remove them from your diet.

Food Labeling Requirements

To help Americans avoid the health risks posed by food allergens, Congress passed the Food Allergen Labeling and Consumer Protection Act of 2004 (FALCPA). The law applies to all foods whose labeling is regulated by the U.S. Food and Drug Administration (FDA), both domestic and imported.

While more than 160 foods can cause allergic reactions in people with food allergies, the law identifies the eight most common allergenic foods. These foods account for 90 percent of food allergic reactions, and are the food sources from which many other ingredients are derived. These are the eight foods identified by the law:

1. Milk
2. Eggs
3. Fish (for example, bass, flounder, cod)
4. Crustacean shellfish (for example, crab, lobster, shrimp)
5. Tree nuts (for example, almonds, walnuts, pecans)
6. Peanuts
7. Wheat
8. Soybeans

These eight foods, and any ingredient that contains protein derived from one or more of them, are designated as "major food allergens" by FALCPA.

The law requires that food labels identify the food source names of all major food allergens used to make the food. This requirement is met if the common or usual name of an ingredient (for example, buttermilk) that is a major food allergen already identifies that allergen's food source name (that is, milk). Otherwise, the allergen's food source name must be declared at least once on the food label in one of two ways.

The name of the food source of a major food allergen must appear:

1. In parentheses following the name of the ingredient. Examples: "lecithin (soy)," "flour (wheat)," and "whey (milk)"; OR
2. Immediately after or next to the list of ingredients in a "contains" statement. Example: "Contains Wheat, Milk, and Soy."

Source: Excerpted from "Food Allergies: What You Need to Know," U.S. Food and Drug Administration (www.fda.gov), June 2010.

Read Food Labels: You must read the list of ingredients on the label of each prepared food that you are considering eating. Many allergens, such as peanut, egg, and milk, appear in prepared foods you normally would not associate with those foods.

Since 2006, U.S. food manufacturers have been required by law to list the ingredients of prepared foods. In addition, food manufacturers must use plain language to disclose whether their products contain (or may contain) any of the top eight allergenic foods—egg, milk, peanut, tree nuts, soy, wheat, shellfish, and fish.

Keep Clean: Simple measures of cleanliness can remove most allergens from the environment of a person with food allergy. For example, simply washing your hands with soap and water will remove peanut allergens, and most household cleaners will remove allergens from surfaces.

How are food allergy reactions treated?

When you have food allergies, you must be prepared to treat an unintentional exposure. Talk to your healthcare professional and develop a plan to protect yourself in case of an unintentional exposure to the food. For example, a plan may include these steps:

- Wear a medical alert bracelet or necklace

- Carry an auto-injector device containing epinephrine (adrenaline)

- Seek medical help immediately

Mild Symptoms: Talk to your healthcare professional to find out what medicines may relieve mild food allergy symptoms that are not part of an anaphylactic reaction. However, be aware that it is very hard for you to know which reactions are mild and which may lead to anaphylaxis.

Food Allergen "Advisory" Labeling

Food Allergen Labeling and Consumer Protection Act of 2004 (FALCPA) labeling requirements do not apply to the potential or unintentional presence of major food allergens in foods resulting from "cross-contact" situations during manufacturing, for example, because of shared equipment or processing lines. In the context of food allergens, "cross-contact" occurs when a residue or trace amount of an allergenic food becomes incorporated into another food not intended to contain it.

U.S. Food and Drug Administration (FDA) guidance for the food industry states that food allergen advisory statements, for example, "may contain [allergen]" or "produced in a facility that also uses [allergen]" should not be used as a substitute for adhering to current good manufacturing practices and must be truthful and not misleading. FDA is considering ways to best manage the use of these types of statements by manufacturers to better inform consumers.

Source: Excerpted from "Food Allergies: What You Need to Know," U.S. Food and Drug Administration (www.fda.gov), June 2010.

Chapter 53

Dealing With Lactose Intolerance

What is lactose intolerance?

Lactose intolerance is the inability or insufficient ability to digest lactose, a sugar found in milk and milk products. Lactose intolerance is caused by a deficiency of the enzyme lactase, which is produced by the cells lining the small intestine. Lactase breaks down lactose into two simpler forms of sugar called glucose and galactose, which are then absorbed into the bloodstream.

Not all people with lactase deficiency have digestive symptoms, but those who do may have lactose intolerance. Most people with lactose intolerance can tolerate some amount of lactose in their diet.

People sometimes confuse lactose intolerance with cow milk allergy. Milk allergy is a reaction by the body's immune system to one or more milk proteins and can be life threatening when just a small amount of milk or milk product is consumed. Milk allergy most commonly appears in the first year of life, while lactose intolerance occurs more often in adulthood.

What causes lactose intolerance?

The cause of lactose intolerance is best explained by describing how a person develops lactase deficiency.

Primary lactase deficiency develops over time and begins after about age two when the body begins to produce less lactase. Most children who have lactase deficiency do not experience symptoms of lactose intolerance until late adolescence or adulthood.

About This Chapter: Excerpted from "Lactose Intolerance," National Digestive Disease Information Clearinghouse (http://digestive.niddk.nih.gov), June 2009.

Researchers have identified a possible genetic link to primary lactase deficiency. Some people inherit a gene from their parents that makes it likely they will develop primary lactase deficiency. This discovery may be useful in developing future genetic tests to identify people at risk for lactose intolerance.

Secondary lactase deficiency results from injury to the small intestine that occurs with severe diarrheal illness, celiac disease, Crohn disease, or chemotherapy. This type of lactase deficiency can occur at any age but is more common in infancy.

Who is at risk for lactose intolerance?

Lactose intolerance is a common condition that is more likely to occur in adulthood, with a higher incidence in older adults. Some ethnic and racial populations are more affected than others, including African Americans, Hispanic Americans, American Indians, and Asian Americans. The condition is least common among Americans of northern European descent.

Infants born prematurely are more likely to have lactase deficiency because an infant's lactase levels do not increase until the third trimester of pregnancy.

What are the symptoms of lactose intolerance?

People with lactose intolerance may feel uncomfortable 30 minutes to two hours after consuming milk and milk products. Symptoms range from mild to severe, based on the amount of lactose consumed and the amount a person can tolerate. Common symptoms include abdominal pain, abdominal bloating, gas, diarrhea, and nausea.

How is lactose intolerance diagnosed?

Lactose intolerance can be hard to diagnose based on symptoms alone. People may think they suffer from lactose intolerance because they have digestive symptoms; however, other conditions such as irritable bowel syndrome can cause similar symptoms. After taking a medical history and performing a physical examination, the doctor may first recommend eliminating all milk and milk products from the person's diet for a short time to see if the symptoms resolve. Tests may be necessary to provide more information.

Two tests are commonly used to measure the digestion of lactose:

Hydrogen Breath Test: The person drinks a lactose-loaded beverage and then the breath is analyzed at regular intervals to measure the amount of hydrogen. Normally, very little hydrogen is detectable in the breath, but undigested lactose produces high levels of hydrogen. Smoking and some foods and medications may affect the accuracy of the results. People should check with their doctor about foods and medications that may interfere with test results.

Stool Acidity Test: The stool acidity test is used for infants and young children to measure the amount of acid in the stool. Undigested lactose creates lactic acid and other fatty acids that can be detected in a stool sample. Glucose may also be present in the stool as a result of undigested lactose.

How is lactose intolerance managed?

Although the body's ability to produce lactase cannot be changed, the symptoms of lactose intolerance can be managed with dietary changes. Most people with lactose intolerance can tolerate some amount of lactose in their diet. Gradually introducing small amounts of milk or milk products may help some people adapt to them with fewer symptoms. Often, people can better tolerate milk or milk products by taking them with meals.

The amount of change needed in the diet depends on how much lactose a person can consume without symptoms. For example, one person may have severe symptoms after drinking a small glass of milk, while another can drink a large glass without symptoms. Others can easily consume yogurt and hard cheeses such as cheddar and Swiss but not milk or other milk products.

People With Lactose Intolerance Can Still Have Dairy Products

Most people with lactose intolerance do not require a completely lactose-free diet. Studies show that there are some things people with lactose intolerance can do to have fewer symptoms of lactose intolerance:

- Drink low-fat or fat-free milk in servings of 1 cup or less.
- Drink low-fat or fat-free milk with other food, such as with breakfast cereal, instead of by itself.
- Eat dairy products other than milk, such as low-fat or fat-free hard cheeses or cottage cheese, or low-fat or fat-free ice cream or yogurt. These foods contain a lower amount of lactose per serving compared with milk and may cause fewer symptoms.
- Choose lactose-free milk and milk products, which have the same amount of calcium as regular milk.
- Use over-the-counter pills or drops that contain lactase, which can eliminate symptoms altogether

Source: Excerpted from "Lactose Intolerance," National Institute of Child Health and Human Development (www.nichd.nih.gov), February 19, 2007.

The *Dietary Guidelines for Americans* recommend that people with lactose intolerance choose milk products with lower levels of lactose than regular milk, such as yogurt and hard cheese.

Lactose-free and lactose-reduced milk and milk products, available at most supermarkets, are identical to regular milk except that the lactase enzyme has been added. Lactose-free milk remains fresh for about the same length of time or longer than regular milk if it is ultra-pasteurized. Lactose-free milk may have a slightly sweeter taste than regular milk. Soy milk and other products may be recommended by a health professional.

People who still experience symptoms after dietary changes can take over-the-counter lactase enzyme drops or tablets. Taking the tablets or a few drops of the liquid enzyme when consuming milk or milk products may make these foods more tolerable for people with lactose intolerance.

What about lactose intolerance and calcium intake?

Milk and milk products are a major source of calcium and other nutrients. Calcium is essential for the growth and repair of bones at all ages. A shortage of calcium intake may lead to fragile bones that can easily fracture later in life, a condition called osteoporosis.

The amount of calcium a person needs to maintain good health varies by age. Recommendations are shown in Table 53.1.

Getting enough calcium is important for people with lactose intolerance when the intake of milk and milk products is limited. Many foods can provide calcium and other nutrients the body needs. Non-milk products that are high in calcium include fish with soft bones such as salmon and sardines and dark green vegetables such as spinach. Table 53.2 lists foods that are good sources of dietary calcium.

Table 53.1. Recommended Calcium Intake By Age Group

Age group	Amount of calcium to consume daily, in milligrams (mg)
0–6 months	210 mg
7–12 months	270 mg
1–3 years	500 mg
4–8 years	800 mg
9–18 years	1,300 mg
19–50 years	1,000 mg
51–70+ years	1,200 mg

Source: Adapted from Dietary Reference Intakes, 2004, Institute of Medicine, National Academy of Sciences.

Yogurt made with active and live bacterial cultures is a good source of calcium for many people with lactose intolerance. When this type of yogurt enters the intestine, the bacterial cultures convert lactose to lactic acid, so the yogurt may be well-tolerated due to a lower lactose content than yogurt without live cultures. Frozen yogurt does not contain bacterial cultures, so it may not be well tolerated.

Calcium is absorbed and used in the body only when enough vitamin D is present. Some people with lactose intolerance may not be getting enough vitamin D. Vitamin D comes from food sources such as eggs, liver, and vitamin D-fortified milk and yogurt. Regular exposure to sunlight also helps the body naturally absorb vitamin D. Talking with a doctor or registered dietitian may be helpful in planning a balanced diet that provides an adequate amount of nutrients—including calcium and vitamin D—and minimizes discomfort. A health professional can determine whether calcium and other dietary supplements are needed.

Table 53.2. Calcium Content In Common Foods

Non-Milk Products	Calcium Content
Rhubarb, frozen, cooked, 1 cup	348 mg
Sardines, with bone, 3 oz.	325 mg
Spinach, frozen, cooked, 1 cup	291 mg
Salmon, canned, with bone, 3 oz.	181 mg
Soy milk, unfortified, 1 cup	61 mg
Orange, 1 medium	52 mg
Broccoli, raw, 1 cup	41 mg
Pinto beans, cooked, 1/2 cup	40 mg
Lettuce greens, 1 cup	20 mg
Tuna, white, canned, 3 oz.	12 mg
Milk and Milk Products	
Yogurt, with active and live cultures, plain, low-fat, vitamin D-fortified, 1 cup	415 mg
Milk, reduced fat, vitamin D-fortified, 1 cup	285 mg
Swiss cheese, 1 oz.	224 mg
Cottage cheese, 1/2 cup	87 mg
Ice cream, 1/2 cup	84 mg

Source: Adapted from U.S. Department of Agriculture, Agricultural Research Service. 2008. USDA National Nutrient Database for Standard Reference, Release 21.

What other products contain lactose?

Milk and milk products are often added to processed foods—foods that have been altered to prolong their shelf life. People with lactose intolerance should be aware of the many food products that may contain even small amounts of lactose, such as the following:

- Bread and other baked goods
- Waffles, pancakes, biscuits, cookies, and mixes to make them
- Processed breakfast foods such as doughnuts, frozen waffles and pancakes, toaster pastries, and sweet rolls
- Processed breakfast cereals
- Instant potatoes, soups, and breakfast drinks
- Potato chips, corn chips, and other processed snacks
- Processed meats, such as bacon, sausage, hot dogs, and lunch meats
- Margarine
- Salad dressings
- Liquid and powdered milk-based meal replacements
- Protein powders and bars
- Candies
- Non-dairy liquid and powdered coffee creamers
- Non-dairy whipped toppings

Checking the ingredients on food labels is helpful in finding possible sources of lactose in food products. If any of the following words are listed on a food label, the product contains lactose:

- Milk
- Lactose
- Whey
- Curds
- Milk by-products
- Dry milk solids
- Non-fat dry milk powder

Lactose is also used in some prescription medicines, including birth control pills, and over-the-counter medicines like products to treat stomach acid and gas. These medicines most often cause symptoms in people with severe lactose intolerance.

Points To Remember

- Lactose intolerance is the inability or insufficient ability to digest lactose, a sugar found in milk and milk products.
- Lactose intolerance is caused by a deficiency of the enzyme lactase, which is produced by the cells lining the small intestine.
- Not all people with lactase deficiency have digestive symptoms, but those who do may have lactose intolerance.
- Most people with lactose intolerance can tolerate some amount of lactose in their diet.
- People with lactose intolerance may feel uncomfortable after consuming milk and milk products. Symptoms can include abdominal pain, abdominal bloating, gas, diarrhea, and nausea.
- The symptoms of lactose intolerance can be managed with dietary changes.
- Getting enough calcium and vitamin D is a concern for people with lactose intolerance when the intake of milk and milk products is limited. Many foods can provide the calcium and other nutrients the body needs.
- Talking with a doctor or registered dietitian may be helpful in planning a balanced diet that provides an adequate amount of nutrients—including calcium and vitamin D—and minimizes discomfort. A health professional can determine whether calcium and other dietary supplements are needed.
- Milk and milk products are often added to processed foods. Checking the ingredients on food labels is helpful in finding possible sources of lactose in food products.

Source: National Digestive Disease Information Clearinghouse, June 2009.

Chapter 54

Understanding Foodborne Illness

What are foodborne illnesses?

Foodborne illnesses are caused by eating food or drinking beverages contaminated with bacteria, parasites, or viruses. Harmful chemicals can also cause foodborne illnesses if they have contaminated food during harvesting or processing. Foodborne illnesses can cause symptoms that range from an upset stomach to more serious symptoms, including diarrhea, fever, vomiting, abdominal cramps, and dehydration. Most foodborne infections are undiagnosed and unreported, though the Centers for Disease Control and Prevention estimates that every year about 76 million people in the United States become ill from pathogens, or disease-causing substances, in food. Of these people, about 5,000 die.

What are the causes of foodborne illnesses?

Harmful bacteria are the most common cause of foodborne illnesses. Some bacteria may be present on foods when you purchase them. Raw foods are the most common source of foodborne illnesses because they are not sterile; examples include raw meat and poultry that may have become contaminated during slaughter. Seafood may become contaminated during harvest or through processing. One in 10,000 eggs may be contaminated with *Salmonella* inside the eggshell. Produce such as spinach, lettuce, tomatoes, sprouts, and melons can become contaminated with *Salmonella*, *Shigella*, or *Escherichia coli* (*E. coli*) *O157:H7*. Contamination can occur during growing, harvesting, processing, storing, shipping, or final preparation. Sources of produce contamination are varied as these foods are grown in soil and can become contaminated during growth or through processing and distribution. Contamination may also

About This Chapter: Excerpted from "Bacteria and Foodborne Illness," National Digestive Diseases Information Clearinghouse, March 2007.

occur during food preparation in a restaurant or a home kitchen. The most common form of contamination from handled foods is the calicivirus, also called the Norwalk-like virus.

When food is cooked and left out for more than two hours at room temperature, bacteria can multiply quickly. Most bacteria grow undetected because they don't produce a bad odor or change the color or texture of the food. Freezing food slows or stops bacteria's growth but does not destroy the bacteria. The microbes can become reactivated when the food is thawed. Refrigeration also can slow the growth of some bacteria. Thorough cooking is needed to destroy the bacteria.

What are the symptoms of foodborne illnesses?

In most cases of foodborne illnesses, symptoms resemble intestinal flu and may last a few hours or even several days. Symptoms can range from mild to serious and include the following:

- Abdominal cramps
- Nausea
- Vomiting
- Diarrhea, which is sometimes bloody
- Fever
- Dehydration

What are the risk factors of foodborne illnesses?

Some people are at greater risk for bacterial infections because of their age or an unhealthy immune system. Young children, pregnant women, and older adults are at greatest risk.

What are the complications of foodborne illnesses?

Some micro-organisms, such as *Listeria monocytogenes* and *Clostridium botulinum*, cause far more serious symptoms than vomiting and diarrhea. They can cause spontaneous abortion or death.

In some people, especially children, hemolytic uremic syndrome (HUS) can result from infection by a particular strain of bacteria, *E. coli O157:H7*, and can lead to kidney failure and death. HUS is a rare disorder that affects primarily children between the ages of one and 10 years old and is the leading cause of acute renal failure in previously healthy children. A child may become infected after consuming contaminated food or beverages, such as meat, especially undercooked ground beef; unpasteurized juices; contaminated water; or through contact with an infected person.

The most common symptoms of HUS infection are vomiting, abdominal pain, and diarrhea, which may be bloody. In 5% to 10% of cases, HUS develops about five to 10 days after the onset of illness. This disease may last from one to 15 days and is fatal in 3% to 5% of cases. Other symptoms of HUS include fever, lethargy or sluggishness, irritability, and paleness or pallor. In about half the cases, the disease progresses until it causes acute renal failure, which means the kidneys are unable to remove waste products from the blood and excrete them into the urine. A decrease in circulating red blood cells and blood platelets and reduced blood flow to organs may lead to multiple organ failure. Seizures, heart failure, inflammation of the pancreas, and diabetes can also result. However, most children recover completely.

See a doctor right away if you have any of the following symptoms with diarrhea:

- High fever, temperature over 101.5° F, measured orally
- Blood in the stools
- Diarrhea that lasts more than three days
- Prolonged vomiting that prevents keeping liquid down and can lead to dehydration
- Signs of severe dehydration, such as dry mouth, sticky saliva, decreased urination, dizziness, fatigue, sunken eyes, low blood pressure, or increased heart rate and breathing rate
- Signs of shock, such as weak or rapid pulse or shallow breathing
- Confusion or difficulty reasoning

How are foodborne illnesses diagnosed?

Your doctor may be able to diagnose foodborne illnesses from a list of what you've eaten recently and from results of appropriate laboratory tests. Diagnostic tests for foodborne illnesses should include examination of the feces. A sample of the suspected food, if available, can also be tested for bacterial toxins, viruses, and parasites.

How are foodborne illnesses treated?

Most cases of foodborne illnesses are mild and can be treated by increasing fluid intake, either orally or intravenously, to replace lost fluids and electrolytes. People who experience gastrointestinal or neurologic symptoms should seek medical attention.

In the most severe situations, such as HUS, hospitalization may be needed to receive supportive nutritional and medical therapy. Maintaining adequate fluid and electrolyte balance and controlling blood pressure are important. Doctors will try to minimize the impact of reduced kidney function. Dialysis may be needed until the kidneys can function normally. Blood transfusions also may be needed.

How are foodborne illnesses prevented?

Most cases of foodborne illnesses can be prevented through proper cooking or processing of food, which kills bacteria. In addition, because bacteria multiply rapidly between 40° F and 140° F, food must be kept out of this temperature range.

Follow these tips to prevent harmful bacteria from growing in food:

- **Refrigerate foods promptly:** If prepared food stands at room temperature for more than two hours, it may not be safe to eat. Set your refrigerator at 40° F or lower and your freezer at 0° F.

- **Cook food to the appropriate internal temperature:** 145° F for roasts, steaks, and chops of beef, veal, and lamb; 160° F for pork, ground veal, and ground beef; 165° F for ground poultry; and 180° F for whole poultry. Use a meat thermometer to be sure. Foods are properly cooked only when they are heated long enough and at a high enough temperature to kill the harmful bacteria that cause illnesses.

- **Prevent cross-contamination:** Bacteria can spread from one food product to another throughout the kitchen and can get onto cutting boards, knives, sponges, and countertops. Keep raw meat, poultry, seafood, and their juices away from all ready-to-eat foods.

- **Wash utensils and surfaces before and after use with hot, soapy water:** Better still, sanitize them with diluted bleach (one teaspoon of bleach to 1 quart of hot water).

- **Handle food properly:** Always wash your hands for at least 20 seconds with warm, soapy water before and after handling raw meat, poultry, fish, shellfish, produce, or eggs.

- **Never defrost food on the kitchen counter:** Use the refrigerator, cold running water, or the microwave oven.

- **Do not pack the refrigerator:** Cool air must circulate to keep food safe.

There are a many things you could do to help keep harmful bacteria from growing in food. The following guidelines can help ensure your safety:

- Wash your hands after using the bathroom, changing diapers, or touching animals.

- Wash sponges and dish towels weekly in hot water in the washing machine.

- Keep cold food cold and hot food hot.

- Maintain the temperature of hot cooked food at 140° F or higher.

- Reheat cooked food to at least 165° F.

- Refrigerate or freeze perishables, produce, prepared food, and leftovers within two hours.

- Never let food marinate at room temperature, refrigerate it instead.

- Divide any large amounts of leftovers into small, shallow containers for quick cooling in the refrigerator.

- Remove the stuffing from poultry and other meats immediately and refrigerate it in a separate container.

- Wash all unpackaged fruits and vegetables, and those packaged and not marked "pre-washed," under running water just before eating, cutting, or cooking. Scrub firm produce such as melons and cucumbers with a clean produce brush. Dry all produce with a paper towel to further reduce any possible bacteria.

Tips For Preventing Foodborne Illnesses

You can prevent foodborne illnesses by taking the following precautions:

- Wash your hands with warm, soapy water before and after preparing food and after using the bathroom or changing diapers.
- Keep raw meat, poultry, seafood, and their juices away from ready-to-eat foods.
- Make sure to cook foods properly and at a high enough temperature to kill harmful bacteria.
- Always refrigerate foods within two hours or less after cooking because cold temperatures will help keep harmful bacteria from growing and multiplying.
- Clean surfaces well before and after using them to prepare food.

What is food irradiation?

Food irradiation is the treatment of food with high energy such as gamma rays, electron beams, or x-rays as a means of cold pasteurization, which destroys living bacteria to control foodborne illnesses. The United States relies exclusively on the use of gamma rays, which are similar to ultraviolet light and microwaves and pass through food leaving no residue. Food irradiation is approved for wheat, potatoes, spices, seasonings, pork, poultry, red meats, whole fresh fruits, and dry or dehydrated products. Although irradiation destroys many bacteria, it does not sterilize food. Even if you're using food that has been irradiated by the manufacturer, you must continue to take precautions against foodborne illnesses—through proper refrigeration and handling—to safeguard against any surviving organisms. If you are traveling with food, make sure perishable items such as meats are wrapped to prevent leakage. Be sure to fill the cooler with plenty of ice and store it in the car, not the trunk. If any food seems warmer than 40° F, throw it out.

Are there other disorders related to foodborne illness?

Scientists suspect that foodborne pathogens are linked to chronic disorders and can even cause permanent tissue or organ destruction. Research suggests that when some people are infected by foodborne pathogens, the activation of their immune system can trigger an inappropriate autoimmune response, which means the immune system attacks the body's own cells. In some people, an autoimmune response leads to a chronic health condition. Chronic disorders that may be triggered by foodborne pathogens include the following:

- Arthritis
- Kidney failure
- Autoimmune disorders
- Inflammatory bowel disease
- Guillain-Barré syndrome

Further research is needed to explain the link between these disorders and foodborne illnesses.

What are common sources of foodborne illness?

Sources of illness: Raw and undercooked meat and poultry

- **Symptoms:** Abdominal pain, diarrhea, nausea, and vomiting
- **Bacteria:** *Campylobacter jejuni*, *E. coli O157:H7*, *L. monocytogenes*, *Salmonella*

Sources of illness: Raw foods, unpasteurized milk and dairy products, such as soft cheeses

- **Symptoms:** Nausea, vomiting, fever, abdominal cramps, and diarrhea
- **Bacteria:** *L. monocytogenes*, *Salmonella*, *Shigella*, *Staphylococcus aureus*, *C. jejuni*

Sources of illness: Raw and undercooked eggs (often used in foods such as homemade hollandaise sauce, caesar and other salad dressings, tiramisu, homemade ice cream, homemade mayonnaise, cookie dough, and frostings)

- **Symptoms:** Nausea, vomiting, fever, abdominal cramps, and diarrhea
- **Bacterium:** *Salmonella enteritidis*

Sources of illness: Raw and undercooked shellfish

- **Symptoms:** Chills, fever, and collapse

- **Bacteria:** *Vibrio vulnificus*, *Vibrio parahaemolyticus*

Sources of illness: Improperly canned goods, smoked or salted fish

- **Symptoms:** Double vision, inability to swallow, difficulty speaking, and inability to breathe. Seek medical help right away if you experience any of these symptoms.

- **Bacterium:** *C. botulinum*

Sources of illness: Fresh or minimally processed produce, contaminated water

- **Symptoms:** Bloody diarrhea, nausea, and vomiting

- **Bacteria:** *E. coli O157:H7*, *L. monocytogenes*, *Salmonella*, *Shigella*, *Yersinia enterocolitica*, viruses, and parasites

Points To Remember

Foodborne illnesses result from eating food or drinking beverages that are contaminated with bacteria, viruses, or parasites. Young children, pregnant women, older adults, and people with lowered immunity are at greater risk for foodborne illnesses. Symptoms usually resemble intestinal flu.

See a doctor immediately if you have more serious problems or do not seem to be improving as expected. Treatment may range from replacement of lost fluids and electrolytes for mild cases of foodborne illnesses to hospitalization for severe conditions such as hemolytic uremic syndrome.

Chapter 55

Understanding Eating Disorders

Eating Disorders

An eating disorder is marked by extremes. It is present when a person experiences severe disturbances in eating behavior, such as extreme reduction of food intake or extreme overeating, or feelings of extreme distress or concern about body weight or shape.

A person with an eating disorder may have started out just eating smaller or larger amounts of food than usual, but at some point, the urge to eat less or more spirals out of control. Eating disorders are very complex, and despite scientific research to understand them, the biological, behavioral and social underpinnings of these illnesses remain elusive.

The two main types of eating disorders are anorexia nervosa and bulimia nervosa. A third category is "eating disorders not otherwise specified (EDNOS)," which includes several variations of eating disorders. Most of these disorders are similar to anorexia or bulimia but with slightly different characteristics. Binge eating disorder, which has received increasing research and media attention in recent years, is one type of EDNOS.

Eating disorders frequently appear during adolescence or young adulthood, but some reports indicate that they can develop during childhood or later in adulthood. Women and girls are much more likely than males to develop an eating disorder. Men and boys account for an estimated 5% to 15% of patients with anorexia or bulimia and an estimated 35% of those with binge eating disorder. Eating disorders are real, treatable medical illnesses with complex

About This Chapter: Excerpted from "Eating Disorders," National Institute of Mental Health (www.nimh.nih.gov), 2010; "Anorexia Nervosa," and "Bulimia Nervosa," National Women's Health Information Center (www.womenshealth.gov), March 2010; and "Binge Eating Disorder," National Institute of Diabetes and Digestive and Kidney Diseases (www.niddk.nih.gov), June 2008.

underlying psychological and biological causes. They frequently co-exist with other psychiatric disorders such as depression, substance abuse, or anxiety disorders. People with eating disorders also can suffer from numerous other physical health complications, such as heart conditions or kidney failure, which can lead to death.

How are men and boys affected?

Although eating disorders primarily affect women and girls, boys and men are also vulnerable. One in four preadolescent cases of anorexia occurs in boys, and binge-eating disorder affects females and males about equally.

Like females who have eating disorders, males with the illness have a warped sense of body image and often have muscle dysmorphia, a type of disorder that is characterized by an extreme concern with becoming more muscular. Some boys with the disorder want to lose weight, while others want to gain weight or "bulk up." Boys who think they are too small are at a greater risk for using steroids or other dangerous drugs to increase muscle mass.

Boys with eating disorders exhibit the same types of emotional, physical and behavioral signs and symptoms as girls, but for a variety of reasons, boys are less likely to be diagnosed with what is often considered a stereotypically "female" disorder.

Anorexia Nervosa

Anorexia nervosa, or anorexia, is a type of eating disorder that mainly affects adolescent girls and young women. A person with this disease has an intense fear of gaining weight and limits the food she eats. She typically has a low body weight, refuses to keep a normal body weight, is extremely afraid of becoming fat, and believes she is fat even when she's very thin. She misses three (menstrual) periods in a row (for girls/women who have started having their periods).

Eating Disorders Are Treatable Diseases

Psychological and medicinal treatments are effective for many eating disorders. However, in more chronic cases, specific treatments have not yet been identified.

In these cases, treatment plans often are tailored to the patient's individual needs that may include medical care and monitoring, medications, nutritional counseling, and individual, group and/or family psychotherapy. Some patients may also need to be hospitalized to treat malnutrition or to gain weight, or for other reasons.

Source: National Institute of Mental Health (www.nimh.nih.gov), 2010.

Characteristics Of Anorexia Nervosa

Anorexia nervosa is characterized by emaciation, a relentless pursuit of thinness and unwillingness to maintain a normal or healthy weight, a distortion of body image and intense fear of gaining weight, a lack of menstruation among girls and women, and extremely disturbed eating behavior. Some people with anorexia lose weight by dieting and exercising excessively—others lose weight by self-induced vomiting, or misusing laxatives, diuretics, or enemas.

Many people with anorexia see themselves as overweight, even when they are starved or are clearly malnourished. Eating, food and weight control become obsessions. A person with anorexia typically weighs herself or himself repeatedly, portions food carefully, and eats only very small quantities of only certain foods. Some who have anorexia recover with treatment after only one episode. Others get well but have relapses. Still others have a more chronic form of anorexia, in which their health deteriorates over many years as they battle the illness.

According to some studies, people with anorexia are up to ten times more likely to die as a result of their illness compared to those without the disorder. The most common complications that lead to death are cardiac arrest, and electrolyte and fluid imbalances. Suicide also can result.

Source: National Institute of Mental Health (www.nimh.nih.gov), 2010.

Anorexia affects your health because it can damage many parts of your body. A person with anorexia will have many of these signs:

- Loses a lot of weight

- Talks about weight and food all the time

- Moves food around the plate; doesn't eat it

- Weighs food and counts calories

- Follows a strict diet

- Fears gaining weight

- Won't eat in front of others

- Ignores/denies hunger

- Uses extreme measures to lose weight (self-induced vomiting, laxative abuse, diuretic abuse, diet pills, fasting, excessive exercise)

- Thinks she's fat when she's too thin

- Gets sick a lot

- Weighs self several times a day

- Acts moody

- Feels depressed

- Feels irritable

- Doesn't socialize

- Wears baggy clothes to hide appearance

How is anorexia treated?

The good news is that people with this disease can get better. The treatment depends on what the person needs, but the person must get back to a healthy weight.

A health care team of doctors, nutritionists, and therapists will help the patient get better. They will help bring the person back to a normal weight and treat any psychological issues related to anorexia. They will also help the person get rid of any actions or thoughts that cause the eating disorder.

Some research suggests that the use of medicines—such as antidepressants, antipsychotics, or mood stabilizers—may sometimes work for anorexic patients. It is thought that these medicines help the mood and anxiety symptoms that often co-exist with anorexia. Other recent studies, however, suggest that antidepressants may not stop some patients with anorexia from relapsing. Also, no medicine has shown to work 100% of the time during the important first step of restoring a patient to healthy weight. So, it is not clear if and how medications can help anorexic patients get better, but research is still on-going.

Some forms of psychotherapy can help make the psychological reasons for anorexia better. Psychotherapy is sometimes known as "talk therapy." It uses different ways of communicating to change a patient's thoughts or behavior. This kind of therapy can be useful for treating eating disorders in young patients who have not had anorexia for a long time.

Individual counseling can help someone with anorexia. If the patient is young, counseling may involve the whole family. Support groups may also be a part of treatment. In support groups, patients, and families meet and share what they've been through.

Some researchers point out that prescribing medicines and using psychotherapy designed just for anorexic patients works better at treating anorexia than just psychotherapy alone. Whether or not a treatment works, though, depends on the person involved and his or her situation. Unfortunately, no one kind of psychotherapy always works for treating anorexia.

Bulimia Nervosa

Bulimia nervosa, or bulimia, is a type of eating disorder. Someone with bulimia eats a lot of food in a short amount of time (bingeing) and then tries to get rid of the calories by purging. Purging might be done in these ways:

- Making oneself throw up

- Taking laxatives (pills or liquids that increase how fast food moves through your body and leads to a bowel movement)

A person with bulimia may also use these ways to prevent weight gain:

- Exercising a lot (more than normal)

FDA Warnings On Antidepressants

Despite the relative safety and popularity of SSRIs and other antidepressants, some studies have suggested that they may have unintentional effects on some people, especially adolescents and young adults. In 2004, the Food and Drug Administration (FDA) conducted a thorough review of published and unpublished controlled clinical trials of antidepressants that involved nearly 4,400 children and adolescents. The review revealed that 4% of those taking antidepressants thought about or attempted suicide (although no suicides occurred), compared to 2% of those receiving placebos.

This information prompted the FDA, in 2005, to adopt a "black box" warning label on all antidepressant medications to alert the public about the potential increased risk of suicidal thinking or attempts in children and adolescents taking antidepressants. In 2007, the FDA proposed that makers of all antidepressant medications extend the warning to include young adults up through age 24. A "black box" warning is the most serious type of warning on prescription drug labeling.

The warning emphasizes that patients of all ages taking antidepressants should be closely monitored, especially during the initial weeks of treatment. Possible side effects to look for are worsening depression, suicidal thinking or behavior, or any unusual changes in behavior such as sleeplessness, agitation, or withdrawal from normal social situations. The warning adds that families and caregivers should also be told of the need for close monitoring and report any changes to the physician.

Results of a comprehensive review of pediatric trials conducted between 1988 and 2006 suggested that the benefits of antidepressant medications likely outweigh their risks to children and adolescents with major depression and anxiety disorders. The study was funded in part by the National Institute of Mental Health.

Source: National Institute of Mental Health (www.nimh.nih.gov), 2010.

- Restricting her eating or not eating at all (like going without food for a day)

- Taking diuretics (pills that make you urinate)

Bulimia is more than just a problem with food. It's a way of using food to feel in control of other feelings that may seem overwhelming. Purging and other behaviors to prevent weight gain are ways for people with bulimia to feel more in control of their lives and to ease stress and anxiety.

Unlike anorexia, when people are severely underweight, people with bulimia may be underweight, overweight, or have a normal weight. This makes it harder to know if someone has this disease. However, someone with bulimia may have these signs:

- Thinks about food a lot

- Binges (normally in secret)

- Throws up after bingeing

- Uses laxatives, diet pills, or diuretics to control weight

- Is depressed

- Is unhappy and/or thinks a lot about her body shape and weight

- Eats large amounts of food quickly

- Goes to the bathroom all the time after she eats (to throw up)

- Exercises a lot, even during bad weather, fatigue, illness, or injury

- Unusual swelling of the cheeks or jaw area

- Cuts and calluses on the back of the hands and knuckles from making herself throw up

- White enamel of teeth wears away making teeth look clear

- Doesn't see friends or participate in activities as much

- Has rules about food — has "good" foods and "bad" foods

How is bulimia treated?

Someone with bulimia can get better. A health care team of doctors, nutritionists, and therapists will help the patient recover. They will help the person learn healthy eating patterns and cope with their thoughts and feelings. Treatment for bulimia uses a combination of options. Whether or not the treatment works depends on the patient.

Characteristics Of Bulimia Nervosa

Bulimia nervosa is characterized by recurrent and frequent episodes of eating unusually large amounts of food (for example, binge-eating), and feeling a lack of control over the eating. This binge-eating is followed by a type of behavior that compensates for the binge, such as purging (for example, vomiting, excessive use of laxatives or diuretics), fasting and/or excessive exercise.

Unlike anorexia, people with bulimia can fall within the normal range for their age and weight. But like people with anorexia, they often fear gaining weight, want desperately to lose weight, and are intensely unhappy with their body size and shape. Usually, bulimic behavior is done secretly, because it is often accompanied by feelings of disgust or shame. The binging and purging cycle usually repeats several times a week. Similar to anorexia, people with bulimia often have coexisting psychological illnesses, such as depression, anxiety and/or substance abuse problems. Many physical conditions result from the purging aspect of the illness, including electrolyte imbalances, gastrointestinal problems, and oral and tooth-related problems.

Source: National Institute of Mental Health (www.nimh.nih.gov), 2010.

To stop a person from binging and purging, a doctor may recommend the patient receive nutritional advice and psychotherapy, especially cognitive behavioral therapy (CBT), and be prescribed medicine.

CBT is a form of psychotherapy that focuses on the important role of thinking in how we feel and what we do. CBT that has been tailored to treat bulimia has shown to be effective in changing binging and purging behavior, and eating attitudes. Therapy for a person with bulimia may be one-on-one with a therapist or group-based.

Some antidepressants, such as fluoxetine (Prozac), which is the only medication approved by the U.S. Food and Drug Administration (FDA) for treating bulimia, may help patients who also have depression and/or anxiety. It also appears to help reduce binge-eating and purging behavior, reduces the chance of relapse, and improves eating attitudes.

Binge Eating Disorder

Most of us overeat from time to time, and some of us often feel we have eaten more than we should have. Eating a lot of food does not necessarily mean that you have binge eating disorder. Experts generally agree that most people with serious binge eating problems often eat an unusually large amount of food and feel their eating is out of control. People with binge eating disorder also may have these characteristics:

- Eat much more quickly than usual during binge episodes

- Eat until they are uncomfortably full

- Eat large amounts of food even when they are not really hungry

- Eat alone because they are embarrassed about the amount of food they eat

- Feel disgusted, depressed, or guilty after overeating

Binge eating also occurs in another eating disorder called bulimia nervosa. Persons with bulimia nervosa, however, usually purge, fast, or do strenuous exercise after they binge eat. Purging means vomiting or using a lot of diuretics (water pills) or laxatives to keep from gaining weight. Fasting is not eating for at least 24 hours. Strenuous exercise, in this case, means exercising for more than an hour just to keep from gaining weight after binge eating. Purging, fasting, and overexercising are dangerous ways to try to control your weight.

How common is binge eating disorder, and who is at risk?

Binge eating disorder is the most common eating disorder. It affects about 3% of all adults in the United States. People of any age can have binge eating disorder, but it is seen more often in adults age 46 to 55. Binge eating disorder is a little more common in women than in men; three women for every two men have it. The disorder affects blacks as often as whites, but it is not known how often it affects people in other ethnic groups.

Although most obese people do not have binge eating disorder, people with this problem are usually overweight or obese. Binge eating disorder is more common in people who are severely obese. Normal-weight people can also have the disorder.

People who are obese and have binge eating disorder often became overweight at a younger age than those without the disorder. They might also lose and gain weight more often, a process known as weight cycling or "yo-yo dieting."

What causes binge eating disorder?

No one knows for sure what causes binge eating disorder. As many as half of all people with binge eating disorder are depressed or have been depressed in the past. Whether depression causes binge eating disorder, or whether binge eating disorder causes depression, is not known.

It is also unclear if dieting and binge eating are related, although some people binge eat after dieting. In these cases, dieting means skipping meals, not eating enough food each day, or avoiding certain kinds of food. These are unhealthy ways to try to change your body shape and weight.

Studies suggest that people with binge eating disorder may have trouble handling some of their emotions. Many people who are binge eaters say that being angry, sad, bored, worried, or stressed can cause them to binge eat.

Characteristics Of Binge Eating Disorder

Binge-eating disorder is characterized by recurrent binge eating episodes during which a person feels a loss of control over his or her eating. Unlike bulimia, binge eating episodes are not followed by purging, excessive exercise, or fasting. As a result, people with binge-eating disorder often are overweight or obese. They also experience guilt, shame and/or distress about the binge-eating, which can lead to more binge eating.

Obese people with binge eating disorder often have coexisting psychological illnesses including anxiety, depression, and personality disorders. In addition, links between obesity and cardiovascular disease and hypertension are well documented.

Source: National Institute of Mental Health (www.nimh.nih.gov), 2010.

Certain behaviors and emotional problems are more common in people with binge eating disorder. These include abusing alcohol, acting quickly without thinking (impulsive behavior), not feeling in charge of themselves, not feeling a part of their communities, and not noticing and talking about their feelings.

Researchers are looking into how brain chemicals and metabolism (the way the body uses calories) affect binge eating disorder. Other research suggests that genes may be involved in binge eating, since the disorder often occurs in several members of the same family. This research is still in the early stages.

What are the complications of binge eating disorder?

People with binge eating disorder are usually very upset by their binge eating and may become depressed. Research has shown that people with binge eating disorder report more health problems, stress, trouble sleeping, and suicidal thoughts than do people without an eating disorder. Other complications from binge eating disorder could include joint pain, digestive problems, headache, muscle pain, and menstrual problems.

People with binge eating disorder often feel bad about themselves and may miss work, school, or social activities to binge eat.

People with binge eating disorder may gain weight. Weight gain can lead to obesity, and obesity puts people at risk for many health problems, including type 2 diabetes, high blood pressure, high blood cholesterol levels, gallbladder disease, heart disease, and certain types of cancer.

Most people who binge eat, whether they are obese or not, feel ashamed and try to hide their problem. Often they become so good at hiding it that even close friends and family members do not know that their loved one binge eats.

Should people with binge eating disorder try to lose weight?

People with binge eating disorder should get help from a health professional such as a psychiatrist, psychologist, or clinical social worker.

Many people with binge eating disorder are obese and have health problems because of their weight. They should try to lose weight and keep it off; however, research shows that long-term weight loss is more likely when a person has long-term control over his or her binge eating.

People with binge eating disorder who are obese may benefit from a weight-loss program that also offers treatment for eating disorders. However, some people with binge eating disorder may do just as well in a standard weight-loss program as people who do not binge eat.

People who are not overweight should avoid trying to lose weight because it may make their binge eating worse.

How can people with binge eating disorder be helped?

People with binge eating disorder should get help from a health care professional such as a psychiatrist, psychologist, or clinical social worker. There are several different ways to treat binge eating disorder.

- Cognitive behavioral therapy teaches people how to keep track of their eating and change their unhealthy eating habits. It teaches them how to change the way they act in tough situations. It also helps them feel better about their body shape and weight.

- Interpersonal psychotherapy helps people look at their relationships with friends and family and make changes in problem areas.

- Drug therapy, such as antidepressants, may be helpful for some people.

The methods mentioned here seem to be equally helpful. Researchers are still trying to find the treatment that is the most helpful in controlling binge eating disorder. Combining drug and behavioral therapy has shown promising results for treating overweight and obese individuals with binge eating disorder. Drug therapy has been shown to benefit weight management and promote weight loss, while behavioral therapy has been shown to improve the psychological components of binge eating.

Other therapies being tried include dialectical behavior therapy, which helps people regulate their emotions; drug therapy with the anti-seizure medication topiramate; weight-loss surgery (bariatric surgery); exercise used alone or in combination with cognitive behavioral therapy; and self-help. Self-help books, videos, and groups have helped some people control their binge eating.

Part Seven
If You Need More Information

Chapter 56

Cooking Tips And Resources

Food Safety

A critical part of healthy eating is keeping foods safe. Food may be handled numerous times as it moves from the farm to homes. Individuals in their own homes can reduce contaminants and keep food safe to eat by following safe food handling practices. Four basic food safety principles work together to reduce the risk of foodborne illness: clean, separate, cook, and chill. These four principles are the cornerstones of Fight BAC!®, a national food safety education campaign (visit www.fightbac.org).

Clean

Microbes, such as bacteria and viruses, can be spread throughout the kitchen and get onto hands, cutting boards, utensils, countertops, reusable grocery bags, and foods. This is called "cross-contamination." Hand washing is key to preventing contamination of food with microbes from raw animal products (for example, raw seafood, meat, poultry, and eggs) and from people (for example, cold, flu, and Staph infections). Frequent cleaning of surfaces is essential in preventing cross-contamination. To reduce microbes and contaminants from foods, all

About This Chapter: "Food Safety," is excerpted from *Dietary Guidelines for Americans 2010*, U.S. Department of Agriculture, December 2010. Text under the heading "Online Recipe Resources" is excerpted from "Eating Smart: A Nutrition Resource List for Consumers," Food and Nutrition Information Center (http://www.nal.usda.gov/fnic), September 2010. Text under the heading "Tips for Holiday Time" was excerpted and compiled from "Tasty Holiday Tips to Help Your Family Celebrate and Maintain a Healthy Weight," an undated fact sheet produced by the National Heart Lung and Blood Institute (www.nhlbi.nih.gov); and "It's Turkey Time: Safely Prepare Your Holiday Meal," Centers for Disease Control and Prevention, May 26, 2011.Additional resources were compiled from other sources deemed accurate. Inclusion does not constitute endorsement and there is no implication associated with omission. All website information was verified in April 2011.

produce, regardless of where it was grown or purchased, should be thoroughly rinsed. This is particularly important for produce that will be eaten raw.

Foodborne Illnesses

Every year, foodborne illness affects more than 76 million individuals in the United States, leading to 325,000 hospitalizations and 5,000 deaths.

Source: U.S. Department of Agriculture, December 2010.

Hands: Hands should be washed before and after preparing food, especially after handling raw seafood, meat, poultry, or eggs, and before eating. In addition, hand washing is recommended after going to the bathroom, changing diapers, coughing or sneezing, tending to someone who is sick or injured, touching animals, and handling garbage. Hands should be washed using soap and water. Soaps with antimicrobial agents are not needed for consumer hand washing, and their use over time can lead to growth of microbes resistant to these agents. Alcohol-based (60% or more), rinse-free hand sanitizers should be used when hand washing with soap is not possible.

Wash Hands With Soap And Water

- Wet hands with clean running water and apply soap. Use warm water if it is available.
- Rub hands together to make a lather and scrub all parts of the hands for 20 seconds.
- Rinse hands well under running water.
- Dry hands using a clean paper towel. If possible, use a paper towel to turn off the faucet.

Source: U.S. Department of Agriculture, December 2010.

Surfaces: Surfaces should be washed with hot, soapy water. A solution of 1 tablespoon of unscented, liquid chlorine bleach per gallon of water can be used to sanitize surfaces. Many surfaces should be kept clean, including tables, countertops, sinks, utensils, cutting boards, and appliances. For example, the insides of microwaves easily become soiled with food, allowing microbes to grow. They should be cleaned often.

Clean the inside and the outside of appliances. Pay particular attention to buttons and handles where cross-contamination to hands can occur. Wipe up spills immediately—clean food contact surfaces often. At least once a week, throw out refrigerated foods that should no longer be eaten. Cooked leftovers should be discarded after four days; raw poultry and ground meats, one to two days.

Foods: All produce, regardless of where it was grown or purchased, should be thoroughly rinsed. Many precut packaged items, like lettuce or baby carrots, are labeled as prewashed and ready-to-eat. These products can be eaten without further rinsing.

Raw seafood, meat, and poultry should not be rinsed. Bacteria in these raw juices can spread to other foods, utensils, and surfaces, leading to foodborne illness.

Produce Safety

- Rinse fresh vegetables and fruits under running water just before eating, cutting, or cooking.
- Do not use soap or detergent; commercial produce washes are not needed.
- Even if you plan to peel or cut the produce before eating, it is still important to thoroughly rinse it first to prevent microbes from transferring from the outside to the inside of the produce.
- Scrub firm produce, such as melons and cucumbers, with a clean produce brush while you rinse it.
- Dry produce with a clean cloth towel or paper towel to further reduce bacteria that may be present. Wet produce can allow remaining microbes to multiply faster.

Source: U.S. Department of Agriculture, December 2010.

Separate

Separating foods that are ready-to-eat from those that are raw or that might otherwise contain harmful microbes is key to preventing foodborne illness. Attention should be given to separating foods at every step of food handling, from purchase to preparation to serving.

When preparing and serving food, always use a clean cutting board for fresh produce and a separate one for raw seafood, meat, and poultry. Always use a clean plate to serve and eat food, and never place cooked food back on the same plate or cutting board that previously held raw food.

Cook And Chill

Seafood, meat, poultry, and egg dishes should be cooked to the recommended safe minimum internal temperature to destroy harmful microbes (see Table 56.1). It is not always possible to tell whether a food is safe by how it looks. A food thermometer should be used to ensure that food is safely cooked and that cooked food is held at safe temperatures until eaten. In general, the food thermometer should be placed in the thickest part of the food, not touch-

Table 56.1. Recommended Safe Minimum Internal Cooking Temperatures (use a food thermometer)

Food	Degrees Fahrenheit (°F)
Ground meat and meat mixtures	
Beef, pork, veal, lamb	160
Turkey, chicken	165
Fresh beef, veal, lamb	
Steaks, roasts, chops	145
Poultry	
Chicken and turkey, whole	165
Poultry breasts, roasts	165
Poultry thighs, wings	165
Duck and goose	165
Stuffing (cooked alone or in bird)	165
Fresh pork	160
Ham	
Fresh (raw)	160
Pre-cooked (to reheat)	140
Eggs and egg dishes	
Eggs	Cook until yolk and white are firm.
Egg dishes	160
Seafood	
Fish	145, Cook fish until it is opaque (milky white) and flakes with a fork.
Shrimp, lobster, scallops	Cook until the flesh of shrimp and lobster are an opaque color. Scallops should be opaque and firm.
Clams, mussels, oysters	Cook until their shells open. This means that they are done. Throw away any that were already open before cooking as well as ones that did not open after cooking.
Casseroles and reheated leftovers	165

ing bone, fat, or gristle. The manufacturer's instructions should be followed for the amount of time needed to measure the temperature of foods. Food thermometers should be cleaned with hot, soapy water before and after each use.

Temperature rules also apply to microwave cooking. Microwave ovens can cook unevenly and leave "cold spots" where harmful bacteria can survive. When cooking using a microwave, foods should be stirred, rotated, and/or flipped periodically to help them cook evenly. Microwave cooking instructions on food packages always should be followed.

Keep Foods At Safe Temperatures: Hold cold foods at 40° F or below. Keep hot foods at 140° F or above. Foods are no longer safe to eat when they have been in the danger zone of 40–140°F for more than two hours (one hour if the temperature was above 90° F).

- When shopping, the two-hour window includes the amount of time food is in the grocery basket, car, and on the kitchen counter.

- As soon as frozen food begins to thaw and become warmer than 40°F, any bacteria that may have been present before freezing can begin to multiply. Use one of the three safe ways to thaw foods: (1) in the refrigerator, (2) in cold water (that is, in a leakproof bag, changing cold water every 30 minutes), or (3) in the microwave. Never thaw food on the counter.

Keep your refrigerator at 40° F or below. Keep your freezer at 0° F or below. Monitor these temperatures with appliance thermometers.

Tips For Holiday Time

Follow these suggestions to help reduce the number of calories consumed:

- Use ingredient substitutions. For example, substitute one cup of fat-free evaporated milk for one cup of cream. Replace one cup of butter, margarine, or oil with ½ cup of apple butter or applesauce, and try using a graham cracker crumb crust instead of pastry dough.

- Take a tip from the reindeer and snack on something green at holiday parties. Also ditch the full-fat dips and dressings; instead use fat-free or reduced-fat yogurt in your recipes and for the veggie dip.

- In Santa's chimney-side treats, substitute three tablespoons of unsweetened cocoa powder plus 1 tablespoon of vegetable oil for one ounce of unsweetened baking chocolate. He may "know if you've been bad or good," but he will never know he is eating healthier.

Feasts and Parties

You don't have to give up all of your holiday favorites if you make healthy choices and limit portion sizes. At a party or holiday gathering, follow these tips to avoid overeating and to choose healthy foods.

- If you're at a buffet, fix your plate and move to another room away from the food, if possible.
- Choose smaller portions.
- Choose low-calorie drinks such as sparkling water, unsweetened tea, or diet beverages.
- Watch out for heavy holiday favorites such as hams coated with a honey glaze, turkey swimming in gravy, and side dishes loaded with butter, sour cream, cheese, or mayonnaise. Instead, choose turkey without gravy and trim off the skin or choose other lean meats.
- Look for side dishes and vegetables that are light on butter, dressing, and other extra fats and sugars, such as marshmallows or fried vegetable toppings.
- Watch the salt. Some holiday favorites are made with prepared foods high in sodium. Choose fresh or frozen vegetables that are low in sodium.
- Select fruit instead of pies, cakes, and other desserts high in fat, cholesterol and sugar.
- Focus on friends, family, and activities instead of food. Take a walk after a meal or join in the dancing at a party.

Source: Excerpted from "Managing Diabetes During the Holidays," Centers for Disease Control and Prevention, December 1, 2010.

- Pour yourself a tall glass of fat-free milk. Milk is an excellent source of protein, calcium, and vitamin D. If you prefer eggnog, try sipping on a fat-free or low-fat version.

- Have one or two of your favorite holiday foods (not five or six), and stay as light as your Menorah! Larger portions mean more calories, which can add up to extra pounds.

When preparing a turkey, be aware of the four main safety issues: thawing, preparing, stuffing, and cooking to adequate temperature.

Safe Thawing: Thawing turkeys must be kept at a safe temperature. While frozen, a turkey is safe indefinitely, but as soon as it begins to thaw, bacteria that may have been present before freezing can begin to grow again. There are three safe ways to thaw food: in the refrigerator, in cold water, and in a microwave oven.

Safe Preparation: Bacteria present on raw poultry can contaminate your hands, utensils, and work surfaces as you prepare the turkey. If these areas are not cleaned thoroughly before working with other foods, bacteria from the raw poultry can then be transferred to other foods. After working with raw poultry, always wash your hands, utensils, and work surfaces before they touch other foods.

Safe Stuffing: For optimal safety and uniform doneness, cook the stuffing outside the turkey in a casserole dish. However, if you place stuffing inside the turkey, do so just before cooking, and use a food thermometer. Make sure the center of the stuffing reaches a safe minimum internal temperature of 165° F. Bacteria can survive in stuffing that has not reached 165° F, possibly resulting in foodborne illness.

Online Recipe Resources

American Institute for Cancer Research Test Kitchen

http://www.aicr.org/sitc/PageServer?pagename=reduce_diet_recipes_test_kitchen

Click on links to recipes as well as meal courses including appetizers, soups, salads, and desserts. Each category has dozens of healthy menu options, each with nutrition facts included.

Delicious Decisions American Heart Association

http://www.deliciousdecisions.org

Features heart-healthy recipes, including their nutritional content, in an online searchable database. Multiple search features allow users to browse recipes by category or find recipes by main ingredient, cooking method, cuisine, or a combination of approaches.

Fruits and Veggies—More Matters

Centers for Disease Control and Prevention

http://apps.nccd.cdc.gov/dnparecipe/recipesearch.aspx

Offers searchable recipes with fruits and vegetables as the main ingredient for every course including beverages and desserts. Nutrition facts per serving are included.

Keep the Beat: Deliciously Healthy Eating

National Institutes of Health, National Heart Lung and Blood Institute (NHLBI)

http://hp2010.nhlbihin.net/healthyeating

Provides heart-healthy recipes created for NHLBI by a chef and registered dietitian that can be accessed by ingredient or category search, or by links on the home page. Site includes a Food Preparation Glossary, safe cooking rules, healthy eating video clips, and more.

Mayo Clinic Healthy Recipes Center

http://www.mayoclinic.com/health/healthy-recipes/RecipeIndex

Features recipes organized by preparation method, ingredients, number of servings, and special nutrition modifications (such as low sodium). All recipes include a "Dietitian's Tip" on preparation techniques and food safety. Nutrition facts per serving are included.

Meals Matter Dairy Council of California

http://www.mealsmatter.org

Offers recipes and meal planning tools from shopping lists to cookbooks. Also found on this website are various interactive tools, educational materials, and a blog.

Nutrition.gov Cooking Methods and Recipes

Food and Nutrition Information Center

http://www.nutrition.gov/recipes

Links to cooking and recipe resources from various federal government agencies. Also links to FNIC's Vegetarian Recipes and Meal Planning page.

SNAP-Ed Connection Recipe Finder Database

National Agricultural Library, SNAP-Ed Connection

http://recipefinder.nal.usda.gov

A searchable database of recipes submitted by Supplemental Nutrition Assistance Program (SNAP) nutrition educators. Each recipe provides cost per recipe, cost per serving, nutrition facts, a printable shopping list, and an option to print a 3"x5" recipe card. The search page also offers links to food demo and food safety tips and tips for involving kids in the kitchen. Recipes are also translated into Spanish.

Spend Smart Eat Smart

Iowa State University Extension

http://recipes.extension.iastate.edu

A list of recipes, including main dishes, side dishes, snacks, and dishes that are fast and easy or freeze well. Each recipe includes nutrition facts.

USA.gov American Recipes

http://www.firstgov.gov/Citizen/Topics/Health/Recipes.shtml

Lists links to different types of recipe pages with topics including kids' recipes, cooking for a crowd, and special recipe collections and publications. This unique government site also lists recipes "From Famous Americans" for some historical American cooking ideas.

Teen-Friendly Cookbooks

Cooking Up a Storm: The Teen Survival Cookbook
By Sam Stern
Published by Candlewick Press, 2006

Eat Fresh Food: Awesome Recipes for Teen Chefs
By Rozanne Gold and Phil Mansfield
Published by Bloomsbury USA, 2009

Student's Vegetarian Cookbook For Dummies
By Connie Sarros
Published by John Wiley, 2011

Student's Vegetarian Cookbook: Quick, Easy, Cheap, and Tasty Vegetarian Recipes, Revised Edition
By Carole Raymond
Published by Crown, 2003

Teen Cuisine
By Matthew Locricchio
Published by Marshall Cavendish, 2010

Teens Cook Dessert
By Megan Carle and Jill Carle
Published by Ten Speed Press, 2006

Teens Cook: How to Cook What You Want to Eat
By Meghan Carle, Jill Carle, and Judi Carle
Published by Ten Speed Press, 2004

Teen's Vegetarian Cookbook
By Judy Krizmanic and Matthew Wawiorka
Published by Paw Prints, 2008

Chapter 57

Resources For Dietary Information

American Diabetes Association

1701 North Beauregard Street
Alexandria, VA 22311
Toll-Free: 800-DIABETES (342-2383)
Website: http://www.diabetes.com

American Dietetic Association

120 S. Riverside Plaza
Suite 2000
Chicago, IL 60606-6995
Toll-Free: 800-877-1600
Fax: 312-899-4899
Website: http://www.eatright.org
E-mail: hotline@eatright.org

American Heart Association

7272 Greenville Avenue
Dallas, TX 75231-4596
Toll-Free: 800-AHA-USA1 (242-8721)
Website: http://www.americanheart.org

Asthma and Allergy Foundation of America

8201 Corporate Drive
Suite 1000
Landover, MD 20785
Toll-Free: 800-7-ASTHMA (727-8462)
Website: http://www.aafa.org
E-mail: info@aafa.org

Celiac Disease Foundation

13251 Ventura Blvd.
Suite 1
Studio City, CA 91604
Phone: 818-990-2354
Fax: 818-990-2379
Website: http://www.celiac.org
E-mail: cdf@celiac.org

About This Chapter: The resources listed in this chapter were compiled from the Food and Nutrition Information Center's Eating Smart resource list, Weight-Control Information Network Resources page, and other sources deemed accurate. Inclusion does not constitute endorsement and there is no implication associated with omission. All contact information was verified in April 2011.

Center for Nutrition Policy and Promotion

3101 Park Center Dr. 10th Floor
Alexandria, VA 22302-1594
Website: http://www.choosemyplate.gov
E-mail: support@cnpp.usda.gov

Center for Science in the Public Interest

1220 L St. NW., Suite 300
Washington, DC 20009
Phone: 202-332-9110
Fax: 202-265-4954
Website: http://www.cspinet.org
E-mail: cspi@cspinet.org

Centers for Disease Control and Prevention (CDC)

Division of Nutrition, Physical Activity,
and Obesity (DNPAO)
1600 Clifton Road
Atlanta, GA 30333
Toll-Free: 800-CDC-INFO (232-4636)
Toll-Free TTY: 888-232-6348
Nutrition Website: http://www.cdc.gov/
nutrition/index.html
E-mail: cdcinfo@cdc.gov

Eating Disorder Referral and Information Center

2923 Sandy Pointe, Suite 6
Del Mar, CA 92014-2052
Phone: 858-792-7463
Fax: 858-220-7417
Website: http://www.edreferral.com
E-mail: edreferral@aol.com

Food Allergy and Anaphylaxis Network

11781 Lee Jackson Hwy.
Suite 160
Fairfax, VA 22033
Toll-Free: 800-929-4040
Website: http://www.foodallergy.org
E-mail: faan@foodallergy.org

Food and Nutrition Information Center

USDA Agriculture Research Service
10301 Baltimore Ave.
Beltsville, MD 20705-2351
Phone: 301-504-5719
Website: http://www.nal.usda.gov/fnic
E-mail: fnic@nal.usda.gov

Food Safety and Inspection Service

United States Department of Agriculture
1400 Independence Ave., SW
Room 2932-S
Washington, DC 20250-3700
Website: http://www.fsis.usda.gov
E-mail: fsis@usda.gov

Institute of Food Technologists

525 West Van Buren
Suite 1000
Chicago, IL 60607
Toll-Free: 800-IFT-FOOD (438-3663)
Website: http://www.ift.org

International Food Information Council Foundation

1100 Connecticut Ave., NW, Suite 430
Washington, DC 20036
Phone: 202-296-6540
Website: http://www.foodinsight.org
E-mail: foodinfo@ific.org

Milk Matters Calcium Education Campaign

31 Center Dr.
Room 2A32
Bethesda, MD 20892-2425
Toll-Free: 800-370-2943
Phone: 301-496-5133
Fax: 301-496-7101
Website: http://www.nichd.nih.gov/milk
E-mail: NICHDMilkMatters@nail.nih.gov

National Association of Anorexia Nervosa and Associated Eating Disorders

Helpline: 630-577-1330
Website: http://www.anad.org
E-mail: anadhelp@anad.org

National Center for Complementary and Alternative Medicine

NCCAM Clearinghouse
P.O. Box 7923
Gaithersburg, MD 20898
Toll-Free: 888-644-6226
TTY: 866-464-3615
Fax: 866-464-3616
Website: http://nccam.nih.gov

National Diabetes Education Program

1 Diabetes Way
Bethesda, MD 20814-9692
Phone: 301-496-3583
Toll-Free: 888-693-6337
(to order materials)
Website: http://www.ndep.nih.gov
E-mail: ndep@mail.nih.gov

National Eating Disorders Association

603 Stewart Street
Suite 803
Seattle, WA 98101
Toll-Free: 800-931-2237
Phone: 206-382-3587
Fax: 206-829-8501
Website:
http://www.nationaleatingdisorders.org
E-mail: info@nationaleatingdisorders.org

National Heart, Lung, and Blood Institute

NHLBI Health Information Center
P.O. Box 30105
Bethesda, MD 20824-0105
Phone: 301-592-8573
TTY: 240-629-3255
Fax: 240-629-3246
Website: http://www.nhlbi.nih.gov
E-mail: nhlbiinfo@rover.nhlbi.nih.gov

National Institute of Child Health and Human Development

P.O. Box 3006
Rockville, MD 20847
Toll-Free: 800-370-2943
Toll-Free TTY: 888-320-6942
Fax: 301-984-1473
Website: http://www.nichd.nih.gov
E-mail: NICHDInformationResource Center@mail.nih.gov

Obesity Society

8757 Georgia Ave., Suite 1320
Silver Spring, MD 20910
Phone: 301-563-6526
Fax: 301-563-6595
Website: http://www.obesity.org
E-mail: fdea@obesity.org

Office of Dietary Supplements

National Institutes of Health
6100 Executive Blvd.
Room 3B01, MSC 7517
Bethesda, MD 20892-7517
Phone: 301-435-2920
Fax: 301-480-1845
Website: http://ods.od.nih.gov
E-mail: ods@nih.gov

U.S. Department of Agriculture

1400 Independence Ave., SW
Washington, DC 20250
Phone: 202-720-2791
Website: http://www.usda.gov
E-mail: agsec@usda.gov

USDA Meat and Poultry Hotline

Phone: 888-MPHotline (888-674-6854)
(10 a.m.–4 p.m. EST)
Recorded messages 24/7
E-mail: MPHotline.fsis@usda.gov

U.S. Food and Drug Administration (FDA)

Consumer Inquiries
10903 New Hampshire Ave.
Silver Spring, MD 20993
Toll-Free: 888-INFO-FDA (463-6332)
Fax: 301-847-8622
Website: http://www.fda.gov
E-mail: ConsumerInfo@fda.hhs.gov

Vegetarian Resource Group

P.O. Box 1463
Baltimore, MD 21203
Phone: 410-366-834
Website: http://www.vrg.org
E-mail: vrg@vrg.org

Weight-Control Information Network

National Institute of Diabetes and Digestive and Kidney Diseases
1 WIN Way
Bethesda, MD 20892-3665
Toll-Free: 877-946-4627
Fax: 202-828-1028
Website: http://win.niddk.nih.gov
E-mail: win@info.niddk.nih.gov

Interactive Tools and Other Online Resources

Ask the Dietitian Calculators
Healthy Eating for Life Plan:
http://www.dietitian.com/calchelp.php
Healthy Body Calculator:
http://www.dietitian.com/calcbody.php

Body and Mind: Food and Nutrition
Centers for Disease Control and Prevention
Website: http://www.bam.gov/
sub_foodnutrition/index.html

Body Mass Index Calculator
National Heart, Lung, and Blood Institute
Website: http://www.nhlbisupport.com/
bmi/bmicalc.htm

Calcium Quiz—What's Your Calcium Intake?
Dairy Council of California
Website: http://www.dairycouncilofca.org/
Tools/CalciumQuiz

Eat Local: Search for Local Produce or Farmers Markets
National Resources Defense Council
Website:
http://www.simplesteps.org/eat-local

Get Moving! Calculate the Number of Calories Burned
Calorie Control Council
Website: http://www.caloriecontrol.org/
exercalc.html

Girl's Health: Nutrition
Office on Women's Health
Website:
 http://www.girlshealth.gov/nutrition

Farmers Market Search
USDA, Agricultural Marketing Service
Website:
http://apps.ams.usda.gov/FarmersMarkets

Fruits and Veggies Matter Interactive Tools
Centers for Disease Control and Prevention
Includes "Analyze My Plate," and "Recipe Remix"
Website: http://www.fruitsandveggies
matter.gov/activities/index.html

Healthy Dining Finder
Website:
http://www.healthydiningfinder.com

Kidnetic
International Food Information Council
Website: http://kidnetic.com

Kidshealth.org
Nemours Foundation
Website: http://www.kidshealth.org

MyPlate
U.S. Department of Agriculture
Website: http://www.choosemyplate.gov

National Dairy Council
Website:
http://www.nutritionexplorations.org

Nutrition.gov
National Agricultural Library
Website: http://www.nutrition.gov

Personal Nutrition Planner from Meals Matter
Dairy Council of California
Website: http://www.mealsmatter.org/
EatingForHealth/Tools/PNP

Rate Your Restaurant Diet
Center for Science in the Public Interest
Website: http://www.cspinet.org/nah/quiz/
index.html

Spark Teens
Website: http://www.sparkteens.com

Books For Teens About Dietary Information

Food and You: A Guide to Healthy Habits for Teens
By Marjolijn Bijlefeld and Sharon K. Zoumbaris
Published by Greenwood Press, 2008

The Teen Weight-Loss Solution: The Safe And Effective Path to Health and Self-Confidence
By Erika Schwartz
Published by William Morrow, 2004

Ultimate Weight Solution for Teens: The 7 Keys to Weight Freedom
By Jay McGraw
Published by Simon and Schuster, 2003

Weighing In: Nutrition and Weight Management
By Lesli J. Favor and Elizabeth Massie
Published by Marshall Cavendish, 2009

Chapter 58

Resources For Fitness Information

Action for Healthy Kids
4711 West Golf Road
Suite 625
Skokie, IL 60076
Toll-Free: 800-416-5136
Fax: 847-329-1849
Website:
http://www.actionforhealthykids.org

Aerobics and Fitness Association of America
15250 Ventura Boulevard
Suite 200
Sherman Oaks, CA 91403
Toll-Free: 877-YOUR-BODY (968-7263),
Mon.–Fri. 6:30 a.m.–6:30 p.m., Sat 9
a.m.–1 p.m. PST
Website: http://www.afaa.com

American Academy of Orthopaedic Surgeons (AAOS)
6300 North River Road
Rosemont, IL 60018-4262
Phone: 847-823-7186
Fax: 847-823-8125
Website: http://www.aaos.org
E-mail: custserv@aaos.org

American Alliance for Health, Physical Education, Recreation, & Dance
1900 Association Drive
Reston, VA 20191-1598
Toll-Free: 800-213-7193
Phone: 703-476-3400
Website: http://www.aahperd.org

The resources listed in this chapter were compiled from many sources deemed accurate. Inclusion does not constitute endorsement and there is no implication associated with omission. All contact information was verified in April 2010.

American College of Sports Medicine (ACSM)

P.O. Box 1440
Indianapolis, IN 46206-1440
Phone: 317-637-9200
Fax: 317-634-7817
Website: http://www.acsm.org

American Council on Exercise (ACE)

4851 Paramount Drive
San Diego, CA 92123
Toll-Free: 888-825-3636
Phone: 858-279-8227
Fax: 858-576-6564
Website: http://www.acefitness.org
E-mail: support@acefitness.org

American Health and Fitness Alliance

P.O. Box 20750
New York, NY 10021
Phone: 212-808-0765
Fax: 212-988-3130
Website: www.health-fitness.org

American Heart Association

7272 Greenville Avenue
Dallas, TX 75231-4596
Toll-Free: 800-AHA-USA1 (242-8721)
Website: www.americanheart.org

American Orthopaedic Society for Sports Medicine (AOSSM)

6300 North River Road
Suite 500
Rosemont, IL 60018
Phone: 847-292-4900
Website: http://www.sportsmed.org
E-mail: aossm@aossm.org

American Physical Therapy Association (APTA)

1111 North Fairfax Street
Alexandria, VA 22314-1488
Toll-Free: 800-999-2782
Phone: 703-684-APTA (684-2782)
TDD: 703-683-6748
Fax: 703-684-7343
Website: http://www.apta.org
E-mail: Research-dept@apta.org

American Physiological Society

9650 Rockville Pike
Bethesda, MD 20814-3991
Phone: 301-634-7164
Fax: 301-634-7241
Website: http://www.the-aps.org

American Running Association (ARA)

4405 East-West Highway
Suite 405
Bethesda, MD 20814
Phone: 800-776-2732 ext. 13 or ext. 12
Fax: 301-913-9520
Website: http://www.americanrunning.org

American Society of Exercise Physiologists

The College of St. Scholastica
1200 Kenwood Avenue
Duluth, MN 55811
Phone: 218-723-6297
Fax: 218-723-6472
Website: http://www.asep.org

Aquatic Exercise Association (AEA)

P.O. Box 1609
Nokomis, FL 34274-1609
Website: http://www.aeawave.com

Centers for Disease Control and Prevention (CDC)

Division of Nutrition, Physical Activity, and Obesity (DNPAO)
1600 Clifton Road
Atlanta, GA 30333
Toll-Free: 800-CDC-INFO (232-4636)
Toll-Free TTY: 888-232-6348
Website: http://www.cdc.gov/nccdphp/dnpao/index.html
E-mail: cdcinfo@cdc.gov

Disabled Sports USA (DS/USA)

451 Hungerford Drive
Suite 100
Rockville, MD 20850
Phone: 301-217-0960
Fax: 301-217-0968
Website: http://www.dsusa.org
E-mail: information@dsusa.org

Fitness Institute Australia

Suite 505/410 Elizabeth Street
Surry Hills 2010
Australia
Phone: +61 02 9212 7185
Fax: +61 02 9211 0002
Website: http://www.fia.com.au
E-mail: admin@fia.com.au

Fitness League

Station Parade
Sunningdale
Berkshire SL5 0EP
UK
Phone: 01344 874787
Fax: 01344 873887
Website: http://www.thefitnessleague.com
E-mail: info@thefitnessleague.com

Girls Health

Website: www.girlshealth.gov

HealthInsite

Phone: [Australia] +61 1-800-022-222
Website: www.healthinsite.gov.au

HealthyWomen

157 Broad Street
Suite 106
Red Bank, NJ 07701
Toll-Free: 877-986-9472
Fax: 732-530-3347
Website: http://www.healthywomen.org

IDEA Health & Fitness Association

10455 Pacific Center Court
San Diego, CA 92121
Toll-Free: 800-999-4332, ext. 7
Phone: 858-535-8979, ext. 7
Fax: 858-535-8234
Website: http://www.ideafit.com
E-mail: contact@ideafit.com

International Fitness Association (IFA)

12472 Lake Underhill Road, #341
Orlando, FL 32828
Toll-Free: 800-227-1976
Phone: 407-579-8610
Website: http://www.ifafitness.com

IHRSA

70 Fargo Street
Boston, MA 02210
Toll-Free: 800-228-4772
Phone: 617-951-0055
Fax: 617-951-0056
Website: http://www.ihrsa.org

Kids.gov

Website: www.kids.gov

Kidshealth.org

Nemours Foundation
Website: http://www.kidshealth.org

National Academy of Sports Medicine

5845 E. Still Circle, Suite #206
Mesa, AZ 85206
Toll-Free 800-460-6276
International: 1-818-595-1200
Website: http://www.nasm.org

National Alliance for Youth Sports (NAYS)

National Headquarters
2050 Vista Parkway
West Palm Beach, FL 33411
Toll-Free: 800-688-KIDS (729-2057)
Phone: 561-684-1141
Fax: 561-684-2546
Website: http://www.nays.org
E-mail: nays@nays.org

National Association for Health and Fitness (NAHF)

c/o Be Active New York State
65 Niagara Square
Room 607
Buffalo, NY 14202
Phone: 716-583-0521
Fax: 716-851-4309
Website: http://www.physicalfitness.org
E-mail: wellness@city-buffalo.org

National Center on Physical Activity and Disability (NCPAD)

University of Illinois at Chicago, Department of Disability and Human Development
1640 W. Roosevelt Road
Chicago, IL 60608-6904
Toll-Free: 800-900-8086
Fax: 312-355-4058
Website: http://www.ncpad.org
E-mail: ncpad@uic.edu

National Coalition for Promoting Physical Activity

1100 H Street, NW, Suite 510
Washington, DC 20005
Phone: 202-454-7521
Fax: 202-454-7598
Website: http://www.ncppa.org
E-mail: info@ncppa.org

National Institute for Fitness and Sport

250 University Blvd.
Indianapolis, Indiana 46202
Phone: (317) 274-3432
Fax: (317) 274-7408
Website: http://www.nifs.org

National Institutes of Health (NIH)

9000 Rockville Pike
Bethesda, MD 20892
Phone: 301-496-4000
TTY: 301-402-9612
Website: http://www.nih.gov
E-mail: NIHinfo@od.nih.gov

National Recreation and Park Association (NRPA)

22377 Belmont Ridge Road
Ashburn, VA 20148-4501
Toll-Free: 800-626-NRPA (626-6772)
Website: http://www.nrpa.org

National Strength and Conditioning Association (NSCA)

1885 Bob Johnson Drive
Colorado Springs, CO 80906
Toll-Free: 800-815-6826
Phone: 719-632-6722
Fax: 719-632-6367
Website: http://www.nsca-lift.org
E-mail: nsca@nsca-lift.org

National Women's Health Information Center

8270 Willow Oaks Corporate Drive
Fairfax, VA 22031
Toll-Free: 800-994-9662
Toll-Free TTD: 888-220-5446
Website: http://www.womenshealth.gov

PE Central

P.O. Box 10262
Blacksburg, VA 24062
1995 South Main Street
Suite 902
Blacksburg, VA 24060
Phone: 540-953-1043
Fax: 540-301-0112
Website: http://www.pecentral.org
E-mail: pec@pecentral.org

President's Council on Fitness, Sports, and Nutrition

Department W
Tower Building
Suite 560
1101 Wootton Parkway
Rockville, MD 20852
Phone: 240-276-9567
Fax: 240-276-9860
Website: http://www.fitness.gov
E-mail: fitness@hhs.gov

Smallstep

U.S. Department of Health and Human Services
 200 Independence Avenue, SW
Washington, D.C. 20201
Toll-Free: 877-696-6775 (HHS Hotline)
Website: http://www.smallstep.gov

Women's Sports Foundation

National Office
Eisenhower Park
1899 Hempstead Turnpike
Suite 400
East Meadow, NY 11554
Toll-Free: 800-227-3988
Phone: 516-542-4700
Fax: 516-542-4716
Website:
http://www.womenssportsfoundation.org
E-mail:
Info@WomensSportsFoundation.org

Index

Index

Page numbers that appear in *Italics* refer to tables or illustrations. Page numbers that have a small 'n' after the page number refer to information shown as Notes at the beginning of each chapter. Page numbers that appear in **Bold** refer to information contained in boxes on that page (except Notes information at the beginning of each chapter).

A